The Clinical Handbook of

# Endocrinology
# and Metabolic
# Disease

To my special loved ones:
My wife Lenore, and our children:
Andrew, Anna, Heather, Jerrold and Josh

The Clinical Handbook of

# Endocrinology and Metabolic Disease

### Noel I. Robin M.D.

Physician-in-Chief
The Stamford Hospital
Stamford, Connecticut

Professor of Medicine and Associate Dean
New York Medical College
Valhalla, New York

## The Parthenon Publishing Group
International Publishers in Medicine, Science & Technology

NEW YORK                                    LONDON

**Published in the USA and Canada by:**
The Parthenon Publishing Group Inc.
One Blue Hill Plaza, PO Box 1564, Pearl River, NY 10965

**Published in Europe by:**
The Parthenon Publishing Group Ltd.
Casterton Hall, Carnforth, Lancs, LA6 2LA, UK

**Library of Congress Cataloging-in-Publication Data**
   Robin, Noel I.
Clinical handbook of endocrinology and metabolic disease / by Noel
   I. Robin.
      p. cm. — (The clinical handbook series)
   Includes bibliographical references and index.
   ISBN 1-85070-637-9
   1. Endocrine glands — Diseases — Handbooks, manuals, etc.
   2. Metabolism — Disorders — Handbooks, manuals, etc. I. Title.
   II. Series.
      [DNLM: 1. Endocrine Diseases — handbooks. 2. Metabolic Diseases —
   handbooks.  3. Endocrine Diseases — outlines.  4. Metabolic Diseases —
   outlines.  WK 39 R655c 1995]
   RC648.R58  1995
   616.4 — dc20
   DNLM/DLC
   for Library of Congress                                        95-30949
                                                                       CIP

**British Library Cataloguing in Publication Data**
Robin, Noel I.
   Clinical Handbook of Endocrinology and
   Metabolic Disease. - (Clinical Handbook
   Series)
   I. Title II. Series
   616.4

ISBN 1-85070-637-9

Typeset by H&H Graphics, Blackburn, UK
Printed and bound in the USA

# Contents

# Introduction

I have thought about the concept of this book many times over the years. The principles and practices within are based on the countless contributions of many individuals and institutions who have bequeathed so much to our present day medical understanding. I have had the wonderful fortune in the clinical practice of medicine to see and utilize many of these concepts. I have also had the privilege to be intimately involved in medical education and to share the excitement, stimulation and joy of clinical medicine with residents, students and fellow colleagues.

I have written this text to provide an integrated compendium of the practice of clinical endocrinology, whereby the infrastructure of physiology and pathophysiology would be meshed with the realities of pragmatic medical practice. I have also tried to make this a review for physicians, residents and students of all levels and interests. In no way can this book duplicate the rich resources and depth of information presently available in outstanding and comprehensive texts of endocrinology. Yet, I feel this book can serve a useful and readable purpose in presenting a spectrum of issues and problems in clinical endocrinology and metabolism, with appropriate depth, background, relevance and resolution. I hope that this book provides the reader with meaningful and succinct information, yet presents it in a way that 'flows'. I hope I have succeeded.

I could not close without expressing deepest gratitude to my many teachers for their patience, dedication and devotion, and to give special thanks to the finest physician I have known, Dr Edward Meilman.

# Section A

# OVERVIEW OF ENDOCRINOLOGY

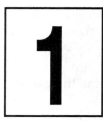

# THE NATURE OF HORMONES

1. Simply stated, hormones are chemical substances produced by tissues that are defined as endocrine in nature. They are secreted directly into the environment, usually the circulation, and produce a wide range of physiologic responses distal from their initial site of production.

2. There are five general categories of function, with overlap, that comprise the domain of endocrinology:

   a. Growth and Development – Securing the full potential and defining the limits of growth of bodily tissues.

   b. Bioregulation – Maintenance of an optimal environment and homeostatic control for orderly tissue function. This can relate to specific organs, functions, systems, or processes that may be singular, diverse, simple, or complex.

   c. Bioenergetics – Providing the appropriate amount, delivery and handling of energy resources to permit functions to proceed in accordance with their physiologic demands.

   d. Reproduction – Insuring not only the survival of the individual, but of the species as well.

   e. Biointegration – Serving as a 'communications link' that integrates seemingly diverse bodily activities.

3. To insure appropriateness of hormonal response based upon a particular need, hormones must be tightly regulated.

   a. The basic pattern of regulation is through a programmed servomechanism. This creates a feedback loop whereby products of synthesis or activity, in turn, determine the pattern and degree of the primal initiating process.

   b. The servomechanism can be complex patterns having multiple 'smaller loops' within the framework of larger patterns.

   c. Regulation can occur through 'traditional' endocrine mechanisms ('circulating' hormones) or through regulation by nerve tissue (neurocrine), surrounding tissues (paracrine), or by the primary tissue itself (autocrine).

4. Hormones can be divided into several major classes based on their chemical structures. These classes tend to have common patterns of target site activity (Table 1-1).

   a. Larger peptide chains. They can be 'pure' proteins (e.g. growth hormone, prolactin) or glycosylated (e.g. follicle stimulating hormone, luteinizing hormone, thyroid stimulating hormone and human chorionic gonadotropin).

   b. Intermediate and smaller peptide chains (e.g insulin, glucagon).

   c. Single amino acids and dipeptide derivatives (e.g. catecholamines and thyroid hormones – both are phenylalanine derivatives).

   d. Steroid hormones.

5. Hormone action requires target site receptivity.

   a. Larger peptides have cell membrane receptor sites.

   b. Thyroid and steroid hormones have intracellular receptor sites.

   c. Hormone–receptor interaction leads to an ultimate biologic response. The role of the receptor is crucial as receptor number and binding affinity is one mechanism of controlling hormonal activity. (Although many, but not all, hormones are transported through the circulation in a 'bound state', this binding does not result in a biologic response even though hormone delivery and concentration may be affected by the degree of binding.)

## TABLE 1-1. CLASSES OF HORMONES

| Hormone Type | Principal Source | Specific Hormones |
|---|---|---|
| Larger Peptide Chains | | |
| Non-glycosylated | Anterior Pituitary Gland | Growth Hormone, Prolactin |
| Glycosylated | Anterior Pituitary Gland | Thyroid Stimulating Hormone, Follicle Stimulating Hormone, Luteinizing Hormone |
| Glycosylated | Placenta | Human Chorionic Gonadotropin |
| Intermediate and Smaller Peptides | Pancreas | Glucagon, Insulin |
| | Thyroid Gland (C-Cells) | Calcitonin |
| Single Amino Acids and Dipeptide Derivatives | Thyroid Gland (Follicular Cells) | Thyroxine, Triiodothyronine |
| | Adrenal Medulla and other Adrenergic sites | Epinephrine, Norepinephrine |
| Steroid Hormones | Adrenal Cortex | Cortisol and related Glucocorticoids, Adrenal Androgens |
| | Testes | Testosterone and related Androgens, |
| | Ovary | Estradiol and related Estrogens, Progesterone |

d.  Hormones that bind to cell membrane receptors bind to a family of effector proteins called 'G' (or Gs) proteins. These proteins have three subunits: an $\alpha$ subunit that is unique to that effector protein and a $\beta$ and $\gamma$ subunit that is common (the $\beta$–$\gamma$ subunit is felt to have an 'anchoring' role). Binding of a hormone to its receptor allows for GTP binding to the 'G' protein. This frees the α subunit to activate adenylate cyclase (a 'second messenger') but also limits the reaction as the α subunit has GTPase activity. This then depletes the GTP and inactivates the process by freeing GDP and allowing the α subunit to re-form with the β and γ. To add to the complexity still further, G proteins can be of an inhibitory or stimulatory nature.

   i. Another 'second messenger' is cyclic GMP. Although also derived from GTP, it is formed by the action of the enzyme guanylate cyclase.

   ii. Still another 'second messenger' is the ionized calcium concentration. It probably exerts its effect by its affinity to the calcium binding protein, calmodulin. A model for this is the action of angiotensin II on stimulation of aldosterone production. It is linked to a G-protein mediated activation of phospholipase C. The resultant hydrolysis of phosphotidylinositol biphosphate produces diacylglycerol and inositol triphosphate, resulting in increased levels of intracellular calcium.

  e. Steroid and thyroid hormones act by ultimately initiating RNA transcription (and new protein synthesis) through eventual nuclear binding. In the case of thyroid hormone, there are additional mitochondrial receptors.

  f. The role of the eicosanoid family of compounds (e.g. prostaglandins, leukotrienes) is assuming increasing importance in relation to hormonally mediated activities.

  g. Because of the target–receptor concept of biologic activation, a single hormone can be responsible for more than one biologic action. Conversely, more than one hormone can 'converge' at the same receptor site resulting in a common biologic response (although differing, at times, in degree).

6. Hormone production, itself, is under genetic control – the rate of production must ultimately result from gene activation and regulation.

  a. Hormones may not be in their 'final packaged form' when initially synthesized – e.g. some hormones are in a 'pre-pro-hormone' or 'pro-hormone' state, while others may be synthesized as part of a 'package' with other active components (e.g. pro-opiomelanocortin).

b. Some hormones undergo peripheral structural changes that result in altered activity (this activity can be augmented as in thyroxine to triiodothyronine conversion, it may be modified as in testosterone to dihydrotestosterone conversion, or it can be changed into a different 'class' of endocrinologic activity as in the case of androgen to estrogen conversion).

c. In steroidogenesis, the products of transcriptionally activated protein synthesis are directed at enzyme production. This enables the steroid 'synthetic cascade' to proceed to final product development.

7. Endocrine disease occurs as a result of either functional or structural derangement. These categories are, by no means, mutually exclusive.

# DISORDERS OF THE HYPOTHALAMUS AND PITUITARY GLAND

# 2

# THE HYPOTHALAMUS AND ANTERIOR PITUITARY GLAND

General Considerations
Cellular Constituents of the Anterior Pituitary
Constituent Hormones of the Anterior Pituitary Gland
    Thyrotropin (TSH)
    Gonadotropins (FSH and LH)
    Growth Hormone (HGH)
    Prolactin (Prl)
    Adrenocorticotropic Hormone (ACTH)

## GENERAL CONSIDERATIONS

1. Any discussion of the pituitary is incomplete without an understanding of the hypothalamus and neuroendocrinology.

2. Hypothalamic function is intimately related to pituitary activity by virtue of close proximity and a specialized circulation.

   a. The primary blood supply to the pituitary is provided by the superior hypophyseal artery, a branch of the internal carotid artery.

   b. The capillaries derived from this artery arborize in the region of the median eminence where a compendium of hypothalamic nuclei are capable of secretion of hypophysiotropic hormones.

   c. These secretions are picked up by capillary venules, but rather than returning directly to the systemic circulation, they are carried down the pituitary stalk into a portal circulation that terminates once again in capillaries. These capillaries are intimately associated with the various cellular constituents of the anterior pituitary and influence hormonal production by the hypothalamic products they carry.

   d. The anterior pituitary secretions are then carried away to the various areas of the body through the internal jugular vein (via the cavernous and petrosal sinuses).

   e. On a per weight basis, no organ receives as much of the cardiac output as the anterior pituitary.

   f. The posterior pituitary, which directly produces (better said, 'transports') the products of hypothalamic nuclei secretion, does not require a portal circulation and receives its blood supply directly from the middle and inferior hypophyseal arteries.

3. Known hypothalamic hormones include:

   a. Those directly secreting into the posterior pituitary gland:

      i. Arginine vasopressin, and

      ii. Oxytocin.

b. Mediators of Anterior Pituitary Function:

   i. Corticotropin releasing factor (CRH),

   ii. Growth hormone releasing hormone (GRH),

   iii. Gonadotropin releasing hormone (GnRH – formerly, LHRH),

   iv. Somatostatin (formerly growth hormone inhibiting hormone),

   v. Prolactin inhibitory hormone (synonymous with dopamine) – it is also referred to as prolactin inhibitory factor, and

   vi. Thyrotropin releasing hormone (TRH).

4. While hypothalamic hormones may influence the pituitary in a 'classic' endocrine fashion (secretion of hormones directly into the circulation without a 'duct'), additional regulation of pituitary function (or hypothalamic function, itself) may be done through neurogenic (e.g. catecholaminergic, cholinergic), paracrine (affected by local 'bathing' influences) or other (including non-pituitary) 'classic' hormones as part of the 'feedback loop'. Cell secretions may govern their own regulation (autocrine). The regulatory network is additionally regulated by a 'retrograde' pituitary–hypothalamic circulation (the so-called 'short loop').

5. With assay refinement and genetic probes, hormones and regulators are no longer geographically relegated to their traditional areas but can be found in other parts of the brain and body. Conversely, hormones and biologically active products originally discovered 'outside' the endocrine system are being 'rediscovered' in these sites and in loci within the central nervous system.

## CELLULAR CONSTITUENTS OF THE ANTERIOR PITUITARY

These comprise cellular sources of pituitary hormones. Histologic properties of these cells may reflect physiologic variation as well as changes of overt disease; cellular distribution may affect the likelihood of location of an adenoma of a particular cell type.

1. Thyrotrophs – basophilic; less than 10% of the cellular pool; tendency to anterior distribution; increased in primary hypothyroidism.

2. Gonadotrophs – basophilic; about 10% of the cellular pool; diffusely distributed; increased in sex hormone-privic states (e.g secondary failure as in menopause, mumps orchitis; primary failure as in Turner's syndrome).

3. Somatotrophs – eosinophilic; comprise the majority of the cellular pool; tendency to lateral distribution.

4. Lactotrophs – eosinophilic; about 20% of the cellular pool; diffusely distributed; increased during pregnancy (estrogen effect).

5. Corticotrophs – basophilic; less than 20% of the cellular pool; antero-medial location; increased in primary adrenal insufficiency; undergo degeneration (Crooke's) with glucocorticoid excess irrespective of its source, even if the excessive glucocorticoid arises from an adjacent ACTH-producing adenoma (Cushing's disease) that results in bilateral adrenal hyperplasia.

## CONSTITUENT HORMONES OF THE ANTERIOR PITUITARY GLAND (Table 2-1)

### Thyrotropin (TSH)
1. Chemistry – A two-chain glycoprotein having an $\alpha$ chain common as well to follicle stimulating hormone (FSH), luteinizing hormone (LH) and human chorionic gonadotropin, but a unique $\beta$ chain. MW – 28 000 (89 amino acids in the $\alpha$ chain; 110 amino acids in the $\beta$). Glycosylation of the hormone is post-translational. In some cases of hypopituitarism, there may be a disparity between the immunoassay and the bioactivity of TSH. This is reflected by a depressed serum thyroxine ($T_4$) and Free $T_4$, but an inappropriately 'normal' or 'near-normal' TSH – the 'measured' TSH does not account for the need for glycosylation to render it hormonally effective.

2. Regulation

   a. TRH is the primary regulator but it does so not by a change in its concentration, but rather by the ability of thyroid hormone (either circulating triiodothyronine ($T_3$) or $T_3$ converted from $T_4$ within pituitary thyrotrophs) to modulate its effect.

    i. Thyrotroph deiodinase is different from peripheral deiodinase in that $T_4$ to $T_3$ conversion is less readily impaired by those same processes which would decrease $T_3$ production peripherally – hence, the tendency to a 'normal' TSH in the 'low $T_3$' syndrome.

    ii. Estrogen augments TRH-mediated TSH stimulation

  b. Pulsatile – within the first few hours of nocturnal sleep.

  c. Inhibited by dopamine and related substances and by somatostatin.

3. Effect – Acts directly on thyroid tissue to promote iodide uptake, organification and thyroid hormone liberation (proteolysis). It has an additional hyperplastic effect on the thyroid gland. Many actions may be 'mimicked' by immunologic thyrotoxic disease (Graves' disease and related entities).

4. Measurement and Evaluation – Direct TSH assay (present assays are second and third generation) – capable of detecting very low values. The TRH stimulation test (with concomitant measurement of the TSH response) is rarely needed – it can sometimes distinguish between pituitary and hypothalamic hypothyroidism, but there is often an overlap (pituitary insufficiency should produce no response; hypothalamic deficiency should produce a response – although in actuality it may be subnormal and delayed).

## Gonadotropins (FSH and LH)

1. Chemistry – Both FSH (MW – 33 000) and LH (MW – 28 000) are glycoproteins (common α chain, unique β chain – the α subunit has 92 amino acids; β subunits have 115 amino acids, each).

2. Regulation

  a. Secretion is both episodic (both sexes) and mediated by regular, 2–4-hourly bursts of GnRH and cyclically patterned in women in concert with the menstrual cycle. In women, both FSH and LH 'peak' prior to ovulation. LH levels are generally low pre- and postovulation but gradually increase up to an LH 'surge' and then decline thereafter (increasing slightly prior to menstruation). FSH levels also increase a few days prior to menstruation and then increase in the early part of

## TABLE 2-1.  CONSTITUENT HORMONES OF THE ANTERIOR PITUITARY GLAND

| Hormone | Structure (Molecular Weight) | Regulators | Major Effect | Most Useful Laboratory Measurement |
|---|---|---|---|---|
| Thyrotropin (TSH) | 2-Chain Glycoprotein (28 000) | **Stimulation** Thyrotropin Releasing Hormone **Inhibition** Dopamine, Somatostatin | Synthesis and Release of Thyroid Hormone | Basal Serum Measurement |
| Follicle Stimulating Hormone (FSH) | 2-Chain Glycoprotein (33 000) | **Stimulation** Gonadotropin Releasing Hormone, Estrogens **Inhibition** Inhibin, Estrogens, Androgens | Stimulates Testicular Growth and Androgen Binding Protein (from Sertoli Cells) in Men; Follicular Development and Estrogen Production in Women | Basal Serum Measurement |
| Luteinizing Hormone (LH) | 2-Chain Glycoprotein (28 000) | **Stimulation** Gonadotropin Releasing Hormone, Estrogens **Inhibition** Estrogens, Androgens | Stimulates Testosterone Production (from Leydig Cells) in Men. Stimulates Ovarian Estrogen and Progesterone in Women | Basal Serum Measurement |
| Growth Hormone (HGH) | 191-Amino Acid Protein (21 500) | **Stimulation** Growth Hormone Releasing Hormone, α-Adrenergic, Cholinergic and Serotoninergic Stimulation; β-Adrenergic Blockade | Mediator of Growth and Protein Anabolism (via Insulin-like Growth Factor-I); Lipolysis; Insulin Antagonism | Stimulation assessed with Insulin-mediated Hypoglycemia; Suppression Assessed after glucose load |

*(continued)*

THE HYPOTHALAMUS AND ANTERIOR PITUITARY GLAND

## TABLE 2-1. CONTINUED

| Hormone | Structure (Molecular Weight) | Regulators | Major Effect | Most Useful Laboratory Measurement |
|---|---|---|---|---|
| | | **Inhibition** Somatostatin; β-Adrenergic Stimulation. α-Adrenergic, Serotonin, Dopamine, and Acetyl Choline blocking agents | | |
| Prolactin | 198-Amino Acid Protein (22 500) | **Stimulation** Thyrotropin Releasing Hormone, Estrogens, Vasoactive Intestinal Peptide, Corticotropin Releasing Hormone, Arginine Vasopressin, Serotonin, Opioids, H-1 Stimulation, H-2 Blockade, Dopamine Inhibition **Inhibition** Prolactin Inhibiting Factor, Dopaminergic Agonism | Milk Secretion | Basal Serum Measurement |
| Adrenocorticotropic Hormone (ACTH) | 39-Amino Acid Polypeptide (4500) | **Stimulation** Corticotropin Releasing Hormone, Endogenous Pyrogens, Immune Modulators and 'physiologic stress' inducers **Inhibition** Glucocorticoids, Corticotropin Releasing Hormone | | Stimulation assessed with Insulin-mediated Hypoglycemia; Suppression assessed after Dexamethasone administration |

the follicular phase but decline once estradiol starts to rise. The decline continues until the modest premenstrual upswing, with the exception of the midcycle peak.

b. The progressive preovulatory increase in estradiol has a stimulating effect on the FSH and LH surge. Estrogen deficiency (as in ovarian failure) is also a stimulus to gonadotropin production (e.g. high levels postmenopausal) as are estrogen antagonists (e.g. clomiphene). Conversely, sex steroids (e.g. oral contraceptives) have an inhibitory effect.

c. In males, inhibin (made by Sertoli cells) appears to have a pre-eminent role in FSH (but not LH) feedback. Testosterone inhibits LH production, but can also inhibit FSH.

d. Dopamine (and related substances), serotonin, and opiates are antagonists (this may help explain sex hormone deficiency, including amenorrhea, in highly conditioned athletes). Opiate antagonists, epinephrine and norepinephrine, are stimulatory.

3. Effect

a. In women, FSH stimulates follicular development (hence its mild preovulation elevation) and (with LH) stimulates follicular estrogen production. Both FSH and LH activate ovulation (and production of a progesterone-producing corpus luteum). LH sustains ovarian hormone production postovulation.

b. In men, LH is the primary stimulus to Leydig cell testosterone production. FSH acts mainly on the Sertoli cell to produce a testosterone-binding protein, thus allowing for an 'enriched' testosterone environment to foster spermatogenesis.

4. Measurement and Evaluation

a. Direct measurement of FSH and LH (with testosterone and estradiol).

b. 'Indirect clinical measurement' – normal menses; impotence or libido are relevant, but not of sufficient sensitivity or specificity.

c. GnRH stimulation tests are generally not of discriminating value.

## Growth Hormone (HGH)

1. Chemistry – a long-chained (191 amino acid), non-glycosylated polypeptide (MW – 21 500) derived from a larger precursor molecule (pre-somatotropin) – variant forms and oligomers of HGH also exist and there is an HGH-binding protein in the circulation (unclear significance).

2. Regulation

   a. Episodic – usually occurs in the third to fourth hour (Stages III and IV) of sleep. May be mediated through growth hormone releasing hormone (GRH) because experimentally administered GRH antibody in rats results in loss of 'spike' (but not basal) activity.

      i. GRH activity has been identified in two hypothalamic peptides of 44 and 40 amino acids, respectively.

      ii. GRH has some structural homology to gastrointestinal hormones.

   b. Basal – degree of suppressive effect on HGH by somatostatin appears to be the determinant of the basal level.

      i. Experimentally administered somatostatin antibody to rats increases the HGH 'baseline' but does not alter 'spike activity'.

      ii. Somatostatin is a ubiquitous 14-amino acid peptide that has a wide range of other inhibitory activities – inhibitory to TSH, pancreatic hormones (insulin and glucagon) and gastrointestinal activity (secretin, gastrin and vasoactive intestinal peptide (VIP)). It is also inhibitory to gall bladder contractility.

      iii. Because of these multiple inhibitory effects, a somatostain analog, Octreotide, has found a wide range of clinical applications. These include not only applications as a potent medical therapy for acromegaly, but also for symptomatic control of carcinoid syndrome, VIP-producing tumors, and diabetic diarrhea. Radioscintigraphy, using labelled somatostatin, has also been an adjunctive tool for tumor localization (e.g. ectopic ACTH production).

    c. α-adrenergic, dopaminergic, cholinergic and serotoninergic influences and β blocking agents stimulate HGH release.

    d. α-adrenergic-blocking agents (e.g. dibenzyline, phentolamine), dopaminolytic agents (e.g. phenothiazides), anti-serotonin agents (cyproheptadine, methysergide), anticholinergic agents and β agonists are inhibitory.

    e. Metabolic Influences – Stimulated by hypoglycemia, amino acids (especially arginine and leucine), and decreased free fatty acids; suppressed by obesity, hyperglycemia and increased free fatty acids.

    f. Hormonal – Stimulated by estrogens, glucagon, and vasopressin; inhibited by progestins and glucocorticoids – increased, however, in stress and exercise (this may represent overriding α-adrenergic action).

3. Effect

    a. Major metabolic effects are lipolytic (with resultant increased acetyl coenzyme A – an important source of energy for other anabolic effects); insulin antagonism (post-receptor) promoting tendency to hyperglycemia.

    b. Actual growth is mediated through synthesis of a somatomedin – originally called 'sulfation factor', then somatomedin C, but its preferred name is insulin-like growth factor I (IGF-I).

       i. Structurally rather homologous to pro-insulin; liver is the richest source but other tissues are capable of production (probably for local use).

      ii. There is a second important somatomedin, somatomedin A or IGF-II. (Somatomedin B is not a separate entity but a portion of the somatomedin A molecule.) Before the acceptance of the term somatomedin, a common generic term was 'non-suppressible insulin-like activity' because of its ability to bind to insulin receptors and exert an insulin-like action.

     iii. HGH and IGF-I comprise an important feedback loop. HGH is elevated when IGF-I levels decrease (e.g. hepatic failure, poor nutritional state, chronic illness, uremia).

IGF-I is elevated in acromegaly (because of the 'non-fluctuation' of IGF-I values, it is a useful laboratory parameter of both the acromegalic state and of growth hormone deficiency – the latter particularly relevant in measurement in adults).

iv. Decreased by estrogen and increased by progesterone and thyroid hormone.

v. The so-called Laron-type dwarfism is a HGH receptor defect with the inability to make IGF-I (growth can be stimulated by IGF-I, directly).

vi. This Laron dwarfism (as well as the HGH resistance that can be seen in the African pygmy, uremia, hepatic failure, and malnutrition) is associated with a decrease in a high-affinity growth hormone binding protein (GHBP). This binding protein may be the extracellular reflection of the cellular receptor. (Another GHBP is not reflective of this receptor and is a low-affinity binder.) Conversely, elevated GHBP is seen in obesity, which is associated with increased tissue responsiveness to HGH.

4. Measurement and Evaluation

   a. To assess for deficiency:

      i. Insulin-mediated hypoglycemia (with serial measurements of HGH) – 0.1–0.15 U/kg body weight, intravenously. It is not the insulin but the hypoglycemia that is the provocateur; adequate hypoglycemia must be achieved. In actuality, many patients may be very sensitive to the insulin because of underlying HGH (and possibly ACTH) deficiency.

      ii. Ancillary provocative tests include L-DOPA and arginine infusion.

      iii. Isolated and random HGH determinations are not useful.

   b. To test for excess:

      i. IGF-I levels (as above)

      ii. HGH levels 2 h postingestion of 100 g of glucose (normals should have values less than 2 ng/ml).

**Prolactin (Prl)**
1.  Chemistry – Non-glycosylated protein; 198 amino acids; MW – 22 500; derived from a large (pre-prolactin) molecule; circulates in multiple forms.

2.  Regulation

    a.  Episodic secretion – multiple daily pulses and during late sleep.

    b.  Physical Factors and Physiologic Stress – Including exercise, nipple and thoracic cage stimulation (e.g. zoster), sexual intercourse, postalimentation.

    c.  Endocrinologic Stimulation

        i.   TRH – May be mechanism (through increased sensitivity to TRH) of hyperprolactinemia in primary hypothryoidism,

        ii.  Estrogen – but not with the estrogen levels of presently used oral contraceptives,

        iii. VIP,

        iv.  CRH, and

        v.   Arginine vasopressin.

    d.  Other physiologic and pharmacologic stimulators

        i.   Opioids

        ii.  Serotonin

        iii. Histamine receptor (H)-1 Stimulation (Hence prolactin is increased with H-2 blockade)

        iv.  Dopamine antagonists or depletors – phenothiazines, butyrophenones, metoclopramide, reserpine, α methyl DOPA.

    e.  Major endogenous regulation of prolactin is inhibitory

        i.   Mediated by prolactin inhibitory factor (Dopamine)

        ii.  Pharmacologically mimicked by dopaminergic agonism – e.g. L-DOPA, bromocriptine, apomorphine, pergolide and carbegoline.

3. Effect – Despite presence of binding sites on other tissues, the major effect of prolactin is on the breast to stimulate production of milk protein (through the initiation of the transcriptional process). Prolactin may also play a role in immunomodulation.

4. Measurement and Evaluation

    a. Although deficiency can be evaluated with a TRH stimulation test (alternatively, the response to chlorpromazine can be measured), a basal level will generally suffice.

    b. Excess states – basal prolactin level (although ambiguity of etiology can occur when levels are closer to the normal limits, values in excess of 200 ng/ml are usually associated with prolactin-secreting tumors).

**Adrenocorticotropic Hormone (ACTH)**
1. Chemistry – A non-glycosylated polypeptide (MW – 4500; 39 amino acids) derived from a larger precursor molecule, pro-opiomelanocortin. ACTH is not produced independent of the associated peptides that this precursor molecule makes. These include: β-lipotropin (which gives rise to γ-lipotropin, resulting ultimately in β-melanocyte-stimulating hormone (MSH), β-endorphin and Met-Enkephalin); ACTH also gives rise to an α-MSH – a clinical corollary is the tendency to hyperpigmentation when ACTH and its parent molecule are stimulated (Figure 2-1).

2. Regulation

    a. CRH – A major stimulator; pulsatile but with diurnal rhythymicity (greatest toward end of sleep, least during late afternoon – diurnal variation does not occur abruptly but is a 'gradual process' during each cycle).

    b. Additional stimuli include physiologic stress, endogenous pyrogens (interleukin 1 is operant), immune modulators (e.g. interleukin 2, interleukin 6, cachectin), and 'physiologic stress' inducers (e.g. cold, mental depression, vasopressin and hypoglycemia).

    c. Feedback inhibition – cortisol (and structural analogs) inhibit CRH; a 'short loop' involves direct ACTH inhibition of CRH.

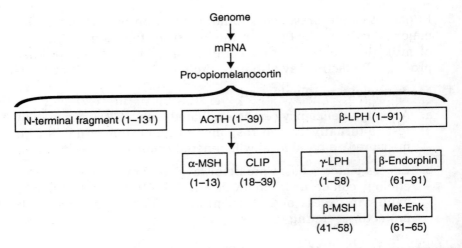

**Figure 2-1.** Biosynthesis of ACTH and Related Peptides: LPH, lipotropin; MSH, melanocyte-stimulating hormone; CLIP, corticotropin-like intermediate lobe peptide. Reproduced with kind permission from *Basic and Clinical Endocrinology*, 4th edn., Greenspan, F.S. and Baxter, J.D. (eds.) Norwalk, CT: Appleton and Lange, 1994, pp. 64–127

3. Effect

   a. Major target site is the adrenal cortex.

   b. Binding to cell membrane initiates activation of c'AMP (mediated by a G protein) resulting in phosphoprotein kinase activation which increases (through phosphorylation) the activity of cholesterol ester hydrolase. The generation of increased free cholesterol serves as a substrate for initiation of adrenal steroidogenesis.

   c. ACTH also enhances the binding of free cholesterol to the P-450 cytochrome enzyme system (the source of subsequent enzymatic participation) and catalyzes the side-chain cleavage of cholesterol (desmolase enzyme) to form pregnenolone.

4. Measurement and Evaluation

   a. Insulin-mediated hypoglycemia – measurement of serum cortisol at 30 and 60 min following intravenous administration of regular insulin, 0.1–0.15 U/kg body weight. With intact pituitary function, insulin should be a potent provocateur of ACTH. This effect would be blunted in both hypothalamic and pituitary disease.

    i. HGH response can be obtained at the same time.

    ii. Caution! – suspected deficiency patients are most vulnerable and sensitive to hypoglycemia.

    iii. The cortisol value at the point of most severe hypoglycemia will have the greatest significance.

b. Metyrapone Stimulation

    i. By blocking the final (11-hydroxylase) step in adrenal steroidogenesis, ACTH is stimulated. A normal stimulated cortisol response requires an intact hypothalamic–pituitary–adrenal axis.

    ii. 11-Deoxycortisol (but not cortisol) response is measured.

c. CRH Stimulation

    i. In patients with cortisol deficiency, basal and post-stimulated ACTH levels are elevated.

    ii. Patients with pituitary insufficiency do not respond. With hypothalamic insufficiency, however, there may be a delayed and protracted response.

d. Suppression Tests

    i. The Dexamethasone Suppression Test is the fundamental generic test for assessment of pituitary autonomy. Patients with pituitary-mediated Cushing's syndrome (Cushing's disease) do no suppress ACTH in response to 'low-dose' dexamethasone (2 mg/day in divided doses), but do exhibit ACTH suppression in response to 'high-dose' dexamethasone (8 mg/day in divided doses).

    ii. Failure to exhibit 'low-dose' suppression forms the basis of the simple, 'overnight' dexamethasone suppression test in which the 08.00 plasma cortisol is measured following administration of 1 mg of dexamethasone between 23.00 and 24.00 of the prior evening. No patient with any form of endogenous Cushing's syndrome should exhibit suppression.

# 3

# HYPOPITUITARISM

**General Principles**
**Etiologies of Hypopituitarism**
**The Empty Sella Syndrome**

## GENERAL PRINCIPLES

1.  The clinical syndrome (Table 3-1) is a composite of:

    a.  General clinical manifestations of the primary disease process (e.g. acromegaly, sarcoidosis, hemochromatosis, radiation therapy).

    b.  The degree to which specific pituitary functions are compromised (growth hormone (HGH) and gonadotropins tend to be affected 'early').

    c.  The effect of involvement of that process in regions adjacent to the pituitary (e.g. optic nerve, chiasm and tract; cavernous sinus involvement affecting cranial nerves III, IV and VI; hypothalamus).

    d.  The abruptness of evolution of that process.

        i.   In general, the more gradual the onset, the more it is 'tolerated'.

        ii.  An extreme case of abrupt onset is pituitary apoplexy.

    e.  The age of the patient.

        i.   HGH deficiency, e.g. has a more obvious structural effect in a prepubertal than a mature person; loss of gonadotropins are more apparent premenopausally.

        ii.  Some diseases are statistically more common in one age group (e.g. craniopharyngioma in childhood; hemochromatosis evolves over many years).

### TABLE 3-1.   FACTORS WHICH AFFECT THE CLINICAL SYNDROME

The Primary Disease Process
Specific Deficiency States
Involvement of Contiguous Structures
Abruptness of Development
Age
Gender
Additional Disease Processes

   f. The gender of the patient – e.g. Sheehan's syndrome occurring in women; prolactin-producing adenomas are generally smaller and diagnosed earlier in women than in men (men are additionally more likely to have 'space-occupying' symptoms – e.g. headache, loss of visual fields); anorexia nervosa (younger women); empty sella syndrome (middle-aged obese women).

   g. Additional Disease Processes – e.g. tuberculosis may be but one manifestation of HIV infection; amyloidosis secondary to myeloma or a chronic inflammatory state; other autoimmune diseases associated with lymphocytic hypophysitis.

2. Although hypothalamic disease (whether primary or secondary) can result in pituitary insufficiency, there are noteworthy features:

   a. Diabetes insipidus is a strong indication of hypothalamic disease (mere 'loss' of the posterior pituitary without concomitant hypothalamic disease – unless there is significant retrograde degeneration – can still result in arginine vasopressin production).

   b. Because prolactin is primarily under tonic inhibition, hyperprolactinemia is a feature of hypothalamic disease (or of impaired hypothalamic–pituitary 'communication').

   c. Some dynamic tests may distinguish between hypothalamic and pituitary disease (e.g. thyrotropin releasing hormone (TRH) and corticotropin releasing hormone (CRH) stimulation), as an 'intact pituitary' may demonstrate a response (albeit it may be delayed and protracted). Note – basal levels of thyroid stimulating hormone (TSH) and gonadotropins in pituitary disease may not be as low as anticipated, because of impaired glycosylation.

   d. Extensive hypothalamic involvement may affect thirst (independent or dependent of overt diabetes insipidus), hunger, behavior, emotion and thermal regulation.

3. While the endocrine deficiency state brought about by hypofunction of a trophic hormone may be similar to the primary deficiency state, there are distinctions:

   a. ACTH deficiency as a cause of Addison's disease is not

associated with hyperpigmentation – hypopigmentation may even be present; there is no associated aldosterone deficiency and thus no overt hyperkalemia. Hyponatremia, however, may be present to a varying degree because of decreased free water clearance.

b. Gonadotropin deficiency as a cause of gonadal failure may not produce 'hot flashes'.

c. TSH deficiency should not produce as severe hypothyroidism as primary hypothyroidism because of a basal 'autonomy' of about 10% of normal thyroid activity.

4. If hypopituitarism is caused by a 'pituitary destructive' condition, prolactin levels will be low. If hypopituitarism is caused by a 'stalk section' or its equivalent, prolactin levels can be elevated and there may be a 'clinical hyperprolactinemic' state.

5. While target organ replacement hormone therapy may obviate the need for specific trophic hormone replacement and may be more practical and cost effective in certain conditions (e.g. thyroxine and hydrocortisone replacement, respectively, for TSH and ACTH deficiency), the desire for fertility clearly dictates a different approach.

6. Despite the 'non-growth' metabolic effects of HGH, its administration is only clearly indicated in those individuals with growth impairment secondary to HGH deficiency. There is a current controversy and debate as to its efficacy in less well-defined conditions:

a. Most children who seek medical counsel for growth deficiency (almost invariably initiated by their concerned parents) have no obvious HGH dysfunction, by endocrinologic testing – these children comprise a variety of 'syndromes' variously called 'constitutional short stature' and 'delayed maturation', among others.

i. While there may be a modest benefit if a regular course of HGH therapy is administered, it requires frequent parenteral administration and is expensive (Who should pay the bill? Is it purely a 'cosmetic' treatment?)

ii. It may hasten sexual maturation.

b. Women with Turner's syndrome, however, can clearly benefit from HGH administration (augmented when anabolic steroids are additionally used).

c. Children with growth retardation secondary to chronic renal failure, and after renal transplantation, demonstrate a beneficial effect; it can also counteract the catabolic effects of chronic glucocorticoid use.

d. In the aging population, HGH levels decrease (males decline gradually, women more abruptly beginning at menopause, although actual decline in both sexes begins in their thirties). Aging is also associated with an altered bodily composition (decreased protein, increased fat).

   i. HGH administration can clearly alter this without significant overt side-effects (only mild elevation of blood sugar). This was well-demonstrated in a widely publicized 6-month trial, although those individuals selected for treatment had clearly low insulin-like growth factor I (IGF-I) levels at the outset.

   ii. Is it appropriate therapy? Who should pay?

   iii. Growth hormone deficiency in adults may be a subtle laboratory diagnosis to make, although stimulatory testing is more discriminatory than measurement of either IGF-I or its binding protein.

   iv. HGH therapy has no role in the primary treatment of obesity or osteoporosis, nor should it be used for 'body building'.

e. Additional possibilities

   i. HGH reverses the protein catabolic perioperative period by 'switching' to fat metabolism.

   ii. HGH can also sensitize the ovaries to gonadotropins (potential use as an ovulatory agent?)

f. This discussion of therapeutic HGH would not occur without the availability of recombinant HGH and a market-driven economy.

i.  Prior therapeutic HGH was cadaver-derived and was of extremely limited quantity, impure and carried the risk of transmitted infection (including Creutzfeldt–Jacob disease).

ii. It is now known that frequent multiple pulses (generally given six times a week by intramuscular or subcutaneous route) are necessary to mimic normal physiology. The use of a 'pump' may even be better because the most important contribution to growth appears to be the nocturnal pulse.

iii. The clinical use of IGF-I also has therapeutic potential (e.g. to improve bone density in age-related osteoporosis).

## ETIOLOGIES OF HYPOPITUITARISM (Table 3-2)

1. Neoplasia

   a. Pituitary Adenomas – Usually endocrinologically active whether or not the clinical syndrome is overt.

   b. Craniopharyngioma

      i.  Arises from Rathke's pouch (embryonic 'rest cells').

      ii. Most common hypothalamic–pituitary tumor in children and seen primarily in the pre-pubertal age group, but it can occur at any age.

      iii. Usually suprasellar with visual field impairment.

### TABLE 3-2.  ETIOLOGIES OF HYPOPITUITARISM

Neoplasia
Infiltrative Disease
Infectious Disease
Vascular Disease
Structural Abnormalities
Ablative
Selective
Autoimmune

     iv. Cystic matrix (high cholesterol concentration) and calcification (CT and MRI may reveal characteristic patterns).

     v. Treatment is difficult because of the tumor extent and poor response to radiation – it is slow growing, however.

  c. Other hypothalamic tumors – e.g. hypothalamic germinoma or meningioma, pinealoma (may be associated with elevation of human chorionic gonadotropin and α-fetoprotein; suppression of melatonin may be ameliorative), meningioma.

  d. Metastatic tumors (e.g. breast – the actual likelihood of hypopituitarism is substantially less than the finding of metastatic disease in the pituitary).

2. Infiltrative Disease

  a. Hemochromatosis – although primary testicular infiltration can also occur (and liver disease can contribute to testicular dysfunction), pituitary involvement is the most common cause of hypogonadism (this is the most prominent effect on the pituitary). An additional (non-pituitary) endocrinopathy is diabetes mellitus ('bronze diabetes').

  b. Amyloidosis.

  c. Granulomatous disease – may be infectious (e.g. tuberculosis, syphilis) or non-infectious (e.g. sarcoidosis).

  d. Histiocytosis X – comprises the spectrum of eosinophilic granuloma, Hand–Schüller–Christian Disease, and Letterer–Siwe Disease.

3. Infectious Disease

4. Vascular Disease

  a. Carotid Aneurysm – Effect of 'pressure atrophy'.

  b. Pituitary Infarction

     i. Postpartum – Sheehan's syndrome (vasospastic ischemia of hypertrophied gland?); Simmond's disease is a name associated with persistent chronic hypopituitarism secondary to antecedent infarction – the cachectic state of the 'index case' however is unclear (anorexia nervosa?) as the patient originally described had a normal pituitary gland at post-mortem.

    ii.  Pituitary Apoplexy – hemorrhagic infarction; acute fulminant syndrome if extensive (ironically, if localized to a tumor, itself, the patient may be relatively asymptomatic and may additionally have the ameliorative benefits of the correction of a primary hyperfunctioning syndrome). Although tumor is the most common setting, prior radiation therapy, diabetes, hypotension and anticoagulation states are associated risk factors.

    iii. Sickle Cell Disease.

5.  Structural Abnormalities – includes primary pituitary agenesis and basal encephalocele.

6.  Ablative – surgery, radiation therapy – including therapy for non-pituitary brain tumors (the hypothalamus is more vulnerable than the pituitary), trauma, following tuberculous meningitis.

7.  Selective – May be congenital (e.g. Kallman's syndrome – hypogonadotropic hypogonadism associated with anosmia; selective deficiencies of pituitary hormones) or acquired (e.g. hypogonadotropic hypogonadism as might occur with 'physical overconditioning' and anorexia nervosa).

8.  (Autoimmune) Lymphocytic Hypophysitis

    a.  A disease of women during pregnancy or the postpartum period.

    b.  Presents as pituitary hormone deficiency because of lymphocyte and plasma cell replacement of normal tissue (follicles may even be seen on histologic examination) – additionally, a 'mass effect' is exerted (there may therefore be confusion with a pituitary tumor or any other space-occupying infiltrative process) and can produce additional symptoms such as visual field defects and headache.

    c.  While multiple deficiencies may occur, prolactin levels may be decreased (producing agalactia) or increased (producing persistent lactation). Unrecognized (even though it is a rare disorder), it has a high mortality.

    d.  May be associated with other immunologically-mediated endocrine states (e.g. thyroiditis, adrenalitis) and even B-12 deficiency (very rare). Unlike 'postpartum thyroiditis', this disease very rarely remits.

9. Idiopathic – Relegated to those cases of unclear etiologies; may be sporadic or genetic (autosomal recessive, X-linked recessive).

## THE EMPTY SELLA SYNDROME

1. Rarely a cause of hypopituitarism although pituitary contents are 'displaced' and incompletely atrophied by arachnoid herniating from the basilar cistern through an incompetent diaphragmatic sella.

2. May be diagnosed serendipitously (seen in at least 5% of random autopsy cases) or in association with headache and benign intracranial hypertension or rarely other central manifestations – e.g. rhinorrhea, loss of visual fields.

3. When 'plain' skull X-rays were done in the past, an enlarged sella was often seen but was non-diagnostic. CT and MRI can show cerebrospinal fluid within the sella, itself, for diagnostic confirmation.

4. Statistically associated with obesity, female gender, middle age; it is usually 'idiopathic' but can also occur postpartum or following pituitary tumor necrosis. Prolactin can be elevated because of 'stalk traction' or association with a lactotrophic adenoma.

# 4

# ACROMEGALY

1. Etiology

   a. The majority of cases are associated with a primary pituitary adenoma.

   b. Although the increased pulse frequency of growth hormone (HGH) in acromegaly might suggest a hypothalamic etiology (i.e. excess growth hormone releasing hormone (GHRH)), such is probably not the case, even though increased pulse frequency (with normalization of amplitude) can persist post-pituitary surgery and mice rendered transgenic for GHRH can develop pituitary hyperplasia and tumors.

   c. The demonstration of a subset (up to 40%) of acromegalic patients with an abnormal Gs protein that 'continually activates' cAMP (and thus would obviate the need for GHRH) gives additional support to a primary pituitary etiology.

   d. Nonetheless, ectopic GHRH has been demonstrated (albeit as a rare cause) to be etiologic in isolated cases of acromegaly (e.g. pheochromocytoma, islet cell tumor, carcinoid). GHRH-secreting hypothalamic and pituitary gangliocytomas have also been described.

   e. Other etiologies of acromegaly include ectopic pituitary adenoma and ectopic HGH secretion, and the McCune–Albright syndrome.

    f.   The histopathology of the pituitary adenoma is of two types: densely or sparsely granulated; and mixed (usually with prolactin-producing capacity, but occasionally with other hormonal production as well). Abnormal hormone production with variable histologies can also occur.

2.   The syndrome is the result of unregulated HGH production that is both excessive and insensitive to normal feedback inhibition. To the extent that the adenoma also makes other hormones, compromises normal pituitary function, is associated with the multiple endocrine neoplasia type I (MEN-I) syndrome, or produces local effects, there can be ancillary clinical facets.

    a.   The effect of HGH in producing unbridled and distorted ('grotesque') growth is mediated through insulin-like growth factor-I (IGF-I; somatomedin C).

        i.   IGF-I levels 'plateau' at values of HGH less than the HGH-producing capacity of the adenoma.

            (a) This results in a rather comparable degree of acromegalic features in most acromegalics (over the same period of time) independent of HGH levels.

            (b) Conversely, to achieve a clinical 'cure' in most acromegalics generally requires a post-glucose suppression HGH value of less than 5 ng/ml.

        ii.   IGF-I (somatomedin C), because of its long half-life (12–24 hours) maintains a 'sustained' effect on growth – this 'stable' value is also helpful for diagnosis and management in an analogous way to glycosylated hemoglobin levels in diabetics.

        iii.   If IGF-I elevations occur prior to epiphyseal closure, gigantism is a predominant feature; post-closure, acromegaly predominates. In actuality, there may be a combination of the two – further, tumor-mediated hypogonadotropic hypogonadism can delay epiphyseal closure.

        iv.   Specific features include (Table 4-1):

            (a) Acral and soft tissue overgrowth 'spadehand'; – e.g. enlarging shoe, ring, glove and hat sizes; malocclusion; upper airway obstruction (sleep apnea).

## TABLE 4-1.   CLINICAL FEATURES OF ACROMEGALY

Acral and Soft Tissue Overgrowth
Exaggerated Facial Features
Encroachment Syndromes
Dermatologic Changes
Visceromegaly
Lethargy and Fatigue

(b) Large nose, thick lips, exaggeration of facial furrows ('leontine facies'), frontal bossing.

(c) Arthropathy, carpal and tarsal tunnel syndromes (producing parasthesias); kyphosis. Common denominator is 'encroachment'.

(d) Hyperhidrosis and increased skin oiliness, acanthosis, papillomas.

(e) Visceromegaly – heart, liver, kidneys, thyroid; colonic polyps; hypertension.

(f) Lethargy, fatigue, weight gain, sleep apnea.

b.  Direct metabolic effects of excessive HGH include glucose intolerance and insulin resistance.

c.  Relevant laboratory studies include (Table 4-2):

## TABLE 4-2.   LABORATORY AND RADIOLOGIC FEATURES OF ACROMEGALY

Hyperphosphatemia
Impaired Glucose Tolerance
HGH Non-Suppressibility
Elevated IGF-I
Abnormal HGH Responsiveness
Radiologic Enlargement of Sella Turcica
Radiologic Confirmation of Somatic Abormalities

i.  Hyperphosphatemia (secondary to increased tubular reabsorption) and hypercalciuria.

ii. Impaired glucose tolerance and evidence of overt diabetes mellitus (especially if there is an underlying propensity); hyperlipidemia.

iii. Failure of HGH suppression after an oral glucose load (100 g).

   (a) Most acromegalics have basal HGH levels greater than 10 ng/ml, but isolated determinations are not reliable. Failure to suppress to less than 5 ng/ml at 60 minutes is considered diagnostic.

   (b) HGH levels tend to be elevated (but suppressible) in renal failure, uncontrolled diabetes mellitus, anorexia nervosa and malnutrition.

iv. An abnormally elevated IGF-I is also considered diagnostic (because of multiple methodologies in use, each determination has to be compared with its own laboratory control). Note: high levels can be physiologic during adolescence and later pregnancy.

v.  Additional endocrinologic studies (of ancillary interest – not necessary or indicated for diagnosis):

   (a) Loss of nocturnal HGH 'pulse'.

   (b) Thyrotropin releasing hormone (TRH) and gonadotropin releasing hormone stimulation of HGH (no effect in normals).

   (c) L-DOPA (and bromocriptine and related analog) inhibition of HGH (they are usually stimulatory in normal states).

d. Radiologic studies include:

   i.  Studies determining the size and extent of the pituitary lesion – CT is very useful but MRI of the sella is the study of choice.

   ii. Supplementary studies for rarer etiologies (as appropriate) – e.g. for ectopic lesions, McCune–Albright syndrome.

iii. Studies confirmatory of the somatic syndrome (e.g. skull and jaw, hands and feet, frontal and maxillary sinuses) are not necessary or indicated, but will show characteristic changes.

3. Treatment – Ideally should eliminate both the mass effect of the tumor and the metabolic consequences of sustained HGH production, and maximize the potential for resurgence of pituitary reserve.

   a. Surgery (Recommended primary treatment)

      i. Transsphenoidal, if possible (lesions without extrasellar expansion). Initial success rate is up to 80%. Because of macroglossia and kyphosis, there may be anesthesia-related problems and tracheostomy may be necessary.

      ii. Postoperative follow-up requires:

         (a) Evaluation for hormonal deficiencies and appropriate treatment. Technical complications include cerebrospinal fluid leaks, meningitis, and bleeding.

         (b) IGF-I (should normalize) and post-glucose HGH should decrease to less than 2 ng/ml. (TRH stimulation test may be of ancillary benefit here.)

         (c) Indefinite follow-up is required (every 6–12 months, or as clinically required).

   b. Radiation Therapy

      i. Treatment of choice for recurrent disease or for surgical failure.

      ii. Up to 80% response rate, but the effect may not be immediate.

      iii. Conventional therapy appears to be as effective as 'heavy particle' (the latter may work more rapidly, but cannot be used in patients with extrasellar extension).

      iv. Hypopituitarism in up to 50% of cases.

   c. Medical Therapies

      i. Bromocriptine – lowers HGH levels in up to 50% of patients (but a smaller percentage truly 'normalize').

ii. Octreotide (Sandostatin: SMS-201-995)

(a) Can normalize HGH and IGF-I levels in up to two-thirds of patients, and can also induce tumor shrinkage.

(b) Side-effects – steatorrhea, diarrhea, worsening glucose intolerance, gall bladder disease.

(c) Needs to be given parenterally in multiple doses, but high doses offer no added clinical or biochemical benefit.

(d) It is expensive – up to \$35–40 a day.

# 5

# PROLACTIN-
# PRODUCING
# ADENOMA

General Considerations
Diagnostic Evaluation of Amenorrhea With or Without Galactorrhea
Medical Therapy
Surgery
Radiation Therapy

## GENERAL CONSIDERATIONS

1. An extremely common lesion when looked at from the point of view of 'incidental' pituitary adenomas found at autopsy – about 25% of autopsied cases have adenomas, nearly half of which demonstrate prolactin production. Yet, the clinical syndromes associated with hyperprolactinemia are generally not apparent in these patients.

2. Eponymic syndromes of lactation described in earlier medical literatures were likely (by today's understanding) to have been associated with prolactin-producing neoplastic disease:

   a. Chiari–Frommel – Persistent postpartum lactation.

   b. Forbes–Albright Syndrome – Lactation associated with a pituitary tumor.

   c. del Castillo's Syndrome – 'Idiopathic' lactation.

3. The specific clinical syndromes of prolactin-producing adenoma are variable and are manifest differently based on age and gender.

   a. In women of reproductive age, amenorrhea is a common presentation, with or without galactorrhea (amenorrhea can be primary or secondary and may occur following oral contraceptive use or pregnancy).

      i. Galactorrhea may not have been noted by the woman but may be observed by an examining physician on manual expression. Galactorrhea without an elevated prolactin level is a common clinical finding and is associated with increased target organ sensitivity.

      ii. Long-standing amenorrhea may diminish the tendency to galactorrhea because of decreased estrogen production.

      iii. The mechanism of amenorrhea (and decreased estrogen) appears to be gonadotropin releasing hormone inhibition. This deficiency state can lead to peripheral manifestations of estrogen deficiency including decreased libido, vaginal dryness and propensity to osteoporosis. The osteoporosis is a function of the estrogen deficiency – women with hyperprolactinemia with normal menses are not at increased risk.

iv. Women with hyperprolactinemia may also have relative infertility (abnormal luteal phase?) and predilection to polycystic ovary syndrome 'variant' (hirsutism, obesity – perhaps secondary to stimulation of adrenal androgens, as dehydroepiandrosterone sulfate is increased). Depression and anxiety may be hyperprolactinemic concomitants.

b. In men of all ages, there is a higher likelihood of tumors being of larger size and brought to medical attention because of local symptoms – in younger males, sexual dysfunction (decreased libido and potency) and infertility are additional complaints. Testosterone levels are decreased because of hypogonadotropinemia, putting men at increased risk for osteoporosis. It should be noted that exogenous testosterone, in the presence of hyperprolactinemia, usually does not correct the impotence – indicative of an additional peripheral effect of the prolactin.

4. It is important to distinguish prolactinomas from other conditions of prolactin elevation or lactation which may or may not produce comparable clinical syndromes:

   a. Organic disease – e.g. hypothyroidism, renal failure, liver dysfunction, chest wall trauma or disease (e.g. Zoster).

   b. 'Physiologic' – e.g. pregnancy, postpartum state (although prolactin levels decrease despite the capability of persistent lactation – indicative that increased target organ sensitivity is the operant mechanism).

   c. Medications – Previously categorized and include the phenothiazine, butyrophenone and benzisoxazole families; metoclopramide, reserpine, H-2 blockers and α-methyl DOPA.

   d. Although 'pituitary disease' will be demonstrated in patients whose hyperprolactinemia is caused by prolactin inhibitory factor inhibition (e.g. 'stalk compression' by cranio-pharyngioma or metastatic tumor), the pathophysiology and treatment plans are different from that of a true prolactinoma.

## DIAGNOSTIC EVALUATION OF AMENORRHEA WITH OR WITHOUT GALACTORRHEA

1. Patients with amenorrhea or galactorrhea without hyper-prolactinemia rarely have a pituitary tumor (an incidental tumor may

'stain' for prolactin but it is 'functionally immature'). Thus, a tumor work-up is not warranted unless clinically indicated (sequential prolactin levels may be helpful).

2. 'Obvious' clinical reasons for hyperprolactinemia should be considered and confirmed (e.g. pregnancy, hypothyroidism, renal failure, liver disease, medications). Although 'provocative tests' have been devised (e.g. thyrotropin releasing hormone stimulation test – tumors do not increase in prolactin response, while normals do), a basal prolactin determination remains the best discriminant and should be obtained (repeated as necessary).

3. Values greater than 200 ng/ml are almost always associated with prolactinomas. The difficulty lies with values substantially less but still above normal (i.e. greater than 20 ng/ml). MRI (preferred) or CT should be performed in all situations of inexplicable prolactin elevations. Unfortunately, not all microadenomas may be visualized; further, some patients with hyperprolactinemia may have an 'incidental' adenoma ('true–true, unrelated').

4. Based on imaging studies, it is important to categorize tumors according to their size:

   a. Microadenomas – tumors that are intrasellar and less than 1 cm in size; panhypopituitarism is highly unlikely and formal testing of pituitary function is generally not necessary, especially if the hyperprolactinemia along with its clinical manifestations are corrected with bromocriptine.

   b. Macroadenomas – tumors that are greater than 1 cm in size; usually produce some degree of sella enlargement and varying degrees of hypopituitarism, depending on their size. They also tend to be associated with the highest elevation of prolactin.

5. It is also important to define goals as they may be related to correction of amenorrhea and sexual function, fertility and osteoporosis (patients with microadenomas or 'idiopathic' hyperprolactinemia can be followed, at times, without specific therapy – certainly tumor size and local symptomatology must always be considered). Estrogen levels (estradiol) or clinical status (e.g. evidence of estrogen effect on Papanicolaou smear, withdrawal bleeding following medroxyprogesterone administration) and testosterone levels are important in rendering intelligent recommendations (gonadotropin levels may also be useful).

## MEDICAL THERAPY

1. Bromocriptine

   a. Highly effective dopaminergic medication that can normalize serum prolactin levels in the vast majority of patients with both microadenomas and macroadenomatous disease. Tumor size shrinks in the majority of macroadenomas treated with bromocriptine. Certainly, it is the treatment of choice in 'idiopathic' hyperprolactinemia.

   b. Given in divided doses (dose range: 2.5–10 mg/day). Nausea is a common side-effect (other common side-effects can include dizziness and orthostatic hypotension). By gradually 'building up' the dose (initial therapy should be only 2.5 mg, once daily, at bedtime), tolerance generally improves. The prolactin level need not be normal if the clinical goal is achieved.

   c. It can be the primary therapy for microadenoma but probably requires indefinite administration for continued normalcy (hence, long-term costs, side-effects, inconvenience, etc. have to be considered). If pregnancy is a desired goal, bromocriptine can be administered until early pregnancy – the patient will usually be aware of antecedent ovulation by symptomatology (e.g. Mittelschmerz, molimina), basal temperature monitoring or an antecedent menstrual period (conversely, she may go 'directly' from the amenorrhea of hyperprolactinemia to the amenorrhea of pregnancy).

      i. Corollaries are:

         (a) Barrier contraception, from the onset of therapy, is necessary if pregnancy is not desired.

         (b) Regular pregnancy testing is advised, as deemed appropriate.

      ii. There are no ill effects of hyperprolactinemia on the fetus – thus, bromocriptine can be discontinued at the onset of pregnancy.

      iii. Despite the known effect of estrogen as a prolactin stimulus, only a small minority of pregnant women have worsening of their clinical state during the bromocriptine withdrawal (although all women should be advised of the possibility). While prolactin levels may be helpful to follow, visual fields are more clinically meaningful, especially if the primary lesion is a macroadenoma.

iv. If necessary, bromocriptine can be reinstituted during pregnancy (this is not the accepted standard if it can be avoided, but there have been no proven deleterious effects on the fetus).

2. Pergolide (whose action and side-effects are similar to those of bromocriptine) and other agents under investigation may have a more significant role in the future. Indeed, carbegoline can be given less frequently (twice weekly) and is better tolerated than is bromocriptine.

## SURGERY

1. The only possibility for long-term definitive cure.

   a. Cure is dependent on the size and extent of the tumor.

   b. In most studies, cure varies between 60 and 80% for microadenomas (less for macroadenomas) but recurrence (over the long term) is a problem, even if the recurrence is in the form of hyperprolactinemia and not an obvious tumor.

2. May be necessary for correction of local symptoms, even if this results only in an 'incomplete debulking process' and an additional modality of therapy is necessary.

3. Surgical extirpation (particularly in a large tumor) may result in postoperative hypopituitarism, even if it was not present preoperatively (hence the need for endocrine assessment following surgery).

## RADIATION THERAPY

1. Generally considered an adjunct in appropriately selected patients.

2. Delayed response and long-term hypopituitarism are features.

# 6

# OTHER PRIMARY TUMORS OF THE ANTERIOR PITUITARY GLAND

Glycoprotein and 'Non-Functioning' Pituitary Adenomas
Thyrotropin-Producing Adenomas
Gonadotropin-Producing Adenomas
Truly 'Non-Functioning' Adenomas

### GLYCOPROTEIN AND 'NON-FUNCTIONING' PITUITARY ADENOMAS (Table 6-1)

With the advent of sophisticated hormone assays and contemporary molecular biology (heralded with the prolactin assay and the realization that the majority of pituitary tumors are prolactin producers), most pituitary tumors can now be classified. Since acromegaly and Cushing's disease have been long-appreciated endocrinopathies, the most recent advances have been made in glycoprotein (thyroid stimulating hormone (TSH), follicle stimulating hormone (FSH) and luteinizing hormone (LH))-producing adenomas.

Evidence from most tumors suggest intrinsic 'clonal' abnormalities that result from loss of regulation of growth control. These may be 'sporadic' or familial. Gene mutations involving several genes (including oncogenes) may be operant. The role of trophic stimulation as a concomitant has still to be clearly defined (e.g. pituitary enlargement occurs in Klinefelter's syndrome and hypothyroidism but tumor genesis is rare; on the other hand, Nelson's syndrome can occur in adrenalectomized patients treated for their Cushing's syndrome).

### THYROTROPIN-PRODUCING ADENOMAS

1. Thyrotoxicosis associated with elevated thyroid hormone parameters and inappropriate TSH elevation ($\alpha$ subunit production is increased disproportionately to that of the intact

### TABLE 6-1.  GLYCOPROTEIN AND 'NON-FUNCTIONING' PITUITARY ADENOMAS

| Endocrine Type | Clinical Features |
| --- | --- |
| Thyrotropin-Producing Adenoma | Thyrotoxicosis With Elevated TSH |
| Gonadotropin-Producing Adenoma | Gonadotropin Excess (Usually FSH With Uncombined $\alpha$ and $\beta$ Subunits) and Relative Hypogonadism |
| Truly 'Non-Functioning' Adenoma | Syndrome Related to 'Mass Effect' and Deficiency State |

TSH). In distinction, in individuals with pituitary resistance to TSH, the molar ratio of α subunit/TSH is always less than one.

2. Histology – chromophobe.

3. Goiter and thyrometabolic manifestations but no ophthalmopathy or pretibial myxedema.

4. Manifestations also include the mass effect of the tumor and hypopituitarism.

5. Treatment is directed primarily at the tumor – surgery (with adjunctive radiation, as necessary).

6. 'Secondary' treatment of the thyrotoxic state may be necessary but is often difficult (e.g. high-dose multiple [131]Iodine treatments).

7. Octreotide has proven to be beneficial in a majority of patients.

## GONADOTROPIN-PRODUCING ADENOMAS

1. The majority are in men; most tumors produce FSH. More significant is the exuberant production of uncombined α and β subunits. Excess FSH β is a frequently found abnormality, often in excess of α subunit production.

2. The most common clinical manifestations are related to the size and extent of the tumor and not hormone excess (conversely, deficiency states may be noted).

3. Despite gonadotropin elevation, impotence and sexual dysfunction are concomitants – explicable by immunologically reactive but biologically inert gonadotropins. Thus, a better term for this class of adenoma might be 'clinically non-functioning' (although hormone-producing) pituitary adenomas. Unlike TSH-producing tumors, α subunits are not made in excess as often.

4. If prolactin levels are elevated, it is probably due to impairment of dopaminergic inhibition.

5. Unlike the normal state, thyrotropin releasing hormone administration may stimulate gonadotropin production. Another interesting phenomenon is the failure of gonadotropin sensitivity to gonadotropin releasing hormone (GnRH) stimulation, a phenomenon that occurs in normals and that has widespread clinical application.

6. Therapy includes surgery, radiation, bromocriptine and octreotide (GnRH analogs are not consistently helpful). The use of radioactively labelled octreotide to detect somatostatin receptors on these cells may be helpful in predicting future response to therapy.

## TRULY 'NON-FUNCTIONING' ADENOMAS

1. Now relegated to less than 10% of all pituitary adenomas.

2. With improved assay and detection of subunits and variants, many may ultimately demonstrate some 'endocrinologic activity'. Growth hormone- and ACTH-producing adenomas have been noted without corresponding syndromes of target organ hyperactivity. This could represent either poor adenoma differentiation or 'sub-clinical' disease.

3. Nonetheless, some tumors are so de-differentiated (null cell adenomas) that no detectable hormonal markers have been found.

4. Clinical presentation related to mass effect and endocrine deficiency state.

5. Therapy: surgery, radiation therapy, octreotide.

## ANATOMY AND PHYSIOLOGY

1. Nerve endings in the posterior pituitary have their cell bodies located in the supraoptic and paraventricular nuclei. They contain cell types that are a part of a larger magno- and parvocellular system that elaborates peptides for other sites (e.g. to stimulate ACTH).

2. Secretory products made by these cells go through an elaborate synthetic process whereby a pre-prohormone gives rise to a prohormone which ultimately results in a neurophysin–hormone product.

3. Oxytocin and vasopressin are the two posterior pituitary hormones. They are both nine-amino acid structures and each is attached to a complementary neurophysin that is 'shed' into the circulation at the time of hormone release (neurophysin I is associated with oxytocin, neurophysin II with vasopressin).

## ACTIONS OF VASOPRESSIN AND OXYTOCIN

1. The primary action of vasopressin is on the collecting tubule epithelium to increase permeability to water – this is mediated through activation of adenylate cyclase. Aquaporin-2 is a collecting tubule product that appears to be a measure of vasopressin effect.

   a. It is important to emphasize that this effect, visually represented by an increase in 'pore size', only allows for water to be passively reabsorbed. If the adjacent medullary interstitium is hypertonic, then reabsorption occurs. If not, reabsorption of water does not occur.

   b. Vasopressin not only permits water but also urea reabsorption and this increases the hypertonicity of the medullary interstitium by about 50%. A corollary is that long periods of time without vasopressin (e.g. as might occur with long-standing excessive fluid intake) results in a relative interstitial 'washout'. Subsequent fluid deprivation and re-stimulation of vasopressin results in a less concentrated urine than might be expected because the collecting tubule water is not as readily 'drawn' to this less hypertonic medullary interstitium.

2. A lesser secondary effect of vasopressin is cardiovascular – it is both a vasoconstrictor and pressor agent (hence 'vasopressin').

3. Oxytocin will not be covered in depth, but it should be noted that its major actions are on special target smooth muscle (myoepithelial cell contraction to produce milk release; uterine contraction in a 'primed' uterus).

## REGULATION OF VASOPRESSIN

1. Osmotic Stimulation – low-level production of vasopressin until 'threshold' osmolality of 280 mOsm/l – then, the levels increase in a 'linear fashion' as a function of osmolality. Note that in normal individuals, the thirst 'threshold' is about 290 mOsm/l.

2. Volume Stimulation

   a. Low pressure 'sensors' (right heart and left atrium) and high pressure 'baroreceptors' (aortic arch and carotid sinus) – left atrial pressure is probably the most important.

   b. As opposed to a 'linear' osmotic response curve, vasopressin increases exponentially with progressive hypovolemia. Hyperosmolality augments the hypovolemic response curve such that higher vasopressin levels are seen at any given level of hypovolemia.

3. Additional Regulators

   a. Stimulators – β-adrenergic stimulation, cholinergic stimulation, angiotensin II (also a dipsogen), opiates, nicotine, histamine, barbiturates, prostaglandin E group, 'retching' reflex.

   b. Inhibitors – oropharyngeal 'reflex' (both antidiuretic hormone (ADH) and thirst are acutely curtailed with water ingestion, even before water absorption has corrected either hyperosmolality or hypovolemia; more pronounced with cold water). Other inhibitors include α-adrenergic stimulation, atrial natriuretic factor (ANF), dilantin and alcohol (acutely).

## DIABETES INSIPIDUS

A syndrome associated with polyuria of a dilute nature secondary to vasopressin deficiency (central) or to impaired response (nephrogenic). If untreated, it can lead to profound hypovolemia and dehydration. Diabetes insipidus should be distinguished from other causes of urinary frequency in which there is not an inappropriately dilute urine. Osmotic-mediated diuresis (e.g. uncontrolled diabetes mellitus) must also be excluded.

A clinically similar syndrome, although etiologically different, is primary polydipsia.

## Central Diabetes Insipidus (Vasopressin Deficiency)

1. Etiologies include:

   a. Familial – autosomal dominant and attributed to a defective propressophysin gene on chromosome 20, resulting in postnatal neuronal degeneration,

   b. Idiopathic – a subset of this category is associated with lymphocytic infundibuloneurohypophysitis (detectable on MRI and reversible),

   c. Traumatic,

   d. Vascular,

   e. Neoplastic – primary and secondary,

   f. Infection,

   g. Autoimmune,

   h. Non-infectious granulomatous, and

   i. Diabetes insipidus of pregnancy – a rare disorder associated with a relative deficiency of vaspressin that may be exaggerated by increased hormonal degradation.

2. While in some situations the defect may be absolute, in most cases, the deficiency is relative. A cardinal feature is often the activation of thirst prior to elaboration of sufficient vasopressin to prevent severe clinical diabetes insipidus. Increased fluid consumption driven by the thirst mechanism can maintain clinical homeostasis.

## Nephrogenic Diabetes Insipidus (Resistance to Vasopressin)

1. Etiologies include:

   a. Intrinsic Renal Disease – derangement of medullary and/or collecting tubule function (e.g. polycystic renal disease, obstructive uropathy, chronic pyelonephritis),

b. Electrolyte Imbalance – hypokalemia, hypercalcemia,

c. Drugs – Lithium, demethylchlortetracycline (Declomycin), colchicine, fluoride, methoxyflurane,

d. Protein Deprivation – failure of adequate urea production to create an optimal medullary tonicity,

e. Sickle cell disease and trait,

f. Granulomatous Disease (Sarcoid), and

g. Familial (X-linked recessive) – associated with a mutation in the vasopressin V-2 receptor gene.

2. To varying degrees, defects represent relative resistance and may be overcome by supraphysiologic doses of vasopressin (not practical, however, from a therapeutic point of view).

**Primary Polydipsia**
1. Basic mechanism is a primary initiation of fluid intake whether thirst-mediated or not, because of an abnormally low osmotic threshold to fluid-seeking behavior.

2. Etiologies include:

a. Psychiatric Disease – such affected individuals may not be able to give you a good answer as to why they are thirsty, and

b. Central Nervous System Disease – traumatic, degenerative (e.g. multiple sclerosis), infectious, neoplastic, etc. Etiologies can overlap those of both central and nephrogenic diabetes insipidus (e.g. sarcoidosis, lithium). Such affected individuals are 'truly thirsty'. The osmotic threshold for thirst is inappropriately low.

**Diagnosis and Work-up**
1. When appropriate clinical data are available (e.g. history of pituitary surgery, sickle cell disease) the diagnosis is easier to make. On the other hand, such information is often not readily obvious. Further, even if there is relevant clinical data (e.g. sarcoidosis, central nervous system disease), it may not prove discriminating. Imaging studies (e.g. pituitary CT) may be important.

2. Serum Osmolality – although generally elevated in central and nephrogenic diabetes insipidus and depressed in primary polydipsia, there is often not clear-cut basal discrimination.

3. Urine Osmolality – relatively low in all three categories. Theoretically it should normalize after dehydration in primary polydipsia (but not in either form of diabetes insipidus) but:

   a. Medullary 'washout' from chronic fluid ingestion will decrease urine concentrating ability (normalization will occur after about 3 days of 'normal' fluid intake).

   b. Dehydration even with diabetes insipidus can increase urine concentration because:

      i. Central deficiency can be partial and vasopressin can be stimulated, albeit requiring a greater degree of hyperosmolality and hypovolemia to do so.

      ii. Non-ADH mechanisms (decreased glomerular filtration rate and diminished solute delivery to the thick ascending limb of Henle) may be operant in both central and nephrogenic diabetes insipidus.

4. Measurement of plasma vasopressin – can be very discriminating, especially when correlated with urine and plasma osmolality and when performed basally and following water deprivation. (Note: If the patient had received prior therapeutic vasopressin, antibody production by the patient may affect the assay).

5. Hypertonic Saline (with basal and postinfusion vasopressin levels and urine and plasma osmolalities) may be a helpful adjunct but because of potential risks and difficulties, it should not be routinely employed.

6. Vasopressin Trial (aqueous pitressin, 5 U; pitressin tannate in oil, 5 U; desmopressin (DDAVP), 1 µg subcutaneously or 20 µg by nasal insufflation) – ability to concentrate urine seen in central diabetes insipidus (and primary polydipsia) but not nephrogenic diabetes insipidus. A danger of this test in primary polydipsia is the continued tendency to take in excessive fluids (because of the decreased 'set point' of fluid ingestion) in the presence of vasopressin 'on board'. This can result in water intoxication.

7. Note: Concomitant anterior pituitary disease (with thyroid hormone and cortisol deficiency) may diminish the anticipated urine volume and diluteness.

**Therapy**
1. Central Diabetes Insipidus

   a. Desmopressin (DDAVP) – a synthetic analog and the present drug of choice in central diabetes insipidus (it is the only useful preparation in the diabetes insipidus of pregnancy). Convenient and effective, but expensive. The only drug that can be taken intranasally (as well as parenterally), but local irritation and variable absorption may be problematic. While two or three times daily administration is recommended and often necessary, expense may be decreased by bedtime use in patients with only partial deficiency who can compensate for excessive urine output during the day with increased fluid intake.

   b. Pitressin Tannate in Oil – less reliable and more erratic; no longer manufactured.

   c. Lysine Vasopressin (Diapid) – nasal administration; short half-life.

   d. Chlorpropramide – enhances peripheral effect of vasopressin, even in the presence of severe deficiency or vasopressin antibodies. Pre-existing deficiency of ADH appears to augment its effect. Potential risk of hypoglycemia (which can usually be pre-empted).

   e. Thiazide Diuretics – may be a useful adjunct; added bonus if used with chlorpropramide, is its ability to mitigate the tendency to hypoglycemia.

2. Nephrogenic Diabetes Insipidus

   a. Correction of underlying disease (if possible).

   b. 'Overriding' doses of DDAVP (usually not practical or appropriate).

   c. Thiazide and Amiloride Diuretics – directly decrease free water clearance and secondarily produce a relative dehydration with decreased tubular fluid delivery to the distal nephron.

3. Primary polydipsia

   a. Correction of underlying problem (if possible).

   b. Use of DDAVP or related agents may decrease the plasma osmolality below the 'trigger threshold' for thirst, but there is always a danger (episodically or chronically) of water intoxication.

   c. Patient education, 'behavior modification', psychotherapy.

## SYNDROME OF INAPPROPRIATE ADH

Although an important etiology of hyponatremia, it is best appreciated in the context of the various mechanisms by which hyponatremia can occur.

1. Pseudohyponatremia

   a. Occurs when non-sodium-containing volume is 'added' to the intravascular compartment. Included are hyperlipidemia (often obvious on direct observation of the blood or after refrigeration), hyperproteinemia (as in paraproteinemias), isotonic bladder irrigating solutions (even if only a small percentage of the administered solution is absorbed, this may be significant considering the total amount of the administered irrigant), and even hyperimmune globulin (because of its high concentration of maltose).

   b. When significant amounts of solute are administered (e.g. mannitol) or rapidly generated and maintained in the intravascular compartment because of inability to be metabolized (e.g. glucose in uncontrolled diabetes), the resultant serum osmolality may be increased, with a resultant decrease in the relative sodium concentration.

2. For the kidney to be able to regulate 'free water' clearance, thus preventing the potential of a hyponatremic state, the following (alone or in concert) must be operant:

   a. The amount of water ingested must not be so great as to overwhelm the ability to excrete it.

      i. Ingestion of such large amounts of fluid are uncommon because otherwise euvolemic, normal individuals are generally incapable of such an act (without profound thirst suppression, gastric distension, nausea and vomiting).

ii. Large fluid intake, however, can occur when parenteral fluids are administered (e.g. intravenous, gastric lavage with a dextrose and water solution) or if there is an underlying psychiatric disturbance (e.g. compulsive water drinking) abetted by a superimposed drug effect or central nervous system pathology.

b. There must be adequacy of glomerular filtration.

c. There must be adequate solute delivery to the only portion of the kidney where dilute urine is made: the thick ascending limb of the loop of Henle. Dilute urine is made there because it is the only site where solute is absorbed in excess of water. At all other sites, solute and water are absorbed equivalent to the tonicity of the tubular fluid. Thus, tubular fluid ('pre-urine') leaving the thick ascending limb is always hypotonic. Its manufacture is contingent upon delivery of sufficient solute there so that appreciable reabsorption of this solute generates an adequate hypotonic 'pre-urine'. Once this 'pre-urine' continues through the remaining nephron (and after its volume is decreased at the 'cortical diluting site'), it can remain hypotonic throughout its passage through the collecting tubule or it can lose varying degrees of that tonicity (even becoming hypertonic) depending on the amount of water that is absorbed from it (ADH-mediated) during passage through the collecting tubule. Inadequate generation of this hypotonic urine can occur when:

i. The amount of solute ingested (as a function of the amount of water) may be so little that the solute is extensively absorbed before it reaches the thick ascending limb of the loop of Henle and hypotonic tubular fluid is not able to be formed – e.g. 'serious' beer drinking.

ii. There is absolute or relative (e.g. congestive heart failure, nephrotic syndrome, mineralocorticoid deficiency) dehydration.

d. The amount of ADH generated or its peripheral effect must not be inappropriately excessive for the underlying condition.

i.   In many clinical situations where the production of ADH is augmented, relative (e.g. congestive heart failure, liver disease) or absolute (e.g. Addison's disease) hypovolemia is often a provocateur. Even in the absence of hyperosmolality, this hypovolemia may be a sufficient stimulus (especially since the production of ADH rises exponentially as a function of the degree of hypovolemia, as opposed to the 'linear' relationship with hyperosmolality). Furthermore, hypovolemia augments the ability for any given degree of hyperosmolality to stimulate ADH.

ii.  As can be inferred from the prior section, often the effect of increased ADH works in concert with an inability to excrete excessive water because of inadequate solute delivery to the thick ascending limb. If excessive fluid is either ingested or administered, water retention can be augmented.

iii. Thiazides, but not loop diuretics, can produce water retention because:

(a) While both diuretics can produce hypovolemia, thiazides and classical loop diuretics (furosemide, ethacrynic acid) differ in their specific sites of action. By acting on the early, thick ascending portion, loop diuretics not only prevent hypotonic urine, but also hypertonic urine from being generated. They do not allow development of a hypertonic medullary interstitium that can produce a hypertonic urine when collecting tubule fluid equilibrates with the interstitium under the influence of ADH.

(b) Thiazides (and related) diuretics affect the so-called thinner 'diluting segment' which is in the cortex. Prevention of solute absorption here does not affect the hypertonicity of the medulla. Hence, ADH can still increase collecting tubule water reabsorption. Impaired cortical solute reabsorption prevents the urine from become dilute and impairs the ability to clear excess free water.

**TABLE 7-1.  CLINICAL STATES ASSOCIATED WITH SYNDROME OF INAPPROPRIATE ANTIDIURETIC HORMONE**

Neoplastic Disease
Pulmonary Disease
Drugs
Central Nervous System Disease
'Appropriate' ADH Syndromes

**Clinical States Associated with Syndrome of Inappropriate ADH** (Table 7-1)

1.  Neoplastic Disease – most commonly seen with carcinoma of the lung (especially small cell) but also seen (among other tumors) in non-small cell lung cancer, adrenal cortical carcinoma, lymphoma, pancreatic carcinoma and cancer of the prostate.

2.  Pulmonary Disease – seen in diverse etiologies including lobar pneumonia, tuberculosis and lung abscess.

3.  Drugs – chlorpropramide, vinca alkaloids, carbamazepine (Tegretol), cyclophosphamide, phenothiazides, fluoxetine.

4.  Central Nervous System Disease – multiple and diverse etiologies.

5.  When seen in such diverse clinical situations as adrenal cortical insufficiency, hypothyroidism, congestive heart failure, liver disease and with thiazide diuretics, the resultant clinical syndromes (including ADH elaboration) are actually 'appropriate' and consistent with a 'physiologic design', even though the resultant water retention and hyponatremia may be 'clinically inappropriate' and not in the best interest of the individual.

**Clinical and Laboratory Features**
1.  Varying degrees of mental dysfunction leading in its extreme to obtundation and seizure activity. Much depends on the degree and rapidity of onset of the hyponatremia.

2.  Edema (unless part of a primary process) is not a feature.

3.  Although hyponatremia is an important feature, the excessive

water retention 'dilutes out' other components as well (e.g. potassium, blood urea nitrogen, chloride). Sodium is used as a benchmark because of its high concentration and relative contribution to the plasma osmolality. The hallmark of the syndrome is the absence of any other potential cause (e.g. liver, renal, cardiac, adrenal disease) and a disparity between the serum and urine osmolality. In severe cases, the urine osmolality need not be very high, only inappropriately high.

4. Urine sodium excretion is generally commensurate with the intake, once a 'steady state' is achieved.

## Mechanisms of ADH Inappropriateness

1. Erratic and episodic fluctuations of vasopressin production (seen in up to 40% of patients of all types).

2. Resetting of vasopressin 'set point' (about 30% of cases).

3. Sustained vasopressin 'leak' at levels of osmolality when it should be suppressed, although levels in response to stimulation are normal (about 20–30% of cases).

4. Purported increased sensitivity to normal amounts of vasopressin (10%).

## Treatment

1. Chronic states are best treated with voluntary fluid restriction – significant thirst and not 'environmental cues' should determine intake (usually kept to 1 liter/day or less).

2. Chronic demethylchlortetracycline (Declomycin) may be helpful (it is important to follow renal function). Lithium is effective but toxic and the dosage is difficult to regulate in this syndrome. Liberal salt intake with oral furosemide may also be useful.

3. Acute symptomatic hyponatremia should be treated with hypertonic (3%) saline and intravenous furosemide, but the severity of the clinical state must justify such an aggressive tactic.

   a. 'Normal saline' is not effective because it does not 'match' the degree of tonicity of the urine and can thus thwart correction of the hyponatremic state.

b.  Caution is needed to prevent excessive volume overload in vulnerable patients (e.g. those with underlying congestive heart failure) unable to deal with rapid correction of the hypo-osmotic state.

c.  Rapid correction might result in the osmotic demyelination syndrome, previously referred to as central pontine and extrapontine myelinolysis. This is characterized by myelin loss in the central pons and other sites (cerebrum, cerebellum, internal capsule, basal ganglia). Hypokalemic patients may be particularly vulnerable.

# Section C

# DISORDERS OF THE THYROID

# 8

# THE THYROID GLAND – INTRODUCTION AND CLINICAL PHYSIOLOGY

## OVERVIEW

1. Shield-like (*Thyrus* in Greek = Shield) organ derived from pharyngeal epithelium; embryologically present at 4 weeks (but iodide concentrating and thyroid hormone producing ability not apparent until 11th week).

2. Migrates caudally from base of tongue (foramen cecum) to permanent location in lower neck; clinical implications include lingual thyroid, thyroglossal duct cyst and pyramidal lobe exaggeration in hyperplastic states.

3. Maternal and fetal thyroid units are independent with little transplacental transfer of thyroid hormone – sufficient quantities, however, can go to the thyroprivic fetus to prevent intrauterine cretinism, and the fetal brain can convert thyroxine to triiodothyronine, which is why neonatal hypothyroid screening and early postpartum replacement therapy can produce a normal child.

4. The adult gland is 15–20 g (individual lobes are approximately $2.5 \times 4$ cm); a thinner isthmus is noted under the cricoid cartilage (good landmark for palpation) – blood supply by superior (external carotid origin) and inferior (subclavian origin) arteries. Blood flow is twice renal blood flow/g tissue and can be in excess of 1 liter/minute in thyrotoxic states (a clinical corollary is the presence of a bruit).

## THYROID HORMONE SYNTHESIS

1. Iodine metabolism

   a. Average daily ingestion in the USA is 500 mg (higher in Japan, lower in Europe – subject to alterations with regional geography, diet, medications). Intake is matched by excretion (97% in urine).

   b. Kidney and thyroid gland are primary competitors for iodide – the thyroid takes up iodide against a large concentration gradient (ratio can be as high as 500 : 1). Process can be blocked by organic anions, e.g. thiocyanate and perchlorate ($SCN^-$, $ClO_4^-$) – excessive quantities of these may be found in 'natural goitrogens' (Brassicaceae or Cruciferae family;

cassava; cigarette smoke? – smoke is also associated with an increased risk of Graves' disease).

2. Organification

   a. Crucial reaction requires $H_2O_2$ generation and peroxidase (933 amino acids, MW = 107 000) to form iodine from iodide. Iodine is then added to tyrosyl moieties.

   b. Process of iodination takes place within the thyroglobulin (MW = 660 000; 110 tyrosine moieties per molecule).

   c. Coupling brings together two iodotyrosine molecules within the thyroglobulin matrix to form iodothyronines.

   d. Conventional antithyroid drugs (thionamides) act at this site – other inhibitory classes include aminoheterocyclics (e.g. para-aminosalicylic acid) and substituted phenols (e.g. resorcinol). Pharmacologic doses of iodide (Wolff–Chaikoff effect) are also inhibitory, but in healthy glands, there is an escape.

3. Thyroid hormone release

   a. Proteolytic process which cleaves active thyroid hormones (primarily thyroxine ($T_4$)), from thyroglobulin (by endocytosis).

   b. Blocked by pharmacologic doses of iodides and lithium.

   c. The role of iodides in thyroid hormone economy is a curious one. Iodine is obviously a primary constituent of thyroid hormone. Deficiency can result in hypothyroidism but the gland can compensate through hyperplasia (goiter may result), increased trapping and increased triiodothyronine ($T_3$)/$T_4$ ratio. Iodide excess can also produce hypothyroidism by:

      i. The Wolff–Chaikoff effect (the failure to 'escape' occurs with intrinsic thyroid disease such as Hashimoto's thyroiditis, following radioactive iodine therapy or surgery).

      ii. Impairment of proteolysis.

      iii. Inhibition of iodide uptake by an autoregulatory process.

      iv. In persons with underlying goiter (especially in iodide deficient environments), iodides may actually induce thyrotoxicosis (Jod–Basedow phenomenon).

## THYROID HORMONE TRANSPORT

1. Thyroid hormones are intensely bound: $T_4$ is 99.97% bound ($t_{1/2}$ of 7 days), $T_3$ is 99.7% bound ($t_{1/2}$ of 1 day).

   a. Thyroxine binding globulin (TBG; MW=54 000; a glycoprotein) is the most specific (although it has the lowest concentration of all the thyroid hormone binders) and carries about 75% of the circulating thyroxine (it also binds $T_3$). It is subject to increased or decreased synthesis or displacement of $T_4$ by a variety of agents and physiologic states.

   b. TBPA (Transthyretin; MW=55 000; 4-chain tetrapeptide without carbohydrate); it is the next most specific and second most concentrated binder – binds $T_4$ but virtually no $T_3$.

   c. Albumin – least specific binder of both $T_4$ and $T_3$.

## THYROID HORMONE REGULATION

1. While it is the free form of the hormone that is metabolically active and forms the rationale for its measurement (directly or indirectly), some organs may be able to extract the bound form (e.g. the liver is effective in doing this; the brain much less so).

2. While both $T_4$ and $T_3$ are present in the thyroid gland ($T_4$ : $T_3$ ratio = 10 : 1), most of the circulating $T_3$ arises from peripheral deiodination (about 80%). The glandular production is subject to change as trophic stimulation results in disproportionate $T_3$ generation (hence seen in both primary hypothyroidism because of increased thyroid stimulating hormone (TSH) stimulation and Graves' disease because of thyroid stimulating immunoglobulins).

3. Central Regulation – TSH: a glycoprotein (MW=28 000) homologous to follicle stimulating hormone, luteinizing hormone and human chorionic gonadotropin with a common α and unique β chain. Post-translational glycosylation confers activity.

   a. β chain confers hormonal uniqueness but excess of homologous hormones (e.g. human chorionic gonadotropin in choriocarcinoma) can produce sustained TSH activity.

   b. Produced in episodic pulses and in early sleep but primarily under thyrotropin releasing hormone (TRH; 1-Pyro-glutamyl-

L-histidyl-L-proline amide) stimulation. The level of thyroid hormone 'bathing' the pituitary determines the effectiveness of TRH and is the rationale for the TRH stimulation test. Thyroid hormone can also directly affect TSH production.

c. $T_3$ and $T_4$ (by conversion to $T_3$ within the thyrotroph) are feedback regulators.

d. Dopamine (and bromocriptine), glucocorticoids and somatostatin inhibit TSH; $\alpha$-adrenergic stimulation augments it.

e. TSH acts on the thyroid by enhancing trapping, organification, coupling and proteolysis. It also has a trophic effect on thyroid growth.

4. Thyroid Autoregulation

   a. There is a 'basal' thyroid autonomy (about 10%) under no TSH stimulation – corollaries include:

      i. $T_4$ levels will never be undetectable in central hypothyroidism

      ii. To 'test' to see if a person with long-standing thyroid hormone has true primary hypothyroidism, change their medication to $T_3$ (Cytomel) – if there is primary hypothyroidism, $T_4$ levels will be undetectable (blood test not to be done until original thyroid hormone is cleared, about 8 weeks).

   b. Trapping of iodide (increased in iodide deficiency) is regulated by its concentration. Iodide deficiency also increases gland $T_3 : T_4$ production and sensitivity to TSH.

## FUNDAMENTAL EFFECTS OF THYROID HORMONE

1. Biochemical effect is felt to be strongly linked to activation of RNA transcription initiated by binding of thyroid hormone to a specific nuclear receptor (homologous to *erb*-A oncogene seen in avian erythroblastosis).

2. Specific enzyme induction (e.g. mitochondrial malic enzyme and cytosol $\alpha$-glycerophosphate dehydrogenase) is augmented by thyroid hormone).

3. Thyroid hormone can also uncouple oxidative phosphorylation and activate cell membrane Na/K ATPase.

4. Because of its fundamental action, all bodily systems require thyroid hormone for normal growth and physiology – role of thyroid hormone is readily appreciated from manifestations in clinical syndromes resulting from excess or deficiency.

5. The role of $T_4$ versus $T_3$ as the primary hormone has still not been resolved.

   a. Evidence for the importance of $T_3$ is that 30 µg of $T_3$ and 90 µg of $T_4$ are produced each day. As 80% of $T_3$ is derived from $T_4$, 24 µg of $T_4$ is used for $T_3$ synthesis. An equivalent amount of $T_4$ goes to the manufacture of reverse $T_3$ or $rT_3$ (an inactive metabolite resulting from 5 deiodination or inner ring deiodination as opposed to 5' deiodination or outer ring deiodination). While the absolute amount of $T_4$ left is still greater than $T_3$ production, $T_3$ is more nuclear receptor avid and potent than $T_4$.

   b. On the other hand, $T_4$ to $T_3$ conversion is impaired by a wide range of clinical states and medications:

      i. Acute and chronic illness (low $T_3$ is frequently found in hospitalized patients),

      ii. Starvation,

      iii. Iodinated compounds (e.g. radiocontrast, amiodarone),

      iv. Propylthiouracil (PTU) (but not Tapazole), hydrocortisone (and related steroids), β-adrenergic blocking agents.

   c. Yet, there may not be clinical hypothyroidism and TSH levels may be essentially normal in the presence of impaired $T_3$ production.

   d. Further, in clinical hypothyroidism with elevated TSH, $T_3$ levels may be normal.

   e. This paradox may arise from the inability to use a single metabolic parameter as a specific index of the thyrometabolic state. Indeed, some cases of 'sick euthyroidism' may be 'subtle' hypothyroidism brought on by the teleologic need to 'shut down' metabolic function in times of catabolic duress.

Because the pituitary outer ring deiodinase is of the 'type I' with a higher '$K$' (dissociation constant) than the peripheral 'Type II', a 'normal' TSH may signify more pituitary than peripheral capability of $T_4$ to $T_3$ conversion.

## TESTS OF THYROID FUNCTION (Table 8-1)

1. Tests that Measure the Peripheral Effect of the Thyroid Hormone – ideally, the 'truest' index of thyrometabolic activity; in actuality, they have varying sensitivities (some tests are very sensitive), but lack specificity.

   a. Basal Metabolic Rate (BMR) – affected by body surface area (increases it), age (highest in infancy, declines with age), pregnancy, neoplastic disease, high cardiac output states, anxiety, perforated ear drum, etc.

   b. Deep Tendon Reflex Evaluation (especially the relaxation time; 'standardized' with the Achilles Reflex 'photo-motogram').

## TABLE 8-1.   TESTS OF THYROID FUNCTION

| Test Category | Tests | Utility | Pitfalls |
|---|---|---|---|
| Tests That Measure Peripheral Effect of The Hormone | BMR, Deep Tendon Reflexes, Cardio-vascular Indices, Serum Parameters | Adjunctive information; monitoring of clinical response to therapy | Lack of specificity; Cannot be quantified with exactness |
| Tests That Measure Thyroid Gland Economy | 24-Hour Radioactive Iodine Uptake | Distinguishes Hyperthyroid from Non-hyperthyroid etiologies of Thyro-oxicosis; dosimetry for radioactive Iodine therapy | Many potential false positive & negatives; it measures the input of iodide into the manufacturing process and not the thyroid hormone produced |
| TSH Determination | | Reflective of the pituitary 'set point', irrespective of circulating thyroid hormone concentration; excellent screening and monitoring test | Affected by some drugs and disease states |

*(continued)*

## TABLE 8-1.  CONTINUED

| Test Category | Tests | Utility | Pitfalls |
|---|---|---|---|
| Tests That Measure The Concentration of Circulating Thyroid Hormone | Serum Thyroxine $(T_4)$ | Excellent screening test; not affected by non-Thyroidal Iodides | Affected by many states and drugs which alter the TBG concentration and the affinity of thyroid hormone to binding proteins |
| | Resin Uptake Test | In concert with the Serum $T_4$, it gives the calculated Free Thyroxine Index (FTI) | Not useful as an isolated test; direct $FT_4$ measurement has supplanted the importance of the FTI |
| | Free Thyroxine $(FT_4)$ | Direct measurement of the Metabolically Active Thyroid Hormone | Affected by some medications and clinical states |
| | Total Triiodothyronine $(T_3)$ | Diagnosis of Non-Hyperthyroxinemic Thyrotoxicosis | Not useful in diagnosis of hypothyroidism; affected by the same protein-binding abnormalities that affect the total $T_4$ |
| | Reverse Triiodothyronine $(rT_3)$ | Can distinguish between True Hypothyroidism and the 'Euthyroid Sick' Syndrome | Not generally useful in clinical practice |
| Special Tests | Serum Thyroglobulin | Following the course of Thyroid Cancer | Not a useful screening test for thyroid cancer |
| | Anti-Thyroid Antibodies | Helpful adjunct in Immunologic Thyroid Disease; confirmation of Hashimoto's Thyroiditis as the cause of a Goiter | Not always present |
| | Thyroid Stimulating Immunoglobulins | Confirmation of 'Euthyroid Graves' or Graves' Opthalmopathy | Not always present |
| | TSH Stimulation Test | Can distinguish Unilateral Thyroid Agenesis from a 'hot' nodule | Replaced as a test of etiology of hypothyroidism by the TSH assay |
| | Imaging Studies | Structure and function of Neoplastic Tissue | Does not supplant the value of direct tisse examination |
| | Thyroid Biopsy | Direct Cyto-Histopathologic Diagnosis | Limited sampling of tissue; cases must be pre-selected |

c. Cardiovascular Indices – pulse rate, pulse pressure, pre-ejection period/left ventricular ejection time (PEP/LVET), Circulation Time.

d. Serum Parameters:

 i. In hypothyroidism: enzyme elevation (creatine phosphokinase, lactate dehydrogenase, serum aspartate aminotransferase (AST), cholesterol elevation (decreased low-density lipoprotein degradation and increased production), abnormally high carcinoembryonic antigen.

 ii. In hyperthyroidism: enzyme elevation (alkaline phosphatase of both bone and liver origin; angiotensin converting enzyme), increased sex steroid binding globulin; increased urinary cAMP in response to epinephrine, increased ferritin, anti-hemophilic globulin (AHG) and gastrin.

2. Tests That Measure Thyroid Gland Economy

a. Radioactive iodine uptake test (RAIU) is the quintessential test in this category. The rationale is that the thyroid gland and kidney compete for iodide with the thyroid gland taking up about 15–25% of the administered isotope (assuming the isotope is not diluted by an excess of unlabelled iodide)

b. Although any isotope of iodide can theoretically be used, $^{123}$I has a shorter half-life and delivers only 1% of the radiation delivered by $^{131}$I. Hyperthyroidism classically increases the uptake; elevations may also be seen in:

 i. Certain inherited disorders of thyroid hormone synthesis.

 ii. Iodine deficiency states (secondary to dietary inadequacy or pathologic loss of iodide or thyroid hormone in urine or stool – e.g. dehalogenase defect, nephrotic syndrome, soybean or cholestyramine-mediated gastrointestinal binding, diarrhea).

 iii. Post-suppression – e.g. following PTU or subacute thyroiditis. Note: if the RAIU is determined only at 24 hours, values in severe Graves' disease and Hashimoto's thyroiditis may be low (but they may be elevated at 4 hours as they may 'peak' early).

c. Hypothyroidism classically decreases the uptake; decreased values are seen in iodide excess states, inflammatory thyroid disease, antithyroid drug therapy, exogenous thyroid hormone or non-thyroid gland endogenous thyroid hormone source (e.g. struma ovarii, metastatic follicular carcinoma of the thyroid).

d. The thyroid nuclear scan, although a special test obtained for graphic evaluation of glandular configuration, is a specialized type of isotopic uptake procedure. Technetium (pertechnetate) is often used in place of radioactive iodine – because it is not organified, the scan is obtained shortly after injection. However, at times, 'cold' radioactive iodine nodules may appear 'functional' with pertechnetate.

e. Perchlorate discharge test is another RAIU variant – 'positive test' seen with normal trapping but abnormal organification (congenital and acquired – e.g. antithyroid drugs, Hashimoto's thyroiditis).

f. The TSH determination is a valuable *in vitro* test that measures the pituitary limb of the feedback loop.

   i. Most laboratories currently use second generation immunoradiometric (IRMA) assays that detect values as low as 0.05 μU/ml (Normal range: 0.5–5.0 μU/ml) – a problem with the previous assay was in obtaining values sufficiently low to substantiate thyrotoxicosis. A newer third generation assay using chemiluminometric technology is available.

   ii. Because of the ability of TSH to vary in response to the 'thyroid hormone set point' for any given individual, it is the most sensitive assay available for diagnosing subtle thyrometabolic dysfunction. It is the screening test of choice for substantiating gland failure or hyperactivity, or in determining adequacy of thyroid hormone replacement dosage.

   iii. The sensitive TSH assay has significantly lessened the need for the TRH stimulation test. The TRH stimulation test shows a blunted response of TSH to TRH administration in thyrotoxicosis and an augmented response in hypothyroidism. The response is also blunted in pituitary (but not hypothalamic) hypothyroidism, renal failure, glucocorticoid and dopamine therapy and acromegaly. It is of value in assessing the degree of autonomy in functioning 'hot nodules' and in substantiating euthyroid Graves' disease (e.g. when ophthalmopathy presents as a singular entity).

iv. The thyroid hormone suppression test is obsolete as a test of thyroid gland autonomy (it can even be harmful as the administered dose of thyroid hormone will be additive if it is used in a situation of thyroid autonomy). It has been supplanted by direct measurement of TSH.

3. Tests That Measure the Concentration of Circulating Thyroid Hormone

a. Serum Thyroxine ($T_4$) – measures total thyroid hormone (free and bound). Normal range: 4–12 µg/dl. Use of protein-bound iodine (measures all iodides) and butanol-extractable iodine (excludes thyroid gland derivatives of a non-hormonal nature) are now relegated to medical history. The assay has traditionally used an isotopic competitive binding technique (newer technologies include nuclear magnetic resonance imaging, chromatography). $T_4$ levels are elevated in thyrotoxicosis and reduced in thyroid hormone deficiency states.

i. Affected by factors which increase or decrease binding protein concentration or affinity:

(a) Increased binding proteins – estrogenic states (including pregnancy, oral contraceptives, Tamoxifen), congenital increase, liver disease (hepatitis, biliary cirrhosis), drugs (perphenazine, 5-fluorouracil, heroin and methadone), HIV infection, and porphyria.

(b) Decreased binding proteins – hyperandrogenic states (including anabolic steroids), congenital deficiency, nephrotic syndrome, glucocorticoid excess, acromegaly, L-asparaginase.

(c) Displacement of $T_4$ from binding proteins (resulting in decreased $T_4$): dilantin (but this also accelerates the metabolism of $T_4$ to $T_3$ giving rise to normal $T_3$ and TSH values but a reduced $T_4$ and free $T_4$), salicylates and non-steroidal anti-inflammatory drugs (NSAIDs) (phenylbutazone, diclofenac, salsalate and naproxen; the following NSAIDs have no effect: diflunisal, ibuprofen, sulindac, piroxicam, and indomethocin) and furosemide.

ii. Affected by abnormal binding protein states (increased $T_4$): familial dysalbuminemic hyperthyroxinemia, abnormal TBPA, antithyroxine globulins.

iii. Can be abnormally high in an otherwise euthyroid person secondary to psychiatric illness (depression, hyperemesis gravidarum), significant non-thyroidal illness (where $T_3$ is significantly reduced), thyroid hormone resistance states and with drugs (iodinated radiocontrast agents, β blockade, amphetamines, L-thyroxine replacement therapy).

iv. Can be abnormally low in an otherwise euthyroid person secondary to profound illness and production of fatty acid (oleic) 'inhibitors' of $T_4$ binding – effect is exaggerated if there is concomitant hypoalbuminemia.

b. The 'Resin Uptake Test'

i. This is sometimes called the 'Resin $T_3$ Test', a poor choice of name because it uses $T_3$ in the assay but does not directly measure it.

ii. This test is most useful when its value is multiplied by the total $T_4$ to give the Thyroid Hormone Binding Index (THBI) (formerly known as the Free Thyroxine Index or FTI). Any binding protein abnormality will be 'cancelled out' by the product which is proportional to the true free $T_4$. True thyrotoxicosis and thyroid deficiency states will be reflected in appropriately abnormal THBI values.

iii. The 'Resin Uptake Test' is limited by extremes of TBG concentration and by the presence of severe non-thyroidal illness and drug-binding inhibition which affect not only $T_4$ binding to TBG but hormone binding to resin as well.

iv. The 'Resin Uptake Test' is normal in familial

dysalbuminemic hyperthyroxinemia and hyperthyrox-inemia secondary to increased TBPA (hence, THBI will be elevated).

c.  Direct Measurement of Free $T_4$ (FT4) (normal range: 0.9–1.7 ng/dl)

   i.  A variety of technologies are presently available for measurement: non-isotopic tests are gaining favor (e.g. chemiluminescence) because of concerns regarding radioactive waste.

   ii.  Generally correlates well with 'true' thyrometabolic state and is not affected by binding abnormalities. May be elevated despite clinical euthyroid state with: exogenous iodinated compounds (radiocontrast, amiodarone), β blockade (propranolol), severe non-thyroidal illness, thyroid hormone resistance states, and with heparin administration (probably secondary to free fatty acid elevation that inhibits $T_4$ binding). May also be elevated when thyroid hormone replacement therapy is achieved with L-thyroxine. May be decreased with severe non-thyroidal illness (circulating inhibitors) and with certain medications (e.g. phenytoin, rifampin).

d.  Serum $T_3$ Determination (normal range: 70–195 ng/dl)

   i.  Analogous to the Total $T_4$, $T_3$ is characteristically elevated in thyrotoxicosis and decreased in hypothyroidism. Because of increased TSH in primary hypothyroidism, the proportion of the the $T_3$ pool from direct glandular secretion increases and the serum $T_3$ level may not be as low as anticipated.

   ii.  Likewise, it may be disproportionately higher in thyrotoxicosis.

   iii.  In 'pure' $T_4$ toxicosis, it may be normal and in $T_3$ toxicosis, it is elevated with a normal $T_4$.

   iv.  Characteristically depressed in a wide range of non-thyroidal illness (with concomitant increase in $rT_3$).

e.  Reverse $T_3$ ($rT_3$) Determination – characteristically increases when $T_3$ is low due to impaired $T_4$ to $T_3$ conversion. Normal range: 25–75 ng/dl. Its use is limited and hence is rarely employed. May be of value if differential diagnosis of low $T_3$ is non-thyroidal illness versus hypothyroidism (in the former, but not the latter, $rT_3$ will be increased – but so will the TSH if it is primary hypothyroidism)

4. Special Tests

    a.  Thyroglobulin (Tg)

        i.  May be useful as an adjunct for following the course of patients with known thyroid cancer who have had prior extirpative or ablative therapy. Elevations on suppressive hormone therapy are suggestive of relapse.

        ii.  Tg may be elevated in thyroiditis, goiter and Graves' disease. May be useful in distinguishing thyrotoxicosis factitia from intrinsic thyrotoxicosis (Tg suppressed in the latter). The presence of endogenous antibodies, however, may nullify the test.

    b.  Thyroid Stimulating Immunoglobulins – a family of immunoglobulins causally associated with Graves' disease, although neither necessary nor indicated in making the diagnosis of thyrotoxicosis. They can be helpful, by their presence, in supporting a diagnosis of 'euthyroid Graves' Disease' or Graves' ophthalmopathy.

    c.  Antimicrosomal (peroxidase) and Antithyroglobulin antibodies – useful adjuncts for the diagnosis of immunologic thyroid disease. Antimicrosomal antibodies are found in nearly 100% of patients with Hashimoto's thyroiditis, and about 80% of patients with Graves' disease. Antithyroglobulin antibodies are less specific (85% in Hashimoto's thyroiditis, and 30% in Graves' disease).

    d.  TSH Stimulation Test – rarely used because of TSH assay availability (was used in the past to distinguish primary versus central hypothyroidism – analogous to Cortrosyn stimulation test). Can be used to distinguish a congenital single thyroid lobe from a hyperfunctioning nodule.

e. Imaging Studies

   i. Radionuclide Scan – depicts thyroid function in an anatomically graphic manner. Most useful in distinguishing functional from non-functional thyroid tissue.

   ii. Thyroid Ultrasound – useful in delineating structural thyroid disease. It can distinguish between solid and cystic thyroid components. Resolution and structural detail much greater than with radionuclide scan.

   iii. CT and MRI – most useful when knowledge of contiguous structures is desired (e.g. tracheal compression with substernal goiter; extent of neoplasia; tumor recurrence; identification of a parathyroid adenoma).

f. Thyroid Biopsy – a refined technique that can provide cytologic and/or histologic diagnosis. Most helpful in 'ruling in' thyroid cancer although unambiguous benign lesions might also be ruled out. Cases should have prior selection. Proper tissue sampling can be problematic, especially in multinodular goiters.

# 9

# HYPOTHYROIDISM

The syndrome of thyroid hormone deficiency and its associated clinical manifestations

## CLINICAL MANIFESTATIONS

Because of the ubiquitous and indispensable role of thyroid hormone in cellular function intrinsic to all bodily systems, the clinical manifestations of its absence are myriad and pan-systemic.

1. Cutaneous
   a. Boggy but non-pitting edema ('myxedema') in subcutaneous tissue secondary to increase in the glycosaminoglycan content of the connective tissue matrix (ironically, it is histologically similar to the 'pretibial myxedema' associated with the Graves' disease type of thyrotoxicosis).

   b. Atrophy of sweat glands with skin dryness; cold pallor (yellowish tint secondary to hypercarotenemia); hyperkeratosis; increased incidence of vitiligo in some (hypopigmentation in secondary hypothyroidism).

   c. Dry and brittle hair; focal and general scalp alopecia; absent lateral eyebrow hair.

2. Gastrointestinal
   a. Decreased peristaltic activity with constipation and distension (replacing the intestinal contents in the peritoneal cavity following laparotomy may be problematic).

   b. Overt obesity is unusual (a 'myth' about hypothyroidism).

   c. Ascites can occur but usually in association with pleural and pericardial effusion.

   d. Association with achlorhydria and impaired intrinsic factor production.

   e. Abnormal liver function studies (aspartate aminotransferase (AST) elevation) secondary to decreased clearance.

3. Nervous System
   a. Lethargy, mental sluggishness, intellectual impairment, dementia (a reversible cause).

b. Psychiatric manifestations ('myxedema madness') but there may be an underlying diathesis to mental illness.

c. Slow, deliberate, coarse speech (structural changes in mouth and tongue can contribute to dysarthria).

d. Abnormal EEG, elevated cerebrospinal fluid protein.

e. Hearing loss, impaired night vision (abnormal vitamin A metabolism).

f. Delayed deep tendon reflexes (DTRs); carpal tunnel and tarsal tunnel syndromes.

4. Muscular System

a. Muscular cramps, aching and stiffness; pseudohypertrophy (Hoffman's or Kocher–Debre–Demelaigne Syndrome).

b. Decreased urinary creatinine; increased creatine tolerance.

5. Skeletal System

a. Rheumatic symptoms; occasional joint effusions. Increased prevalence of hypothyroidism in gout.

b. Impaired bone growth and maturation if process begins pre-pubertally (decreased bone age; stippled epiphyses on X-ray).

c. Decreased bone turnover; decreased urinary calcium. In adults, bone density may be increased.

6. Cardiovascular System

a. Decreased myocardial inotropic and chronotropic contractility.

b. Hypertension – increased peripheral resistance with decreased blood volume and peripheral blood flow (peripheral hypothermy).

c. Tendency to large flabby heart suggestive of congestive heart failure but heart responds normally to exercise with decreased peripheral resistance and increased cardiac output and to the Valsalva maneuver with a decrease in pulse pressure.

d. Abnormal serum enzymes – creatine phosphokinase (CPK), lactate dehydrogenase (LDH) and serum AST are elevated (these enzymes are listed in descending order of magnitude of change). EKG changes include non-specific ST-T wave abnormalities, PR interval prolongation and low voltage.

   e. Abnormal systolic time intervals (increased pre-ejection period (PEP) and PEP/left ventricular ejection time (LVET) ratios).

   f. Pericardial effusion (rich in protein and glycosaminoglycans) but tamponade is rare.

7. Pulmonary System

   a. Pleural effusions are common but are rarely a primary cause of respiratory embarassment.

   b. Decreased diffusing capacity and voluntary ventilation capacity.

   c. Loss of ventilatory drive and infiltrative respiratory muscle myopathy may lead to central sleep apnea; obstructive sleep apnea is also a complication.

8. Hematopoietic System

   a. Normocytic and normochromic anemia of 'disuse' (comparable marrow changes).

   b. Macrocytic anemia secondary to decreased intrinsic factor (B-12 deficiency), folate deficiency (dietary and/or malabsorption), or as a primary consequence of hypothyroidism.

   c. Hypochromic, microcytic anemia secondary to iron deficiency (hypermenorrhea, decreased iron intake, poor iron absorption).

   d. Decreased factors VIII and IX and decreased platelet adhesion.

9. Renal System (including Fluid and Electrolyte)

   a. Decreased glomerular filtration rate and renal blood flow.

   b. Tendency to hyponatremia is not a true sign of the syndrome of inappropriate antidiuretic hormone (SIADH) but rather secondary to renal hemodynamic impairment – ADH levels are reduced.

10. Endocrine System

   a. Increase in size of the pituitary gland (thyrotropic cell hyperplasia) – rarely of clinical significance.

b.  Increased prolactin level (sometimes with galactorrhea) – probably because of increased lactrotrophic sensitivity to thyrotropin releasing hormone (TRH).

c.  Decreased urinary adrenocortical metabolites with normal serum levels.

d.  Decreased pituitary sensitivity to insulin-induced hypoglycemia.

e.  Decreased cAMP response to catecholamines.

11. Reproductive System

a.  In women, irregular menses (usually hypermenorrhea and polymenorrhea).

b.  In men, hypogonadism (may be primary or secondary).

c.  Decreased sex hormone binding globulin with relative increase in free testosterone and estradiol. Testosterone conversion to etiocholanolone (rather than androsterone) is enhanced.

## ETIOLOGIES OF HYPOTHYROIDISM

Secondary causes are all those etiologies which can produce generalized pituitary or hypothalamic deficiency states or which may rarely produce isolated thyrotrophic hormone deficiency. It is generally easy to distinguish between secondary (central) and primary etiologies in that:

1.  The etiologic event that produces a central deficiency usually affects other aspects of pituitary function – e.g. amenorrhea and breast atrophy, hypopigmentation, loss of pubic and axillary hair.

2.  There may be neurologic consequences of a central etiology – e.g. visual field deficits, 3rd nerve palsy, headache. The clinical scenario may be helpful (e.g. pituitary apoplexy, Sheehan's syndrome).

3.  Certain ancillary tests may be different in primary versus secondary etiologies (e.g. cholesterol elevation generally not pronounced in secondary; anti-thyroid antibody studies negative in secondary).

4. Thyroid stimulating hormone (TSH) levels should be inappropriately low (in presence of low thyroxine ($T_4$)) in secondary – in actuality, TSH may be increased but this is bio-inactive TSH and requires stimulation by TRH to render it biologically active.

## PRIMARY HYPOTHYROIDISM (Table 9-1)

1. Post-Ablative Hypothyroidism
   a. Can occur after surgical extirpation, particularly total thyroidectomy for thyroid cancer (in this setting, there may be other post-thyroidectomy complications).
   b. Can occur even after subtotal thyroidectomy for Graves' disease – this may be a function of the mass of tissue extirpated or the inexorable course of primary immunologic disease as the incidence of hypothyroidism increases over time.
   c. Virtually inevitable response to radioactive iodine therapy for Graves' disease – while hypothyroidism may not be an immediate event, there is probably a 3% cumulative increase in annual incidence.
   d. Sometimes an inadvertant consequence of neck irradiation.
2. Idiopathic (Atrophic) Hypothyroidism
   a. High incidence of circulating antithyroid antibodies (thyroglobulin and microsomal) suggest an immunologic basis (antibodies may be of a destructive or 'TSH block' nature).

## TABLE 9-1.  ETIOLOGIES OF PRIMARY HYPOTHYROIDISM

Post-ablative
Idiopathic (Atrophic)
Developmental Deficiencies
Hashimoto's Thyroiditis
Endemic Goiter
Metabolic Defects
Drug-induced
Non-Hashimoto's Inflammatory Thyroid Disease

b.  The gland becomes shrunken and fibrotic – while having a similar pathophysiology to Graves' disease and Hashimoto's thyroiditis, it is felt to be a separate entity (HLA-associated haplotypes are different: DRw3 and B8 in idiopathic hypothyroidism, DR5 in Hashimoto's).

3.  Developmental Deficiency of the Thyroid Gland

a.  Found in 1 : 4000 to 5000 live births. Even though thyroid hormone was seemingly deficient *in utero*, the combination of apparent diminished hormone need during fetal development and a small (albeit finite) amount of transplacental transport of thyroid hormone from mother to fetus mitigates any cretinous tendency *in utero*. The fetal brain is additionally capable of $T_4$ to $T_3$ conversion.

b.  Early detection with neonatal screening has pre-emptively thwarted the development of subsequent cretinism. If therapy is instituted before 28 days, there is no residual neurologic deficit.

4.  Hashimoto's Thyroiditis

a.  Immunologically-mediated chronic lymphocytic thyroiditis – usually associated with high antithyroid antibody titers. Antimicrosomal (antiperoxidase) antibody titers are generally higher than antithyroglobulin.

b.  Although an ancillary study, the perchlorate discharge is often positive and radioactive iodine uptake test may be increased early in the disease (it will eventually decline when hypothyroidism ensues) – both of these support the role of antimicrosomal antibodies not only as a marker but a source of the pathophysiology. Other antibodies including cytotoxic and TSH-binding inhibitory immunoglobulins may be operant in producing hypothyroidism and ultimate gland failure.

c.  Goiter is a common finding – tendency to 'rubbery texture and pebbly surface' with palpable pyramidal lobe. TSH stimulation, local growth factors and lymphocytic infiltration may all be operant.

d.  Iodine seems to play a significant role in its pathogenesis (the higher the dietary iodide content, the greater the prevalence, as in Japan) and the propensity to develop hypothyroidism.

e. Although perhaps more of a theoretical than a practical issue (it is reasonable to give long-term replacement therapy), some cases of hypothyroidism may not be permanent – a large goiter, high TSH level and a strong family history are favorable factors.

5. Endemic Goiter

   a. While iodine deficiency plays the predominant role, geographic isolation and inbreeding may be operant at some level. No one specific metabolic defect, however, has been uncovered. In some cases, there is gland atrophy rather than goiter although some of the largest known goiters are seen in this entity.

   b. When severe and in early life, goitrous cretinism can be the end result.

6. Metabolic Defects of Thyroid Economy

   a. Defects of hormonogenesis including transport defect, organification defect (when associated with nerve deafness, it is called Pendred Syndrome), coupling defect, dehalogenase defect and abnormal iodoprotein production.

   b. A TSH unresponsive state with thyroid hypoplasia, caused by a mutation in the TSH receptor.

   c. Thyroid hormone resistance states – resistance to both $T_4$ and triiodothyronine ($T_3$). Resistance may be generalized (the clinical syndrome may range from hypothyroid to compensated normal), peripheral resistance only (only one reported case), or selective pituitary resistance (thyrotoxic syndrome). Attention deficit hyperactivity has also been linked to generalized resistance to thyroid hormone. This disorder is almost always autosomal dominant and heterozygotes are equally affected because a point mutation in one of the two receptor chain genes ($\beta$ chain gene on chromosome 3) produces a receptor protein that affects normal receptivity of the $\alpha$–$\beta$ cell receptor – a process known as 'dominant negativity'.

7. Drug-induced Hypothyroidism

   a. Iodide-induced

      i. May be transient in an otherwise normal person, the

so-called Wolff–Chaikoff effect (iodide inhibition of organification). In normals, there is an 'escape' mechanism.

    ii. Disease tends to occur in background of a damaged or vulnerable thyroid gland – e.g. prior thyroid surgery, Graves' disease, Hashimoto's thyroiditis.

    iii. Chronic ingestion of iodide (e.g. KI expectorant use) is a common operant factor.

    iv. Fetal syndromes including strangulation have been described (pregnant women should not receive excessive iodide).

  b. Foods of the family Cruciferae – cabbage, kale, rutabaga and turnips. Cassava ingestion probably augments pre-existing iodine deficiency.

  c. Lithium – blocks thyroid hormone release; thyroid enlargement or goiter may be seen even without overt hypothyroidism.

  d. Other goitrogens include para-aminosalicylic acid, resorcinol and phenylbutazone.

8. 'Reversible' Hypothyroidism

  a. Some patients with initial hypothyroidism may become hyperthyroid at a later time – a change in antibody type is postulated

  b. Described in Japan in patients with underlying Hashimoto's thyroiditis.

  c. Transient hypothyroidism may be seen postpartum (mostly with underlying Hashimoto's), in the early period of time after radioactive iodine therapy for Graves' disease, and in association with cancer immunotherapy (e.g. interleukin, lymphokine activated killer (LAK) cells and interferon).

9. Non-Hashimoto's Inflammatory Thyroid Disease can be associated with a 'thyrotoxic phase' (whether or not overtly clinical), but this may be followed by a hypothyroid phase that is characteristically transient but may also become permanent.

Included are subacute (deQuevain's) thyroiditis and chronic (non-Hashimoto's, painless, subacute lymphocytic, postpartum) thyroiditis.

## SUBCLINICAL HYPOTHYROIDISM

1. That subpopulation of patients with $T_4$ levels in the normal range but with inappropriate elevation of TSH. Not to be confused with the 'perception' of hypothyroidism or 'low metabolism'.

2. Seen in otherwise healthy individuals (incidence increases with age), in individuals with underlying treated or untreated thyroid disease (e.g. Hashimoto's, Graves') and in individuals with other immunologic disease linked to hypothyroidism (e.g. pernicious anemia, type I diabetes mellitus).

3. Some may be symptomatic (e.g. fatigue, cold intolerance, muscle cramps and dry skin) – although features of hypothyroidism, they are not specific.

4. Exogenous thyroid hormone may be beneficial – the dose is titrated to bring the TSH into the normal range.

5. A compelling reason to treat selected patients is the concern about an inevitable hypothyroid state (such patients may not be brought to medical attention until a profoundly hypothyroid state ensues). Alternatively, patients may be followed without specific therapy at no less a frequency than annually (and to report to the physician any interim relevant symptoms).

6. A theoretical concern is 'subliminal medication overdose' and resultant osteoporosis, and risk of atrial fibrillation, but this may be overstated (conversely, the high-density lipoprotein profile can be improved with thyroid hormone, an obviously beneficial effect). The expense of 'unnecessary' medication is also a consideration (even though thyroid hormone is relatively inexpensive compared to other medications).

## THE DIAGNOSIS OF HYPOTHYROIDISM

1. Clinical manifestations suggestive of hypothyroidism warrant specific evaluation. Because hypothyroidism is a common entity, and there are many 'non-specific' and subtle features of

hypothyroidism, pre-emptive laboratory screening has become a standard of preventive medicine. Screening is accepted as a cost-effective modality in both ambulatory and acute care settings.

2. A decreased $T_4$ (free $T_4$ as necessary) in concert with an elevated TSH is the *sine qua non* of diagnosis. (In actuality, an increased TSH alone is an earlier manifestation; the earliest manifestation, though not a commonly performed test, is an increased TSH responsiveness to TRH).

3. $T_3$ levels are not generally helpful (or necessary). While decreased in primary hypothyroidism, the decrease may not be as profound as the $T_4$ decrease because TSH stimulates preferential thyroidal production of $T_3$. Additionally, $T_4$ to $T_3$ conversion is enhanced in the hypothyroid state.

4. Ancillary tests may be either of corroborative help or their initial abnormalities may have generated a search for hypothyroidism: these include serum cholesterol, serum aspartate amino-transferase (AST), lactic dehydrogenase (LDH), carcinoembryonic antigen (all elevated in hypothyroidism). Radioactive iodine uptake test is not of much value.

5. Primary versus secondary hypothyroidism should be reasonably distinguishable.

## TREATMENT OF HYPOTHYROIDISM

1. Five Types of Preparations are Available (Table 9-2):

   a. L-Thyroxine – pure $T_4$

   b. L-Triiodothyronine – pure $T_3$

   c. Synthetic mixture of $T_4/T_3$ in 4 : 1 ratio

   d. Desiccated thyroid – 38 µg of $T_4$ and 9 µg of $T_3$ per grain

   e. Thyroglobulin – 36 µg of $T_4$ and 12 µg of $T_3$ per grain.

2. Absorption of $T_3$ is 100%; absorption of $T_4$ is 70–80%.

3. When euthyroid, individuals on L-thyroxine have a higher serum $T_4/T_3$ ratio. The converse is true for desiccated thyroid ($T_4$ levels

## TABLE 9-2.  AVAILABLE THERAPIES TO TREAT HYPOTHYROIDISM

L-Thyroxine (T$_4$)
L-Triiodothyronine (T$_3$)
Synthetic Mixture of T$_4$ : T$_3$ in a 4 : 1 Ratio
Desiccated Thyroid
Thyroglobulin

are actually below normal when euthyroid – further, there is the 'jolt' effect from the T$_3$ content). Average daily replacement using L-thyroxine is 112–125 μg; for desiccated thyroid, it is 1.5–2 grains.

4. Hypothyroidism following surgery or radioactive iodine therapy generally requires less thyroid hormone replacement initially than primary hypothyroidism. There is presumably some level of persistent autonomy that eventually declines, either as a result of decreased stimulating immunoglobulin titers or as an inexorable progression to more irreversible hypothyroidism.

5. Hypothyroidism decreases the metabolic clearance of thyroid hormone so that dose adjustments may be necessary as the hypothyroid state improves. The TSH level is the most sensitive index of response (ideally, it should be some 'metabolic parameter') with T$_4$ levels obtained for adjunctive assessment.

6. The initial replacement and frequency of dose adjustments are a function of the severity of the hypothyroid state. At one end of the spectrum, an otherwise healthy, mildly hypothyroid young person can have full initial replacement. Conversely, an older person with serious underlying medical illness should be prudently started on 12.5–25 μg of L-thyroxine. Incremental dosing changes in all should probably be no more frequent than every 2–4 weeks. Until the full replacement dose is approached, serial TSH values are redundant.

7. There is a hierarchy of clinical improvement with initial diuresis and regression of edema occurring earliest and gastrointestinal and neurologic changes to follow. Cutaneous changes are generally the last to regress.

8. A variety of factors affect dosing:

   a. Drugs – sucralfate, cholestyramine, aluminum hydroxide and colestipol inhibit absorption, as do soybean or simultaneous ferrous sulfate ingestion; phenytoin, (Dilantin), rifampin and carbamazepine increase clearance. An interesting corollary is the potential treatment of iatrogenic thyrotoxicosis with cholestyramine.

   b. Intestinal disease (e.g. malabsorption, irritable bowel disease) decreases absorption.

   c. Hormone requirements decrease with age.

   d. Pregnancy increases hormone requirements (as much as 40%). A logical explanation is the increased 'reservoir' of thyroxine binding globulin that the hyperestrogenic pregnant state produces. This 'reservoir' is 'thyroid hormone avid'. In the absence of endogenous thyroid function, this can only be met by increasing the exogenous dose. Thyroid hormone needs may additionally increase, as a result of the pregnant state.

   e. Conversely, the L-thyroxine requirement decreases in hypothyroid women who are treated with androgen therapy for breast cancer.

   f. Notwithstanding the utility of total $T_4$ or free $T_4$ measurements, the TSH value will be the most helpful in determining long-term maintenance dosage. As opposed to thyroid hormone therapy in thyroid cancer where the object is to suppress pituitary stimulation of the thyroid, the goal of replacement thyroid hormone in the hypothyroid state is to keep the TSH within the normal range. This can be accomplished because the TSH level is far more sensitive to fluctuations in thyroid hormone concentration than are direct measurements of the $T_4$ or free $T_4$. A normal TSH also reflects 'pituitary satisfaction' with a given level of thyroid hormone, irrespective of its serum concentration.

## IS HYPOTHYROIDISM A DETERRENT TO SURGERY?

1. In mild to moderate hypothyroidism, there is no appreciable hazard, even for cardiac surgery.

2. However, the performance of surgery is a function of the need for the procedure at that time. Elective surgery is best deferred.

## MYXEDEMA COMA

1. The syndrome of exaggerated manifestations of hypothyroidism, especially neurologic (impaired sensorium), hypothermia, hypotension, bradycardia and hypoventilation.

2. Can be precipitated by such factors as trauma, infection, a cardiovascular event, cold exposure, surgery and medication. Patients with hypothyroidism are at a greater risk for these events and/or are less able to respond to their effects.

3. Management:

   a. Establishment of diagnosis by known clinical history and/or new clinical and laboratory evaluation.

   b. Diagnose and treat precipitating medical problems (e.g. infection, myocardial infarction).

   c. General supportive care – e.g. fluid and electrolyte balance; slow reversal of hypothermia, glucocorticoids; cardiovascular, renal and pulmonary monitoring.

   d. Specific therapy – L-thyroxine is the drug of choice (because of variable absorption in myxedema and the clinical state of the patient, do not give orally). Initially, 500 μg, intravenous – 100 μg, intravenous, daily, to follow. Some evidence suggests that a lower initial dose may also be effective.

   e. While there is risk of precipitating a cardiovascular–cerebral event when the patient is given a significant dose of thyroid hormone (you would never give such a high dose in an otherwise stable and responsive patient with hypothyroidism), the risk of mortality is great in myxedema coma unless treatment is instituted. While $T_3$ has recently become available in parenteral preparation, there is less experience with it. Were it to be used, it might also create a thyroid 'surge' (although unlike $T_4$, it does not require peripheral conversion).

# THYROTOXICOSIS

The clinical syndrome associated with thyroid hormone excess and its clinical manifestations. The term, hyperthyroidism is sometimes used interchangeably with thyrotoxicosis but hyperthyroidism connotes an overactive thyroid gland. One can be thyrotoxic without thyroid gland hyperactivity and the thyroid gland may be hyperactive without producing a thyrotoxic state.

## CLINICAL MANIFESTATIONS

Analogous to the clinical manifestations of hypothyroidism which are myriad and pan-systemic, the ubiquitous and indispensable role of thyroid hormone renders all bodily systems vulnerable to excessive quantities.

1. Cutaneous
    a. Warm (increased circulation) and smooth (increased epidermal turnover) skin (a helpful corollary is the inappropriate smoothness of elbows – Selenkow's sign).
    b. Tendency to increased perspiration (response to increased thermogenesis).
    c. Hyperpigmentation (increased ACTH secondary to increased glucocorticoid turnover?).
    d. Vitiligo (association with other autoimmune phenomena).
    e. Erythema (especially palmar – secondary to increased cardiac output and peripheral vasodilatation) – may be manifest as 'salmon-pink facies' (described by Samuel Levine).
    f. Fine, soft hair (difficulty in holding a 'perm') with alopecia.
    g. Onycholysis (separation of nail plate from nail bed) on fingers and toes (Plummer's nails).
    h. Diffuse pruritis.
2. Cardiovascular
    a. Increased cardiac output (inotropy and chronotropy). Sinus tachycardia in young but tendency to atrial flutter and fibrillation in elderly (this may be their only overt manifestation of thyrotoxicosis) with resultant congestive heart failure. Atrial fibrillation may be refractory to attempts at cardioversion and relatively refractory to digoxin.

b. Abnormal systolic time intervals, decreased PEP and PEP/LVET.

c. Higher incidence of mitral valve prolapse. Heart sounds are generally loud with prominent apical impulse. Means–Lerman 'scratch'.

3. Hematopoietic System

   a. Anemia (although not very common) may occur because of:

      i. Pernicious anemia (as another autoimmune disease, this can be seen in association with immunologic thyroid disease).

      ii. Increased menstrual bleeding can lead to iron deficiency (in general, however, menses are usually sparser in thyrotoxicosis). Rarely, if there is a microcytic anemia, it may be secondary to decreased iron incorporation into red blood cells. (Parenthetically, thyroid hormone is a stimulus to ferritin production.)

   b. There may be neutropenia (antibody-mediated?) and a relative lymphocytosis.

4. Neurologic System

   a. Tremor – high frequency, low amplitude. May be obvious when paper is placed on outstretched hands but a tremulousness can be noticed virtually anywhere (e.g. outstretched tongue, in exophthalmic eyes, 'electric motor' sensation to the body).

   b. Hyperkinesis – 'restless energy' may be obvious during history taking and physical examination.

   c. Emotional lability and other psychiatric manifestations. Sometimes there is a disparity between a myriad of ideas and impulses, and the will and stamina to carry them out.

   d. Deep tendon hyperreflexia.

5. Muscular System

   a. Myopathy – especially proximal (e.g. difficulty in putting items on shelves, combing hair and walking up stairs). 'Body climbing' needed to arise from a seated position (Gower's sign).

    b. Association with Hypokalemic Familial Periodic Paralysis (primarily among Asians).

    c. Association with Myasthenia Gravis.

6. Skeletal System

    a. Increased bone turnover (catabolism outweighs anabolism) with net loss of bone mass. This bone loss may be considerable when accrued over time, especially when associated with other risk factors for osteoporosis. Conversely, increased bone mineralization and potential reversibility of thyrotoxic bone disease can follow treatment.

    b. Hypercalciuria is common but clinically important hypercalcemia is rare (even though serum values may be elevated). Parathyroid hormone is suppressed. Vitamin D (and active metabolite) clearance is increased with lower serum levels and diminished calcium absorption.

7. Gastrointestinal System

    a. A common manifestation is increased transit time (with associated hyperdefecation). Overt diarrhea and malabsorption, however, are not very common.

    b. Often, there is increased appetite and polyphagia with difficulty in weight maintenance, or even weight loss. When patients are anorectic, weight loss can be considerable.

    c. Abnormalities of liver function (evaluation of aspartate aminotransferase, alkaline phosphatase – bone alkaline phosphatase may also be elevated because of increased bone turnover). Liver histopathology may be normal, reveal fatty infiltration, or show non-specific abnormalities.

8. Respiratory System

Patients may be dyspneic for multiple reasons (e.g. congestive heart failure, increased $O_2$ consumption, respiratory muscle weakness).

9. Eyes

    a. One type of eye manifestation is seen with all etiologies and is due to increased sensitivity to catecholamines.

       i. Mild exophthalmos and stare, lid retraction, lid and globe lag and ease of pupillary dilatation (Loewi's sign) are features.

ii. An opposite situation occurs in Horner's syndrome where a diminished catecholamine influence results in ptosis, pupillary constriction and enophthalmos.

b. Graves' ophthalmopathy is a special type of infiltrative process.

10. Renal (including Fluid and Electrolyte)

Increased renal blood flow and glomerular filtration rate, with tendency to polyuria.

11. Endocrine–Metabolic

a. Increased glucocorticoid metabolism; blunted growth hormone (HGH) response to hypoglycemia and blunted hyperglycemia-mediated HGH suppression.

b. Tendency to aggravate underlying glucose intolerance; oral glucose tolerance test can also be abnormal in otherwise healthy individuals.

c. Increased lipid turnover; hypocholesterolemia.

d. Irregular menses; increased sex hormone binding globulin with resultant decreased free hormone levels; increased androgen to estrogen conversion (a cause of gynecomastia in men?). Increased conversion of testosterone to androsterone rather than etiocholanalone. (A cause of temporal male-pattern alopecia in women?)

## ETIOLOGIES OF THYROTOXICOSIS (Table 10-1)

1. Graves' Disease and Related Disorders;

2. Autonomous Thyrotoxicosis – associated with both single and multinodular thyroid glands;

3. Thyroid stimulating hormone (TSH)-mediated;

4. Trophoblast-mediated;

5. Iodine-induced;

## TABLE 10-1. ETIOLOGIES OF THYROTOXICOSIS

Graves' Disease
Autonomous Thyrotoxicosis
TSH-mediated
Trophoblast-mediated
Iodine-induced
Inflammatory Thyroid Disease
Extra-Thyroidal Thyrotoxicosis

6. Inflammatory Thyroid Disease

   a. Radiation-induced,

   b. Subacute,

   c. Chronic; and

7. Extra-Thyroidal Thyrotoxicosis:

   a. Endogenous – metastatic thyroid cancer; struma ovarii, and

   b. Exogenous – thyroid preparations; food sources.

## GRAVES' DISEASE AND RELATED DISORDERS

1. The most clinically significant etiology of thyrotoxicosis in patients under age 40.

2. An immunologically mediated disease that has overlapping similarities to chronic thyroiditis and primary hypothyroidism.

   a. All of these diseases may have clinical features of one another at one time in their clinical course despite the greater predominance of some particular aspect.

   b. Histopathology may overlap.

   c. Activated T lymphocytes directed against thyroid tissue is a basic feature.

   d. Presence of anti-thyroid antibodies in all.

      i. Anti-microsomal antibody (mediated against peroxidase) is more commonly seen than anti-thyroglobulin antibodies (among immunologic thyroid diseases, anti-microsomal antibodies are most commonly seen in Hashimoto's thyroiditis, and least commonly in primary hypothyroidism).

    ii. About 80% of patients with Graves' disease have a positive anti-microsomal antibody titer.

3. Seen in association with other immunologically mediated diseases: e.g. type I diabetes mellitus, pernicious anemia, myasthenia gravis, systemic lupus erythematosus, and the sicca (Sjogren's) syndrome.

4. HLA B8 and DR3 statistically associated with Graves' disease in whites (B35 in Japanese, Bw46 in Chinese).

5. A family of circulating IgG immunoglobulins has been associated with its pathogenesis.

    a. LATS (Long Acting Thyroid Stimulator) – initially described by Adams and Purves in 1956, it demonstrated the first association of immunoglobulin-mediated thyroid gland stimulation (done in mouse thyroid – unlike TSH whose effect is short-lived, LATS has a sustained activity).

    b. LATS-P (LATS-Protector) – immunoglobulin which prevents LATS absorption onto thyroid tissue. Why should it be associated with thyroid stimulation? (Mouse versus human?)

    c. TBII (Thyrotropin Binding Inhibitor Immunoglobulins) – Radioreceptor assay demonstrating immunoglobulin ability to prevent TSH binding to human or porcine thyroid cell membranes.

    d. TSI (Thyroid Stimulating Immunoglobulins) – capable of stimulating adenylate cyclase activity in human and rat thyroid tissue.

    e. Although correlation with the diagnosis of Graves' disease and its associated ophthalmopathy and dermopathy is imperfect, there appears to be an association with thyroid autonomy and risk of relapse. They may also be helpful in predicting likelihood of neonatal thyrotoxicosis, in clarifying the etiology of Graves' versus autonomous thyrotoxicosis and in diagnosing non-thyrotoxicosis-associated ophthalmopathy as being Graves' in origin.

    f. A fascinating association is the relationship of *Yersinia enterocolitica* (and possibly other enteric pathogens) and Graves' disease (does infection generate an antibody capable of thyroid binding?).

g. A different type of immunoglobulin G, TSBAb (Thyroid Stimulating Blocking Antibody) may correlate with the propensity to hypothryoidism during the course of Graves' disease, or the propensity to produce transient neonatal hypothyroidism when transplacentally passed.

6. Graves' Ophthalmopathy

   a. Infiltrative – affecting extraocular muscles and connective tissue.

   b. The etiology remains enigmatic, although a prevailing hypothesis is that 'cross-antigenicity' exists between thyroid follicular cells and ocular myocytes and fibroblasts. The exact 'trigger' for immune activation, however, is not known.

   c. Although its contemporary utility has been questioned, the mnemonic, NO SPECS (as championed by Werner and adopted by the American Thyroid Association) is a helpful clinical tool (Table 10-2).

   d. An integral part of clinical folklore, the various manifestations of ophthalmopathy and their associated names add a rich perspective to clinical medicine (Table 10-3).

7. Graves' Dermopathy

   a. Similar histopathology to ophthalmopathy,

   b. Tends to affect pretibial and preulnar regions most often,

   c. Rarely may there be a more generalized thyroid acropachy.

### TABLE 10-2. THE NO SPECS MNEMONIC FOR GRAVES' OPHTHALMOPATHY

| Class | Definition |
|---|---|
| N | No Signs or Symptoms |
| O | Only Signs, No Symptoms |
| S | Soft Tissue Swelling |
| P | Proptosis |
| E | Extraocular Muscle Paresis |
| C | Corneal Involvement |
| S | Sight Loss (Optic Nerve Involvement) |

### TABLE 10-3. SIGNS ASSOCIATED WITH GRAVES' OPHTHALMOPATHY: [Adapted from Physical Diagnosis, Major & Delp. W.B. Saunders Company, 1962].

| Sign | Clinical Manifestation |
| --- | --- |
| Enroth's Sign | Swelling of the eyelids |
| Jellinek's Sign | Brownish pigmentation of the eyelids (especially the upper) |
| Dalrymple's Sign | Lid retraction |
| Kocher's Sign | Increased upper lid retraction on attentive gaze |
| von Graefe's Sign | Lid lag on downward gaze |
| Means' Sign | Globe lag on upward gaze |
| Boston's Sign | Jerky lid lag |
| Suker's Sign | Poor fixation on lateral gaze |
| Cowen's Sign | Jerky pupillary reaction to consensual light |
| Möbius' Sign | Weakness on convergence |
| Stellwag's Sign | Infrequent blinking |
| Gifford's Sign | Difficulty in everting the upper lid |
| Knie's Sign | Unequal pupillary dilatation |
| Joffroy's Sign | Absence of forehead wrinkling on upward gaze |
| Riesman's Sign | Bruit over the closed eye |
| Ballet's Sign | Ocular palsies |
| Loewi's Sign | Pupillary dilatation with weak epinephrine solution |

## AUTONOMOUS THYROTOXICOSIS

1. In contrast to Graves' disease, the pathophysiology and thus the clinical picture generally evolve more slowly and the degree of thyrotoxicosis is usually less severe. Cardiovascular manifestations, however, usually predominate and peripheral myopathy (especially in the elderly) may be significant.

2. Seen generally in the older population (in younger individuals, single 'hot' nodules are seen more often than are multiple nodules). In those aged 60 years or older, suppressed serum TSH is associated with a three times increased risk of atrial fibrillation

3. Tumor pathology ranges from a single nodule to an oligonodular one to a more diffuse almost 'nodular hyperplasia'. Although the etiology is unknown, there may be an immunologic component.

## TSH-MEDIATED THYROTOXICOSIS

1. Two etiologies: TSH-producing tumor and primary TSH hypersecretion

    a. TSH-Producing Tumor:

        i. Distinguishing feature is a disproportionately increased $\alpha$ subunit.

        ii. TSH may be the only hormone produced or it may be produced in concert with others.

    b. Primary TSH Hypersecretion:

        i. A special case of the thyroid hormone resistance syndrome in which there is selective pituitary resistance.

        ii. If 'suppressible', it may be 'overridden' with exogenous thyroid hormone (this is analogous to Cushing's disease although it is obviously not of therapeutic value; a rare cause of this syndrome, however, is impaired thyroxine ($T_4$) to triiodothyronine ($T_3$) conversion and exogenous $T_3$ may be therapeutic).

        iii. A crucial laboratory finding is an 'inappropriate' TSH elevation in the presence of a thyrotoxic state.

## TROPHOBLAST-MEDIATED THYROTOXICOSIS

1. Supraphysiologic elaboration of human chorionic gonadotropin-related protein with non-suppressible TSH-like activity.

2. Seen with hydatidiform mole, choriocarcinoma and metastatic testicular embryonal cell carcinoma.

## IODINE-INDUCED THYROTOXICOSIS

1. Seen in setting of underlying thyroid pathology: iodine deficiency states (Jod–Basedow phenomenon) and nodular goiter (these nodules may be relatively deficient in iodide). Can be seen in diffuse hyperplasia as well.

2. A wide range of sources may be the provocateurs: e.g. saturated solution of potassium iodide (SSKI), Betadine (particularly when

applied to an absorptive surface as in a douche), radiocontrast agents, amiodarone, kelp tablets – even bread.

3. Low radioactive iodine uptake – because of 'dilutional effect'. Urinary iodide excretion is increased. This may render therapy difficult (radioactive iodine will not be effective: there is relative resistance to antithyroid drugs).

## INFLAMMATORY THYROID DISEASE

1. Radiation-induced Thyroiditis

   a. Can result from external neck irradiation or following radioactive iodine therapy.

   b. The clinical effects are the result of release of preformed thyroid hormone. As a result, both TSH and radioactive iodine uptake are suppressed.

2. Subacute (deQuervain's) Thyroiditis

   a. Virus-mediated infectious granulomatous disease of the thyroid gland: mumps, ECHO, coxsackie- and influenza viruses (and others) have been implicated. Females predominantly affected, with the middle age years the time of greatest frequency.

   b. In many ways, a systemic disease with focused effects on the thyroid gland. Symptoms of malaise and lassitude, low-grade fever and anorexia are superimposed on thyrotoxic symptoms (warmth, nervousness, tachycardia). Some cases may be subclinical or borderline clinical. The erythrocyte sedimentation rate is often very elevated.

   c. The inflammation can produce local tenderness and sensitivity (sometimes excruciating), gland enlargement and radiation of pain to unusual areas (jaw, back of neck, ear).

   d. Laboratory tests can classically show increased $T_4$ and $T_3$ with suppressed TSH and radioactive iodine uptake. The disease may pass through phases whereby temporary 'exhaustion' of preformed hormone leads to hypothyroidism (with a 'passing' euthyroid state). As TSH recovers from suppression, it rises as does radioactive iodine uptake (as the damaged gland regains its former function). There may be a glandular 'lag period' whereby TSH (before the gland is capable of a full response) and radioactive iodine uptake (before the gland can efficiently make thyroid hormone, even though it can take up iodide) are both elevated. These values eventually return to normal.

e. Although viral antibodies may be found, anti-thyroid antibodies, if present, are in very low titer.

f. Permanent sequelae are rare, but the course may be protracted. Treatment is usually symptomatic. Non-steroidal anti-inflammatory drugs are often effective, but glucocorticoids may be necessary.

3. Chronic Thyroiditis (Non-Hashimoto's; also known as painless thyroiditis, subacute lymphocytic thyroiditis, postpartum thyroiditis).

a. Relatively recently, appreciated as a distinct entity that can cause transient thyrotoxicosis; more commonly seen in younger women (but seen in men at a greater frequency than is Hashimoto's thyroiditis, with less of a tendency to familial clustering). Women with Type I diabetes mellitus are at a particularly high risk for symptomatic postpartum thyroid dysfunction.

b. Classically associated with elevated $T_4$ and $T_3$ levels, suppressed TSH and radioactive iodine uptake in the thyrotoxic phase. Analogous to subacute thyroiditis, it may go through a hypothyroid phase (with antecedent euthyroidism) before ultimately returning to normal.

c. Propensity to elevated antithyroid antibodies (almost all have positive antithyroglobulin antibody; anti-microsomal antibody is less common – titers are generally less than in Hashimoto's thyroiditis). TSH Binding Inhibitory Immunoglobulin also seen. Less than 50% have goiter.

d. HLA-DR3 and -DR5 associated.

e. Tendency to recurrence (about 10%). A fascinating variant is that seen postpartum which tends to recur following subsequent pregnancies (even therapeutic abortions). This is seen in highest incidence in Japan (about 5% of population).

f. Histopathology reveals lymphocytic infiltration (but no germinal centers or Ashkenazy cells which are features of Hashimoto's thyroiditis); increased B cells and increased T-lymphocyte helper : suppressor (cytotoxic) ratio.

g. Treatment is largely supportive and symptomatic (e.g. β blockade). Only a small percentage have permanent hypothyroidism (about one-third may have permanent goiter), so selectivity is important before committing a patient to long-term thyroid hormone supplement.

## ECTOPIC THYROID HORMONE

1. Endogenous sources can be found in struma ovarii (teratomata) and metastatic follicular thyroid cancer – elevated thyroglobulin levels may be seen in the latter.

2. Exogenous sources include thyroid hormone preparations (serum $T_4$ and $T_3$ levels may vary according to the type and dose of medication). Patients may 'innocently' (e.g. weight control 'pills') or intentionally take such medications. A curious form of thyrotoxicosis was described in 1987 secondary to the inclusion of thyroid tissue in bovine neck meat prepared for hamburger production.

## DIAGNOSIS

1. The previously described clinical manifestations represent the spectrum of manifestations seen in thyrotoxicosis. Variations must be considered in the clinical context of a particular etiology – e.g. ophthalmopathy in Graves' disease, thyrocardiac disease as a more overt (or even singular) manifestation is more likely in an elderly patient with autonomous thyrotoxicosis; postpartum occurrence associated with subacute lymphocytic thyroiditis. Duration of the disease is also a factor in the magnitude of certain symptoms (e.g. weight loss, myopathy).

2. Laboratory Tests

   a. Serum parameters are the gold standard.

   b. In most cases, the total $T_4$ level will be elevated (free $T_4$ if there is any question regarding levels of thyroid hormone-binding proteins or the presence of binding inhibitors; the free thyroxine index can approximate the free $T_4$ in most cases). Causes of non-thyrotoxic hyperthyroxinemia should always be entertained in ambiguous cases but an inappropriately 'normal' TSH should rule these out.

c. Total $T_3$ will be elevated (free $T_3$ as necessary) in thyrotoxicosis except in 'pure' $T_4$ toxicosis. Total $T_3$ may also be 'normal' in the Jod–Basedow phenomenon. Conversely, it may be the only hormone elevation in $T_3$ toxicosis or in selective thyrotoxicosis factitia.

d. TSH suppression should occur in all etiologies of thyrotoxicosis, except for those (e.g. Graves', subacute thyroiditis, subacute lymphocytic thyroiditis) that may have a 'phase' of TSH normalcy or elevation and are not associated with clinical thyrotoxicosis during that phase.

e. Radioactive iodine uptake is not a primary diagnostic test; it is only a helpful adjunct when used appropriately. It can generally divide the etiologies of thyrotoxicosis into hyperthyroidism (overproduction of thyroid hormone) and non-hyperthyroidism (non-overproduction of thyroid hormone) but it is fraught with potential error and variation.

f. Immunologic studies may be helpful in determining etiology.

g. Ancillary tests that measure the clinical effects of thyroid hormone are of additional adjunctive value, but can never be considered primary diagnostic tools.

## THERAPY OF THYROTOXICOSIS (Table 10-4)

1. Antithyroid Agents – Thionamides represent the primary class of antithyroid agents. Other types of drugs, such as perchlorate and thiocyanate, that inhibit uptake, have no clinically useful role.

   a. Thionamides work by decreasing the synthesis of thyroid hormone, primarily at the organification level (also inhibit coupling and proteolysis).

   b. Propylthiouracil (PTU), as opposed to methimazole (Tapazole), additionally inhibits $T_4$ to $T_3$ conversion (these two drugs are the only available antithyroid agents in the USA). PTU is thus useful when more rapid eradication of peripheral manifestations is desired.

## TABLE 10-4. DEFINITIVE THERAPY OF THYROTOXICOSIS

| Modality | Generally Accepted Uses | Pitfalls |
|---|---|---|
| Antithyroid Drugs: Propylthiouracil (PTU), Methimazole (Tapazole) | Initial treatment of Graves' disease in a younger person; pregnancy (propylthiouracil) | Protracted treatment course (generally 1 year) with no guarantee of sustained remission; not curative in autonomous thyrotoxicosis |
| Surgery | Antithyroid drug treatment failure in a person not accepting of, or not a candidate for radioactive iodine; symptomatic or cosmetically unacceptable goiter; solitary 'hot' nodules | Surgical morbidity; subsequent hypothyroidism or persistent thyrotoxicosis; not advisable after prior thyroid surgery or radioactive iodine therapy; the patient must be rendered euthyroid prior to surgery |
| Therapeutic Radioactive Iodine | Adult patients with Graves' disease or autonomous thyrotoxicosis; surgical and antithyroid drug treatment failures | Contraindicated in pregnancy |

c. Controversy – While these drugs may merely 'buy time' in Graves' disease (until a spontaneous remission is achieved), there is evidence that they may affect immune function as well by:

   i. Correction of the T-cell imbalance,

   ii. Greater likelihood of remission with a higher dose, and

   iii. Greater likelihood of remission if given with L-thyroxine.

d. Remission rate in Graves' disease is quite variable (on average, less than 50%) – favorable outcomes occur with females, smaller gland size, less thyrotoxicity, high anti-microsomal antobody titer, absent TSI, $T_3$ toxicosis in a diffuse goiter, early decrease in the size of the gland, and normalization of TSH and thyrotropin releasing hormone (TRH) stimulation test. While also effective in other (non-Graves') thyrotoxic states associated with increased glandular hormone synthesis, long-term remission off medication is unlikely and a more definitive therapy is generally necessary.

e. Transplacental transfer may result in fetal thyroid gland enlargement – usually not mechanically problematic. The neonate may have a goiter (compensatory hyperplasia) but is not generally hypothyroid. The neonate may, in fact, become temporarily thyrotoxic because of transplacental transfer of TSI. PTU is the preferred drug in pregnancy because Tapazole has been associated with cutis aplasia in the fetus (PTU is also preferred in nursing mothers because of its relatively low concentration in breast milk – if possible, nursing is not recommended if the mother is on any medication).

f. Tapazole has a longer half-life (6 hours versus 1.5 hours for PTU) but the biologic effect is even greater such that once daily therapy usually suffices. It is ten times more potent than PTU on a per weight basis. Average daily dose: 100–300 mg/day (PTU), 10–30 mg/day (Tapazole).

g. Toxicities associated with both Tapazole and PTU include liver, skin and arthralgias. Agranulocytosis is uncommon with PTU (0.5%) and both very rare and dose-related with Tapazole.

h. Both drugs are useful as adjunctive therapies (for both surgery and radioactive iodine treatment of Graves' disease).

i. PTU has the additional effect of decreasing $T_4$ to $T_3$ conversion which could theoretically decrease the magnitude of the thyrometabolic state.

2. Surgery

a. While an important modality in the past, its role is secondary today and relegated to antithyroid drug treatment 'failures' (e.g. toxicity, poor compliance), associated symptomatic or cosmetically unacceptable goiters, and for patients in whom radioactive iodine is a relative or absolute contraindication or is unacceptable.

b. With diminished performance, incidence of side-effects is more likely to increase – thyroid storm should never be one of them because this is a function of proper medical preoperative management (e.g. thionamides and iodides; β blockade).

c. Side-effects include hypothyroidism (may be immunologically mediated if a late sequelae), persistent hyperthyroidism, hypoparathyroidism and vocal cord paralysis.

d. Because of increased risk of morbidity, surgery is not advised if prior radioactive iodine therapy was given, or if a previous surgical procedure was performed.

3. Radioactive Iodine

a. A safe and effective, simple and inexpensive modality with increasing popularity and widespread use (especially in the USA).

b. No known long-term adverse genetic or oncogenic effect on the recipients of this therapy or their offspring. It is generally not used, however, in the very young and is absolutely contraindicated in pregnancy.

c. Significant toxicities are:

    i. Acute – pain and local tenderness; in some, discomfort may mimic that seen with subacute thyroiditis; some patients are transiently thyrotoxic and those who are potentially vulnerable to a superimposed thyroid hormone burden should be pretreated with anti-thyroid therapy; and

    ii. Chronic – inevitability of hypothyroidism, irrespective of dose; patients treated with a lower dose have a decreased incidence of immediate hypothyroidism, but they are just as vulnerable to long-term gland failure; hypoparathyroidism is not a problem, but there may be 'diminished parathormone reserve'.

d. Dose is a function of gland size (the larger the gland, the higher the dose), radioactive iodine uptake (the lower the uptake, the higher the dose), and the type of thyrotoxicosis (autonomous requires a higher dose than Graves'). As ultimate response is not tightly linked to dose (a higher dose, however, is corrective in a shorter period of time), there is often an empiric component to dosimetry. Higher doses are used with less trepidation because of the decreased likelihood of recurrence, earlier control and the probable need to replace thyroid hormone in almost all patients, sooner or later.

e. There is a perception that radioactive iodine may increase the risk of worsening exophthalmos, but this is controversial. It should not affect the decision-making process if radioactive iodine is clearly indicated.

f. Antecedent treatment with antithyroid drugs may predispose patients to fail radioactive iodine ablative therapy, and it may result in short-term increases in thyroid hormone levels following radioactive iodine therapy. On the other hand, antithyroid pretreatment is judicious in a vulnerable (e.g. elderly, coronary artery disease) patient, because euthyroidism (even if temporary, prior to the radioactive iodine administration) can be predictably and speedily restored, and there would be less hormone release from the radiation-damaged thyroid gland. Further, higher treatment doses of radioactive iodine in such a pre-treated individual could be more predictably used to obliterate the thyrotoxic state.

4. Medical Adjunctive Therapy

   a. β- Adrenergic Blockade – can control cardiovascular symptoms as well as tremulousness, adrenergic-mediated effects on the eye, and increased perspiration. These drugs also inhibit $T_4$ to $T_3$ conversion. Propranalol and atenolol (the latter can be given as a single daily dose, and is β-1 selective) are the most widely used agents.

   b. Iodides – most useful in augmenting the effect of radioactive iodine, in management prior to thyroidectomy and in the treatment of thyroid storm. They inhibit organification and proteolysis. Agents commonly used are Saturated Solution of Potassium Iodide (SSKI) and radiocontrast agents (ipodate and iopanoic acid). In thyroid storm, iodides may be given intravenously (NaI or KI).

   c. Lithium – inhibits proteolysis. Its toxicity precludes any useful role.

5. Treatment Strategies

   a. Radioactive iodine is generally preferred for treatment of most cases of Graves' disease (reluctance in younger patients or pregnancy are exceptions). Radioactive iodine can be safely given to women planning future pregnancy because they can be euthyroid (with or without the need for exogenous thyroid hormone replacement at that time) when pregnancy does occur.

b.  Radioactive iodine is a very effective and definitive therapy for autonomous nodules (thionamides are only a temporizing measure).

c.  Surgery can be a secondary treatment for Graves' disease or a primary treatment for autonomous nodules – especially if there is a cosmetic or locally symptomatic problem.

d.  Inflammatory processes which result in thyroid hormone excess usually require only supportive and symptomatic therapy.

e.  Iodine-mediated thyrotoxicosis may require thionamides in addition to supportive and symptomatic therapy. (Such thyrotoxicosis, especially if amiodarone-mediated, may be relatively refractory to the thionamides.) Isotope dilution secondary to the larger pool of stable iodine militates against the early use of radioactive iodine therapy.

f.  Thyroid storm requires an aggressive multi-faceted approach including:

   i.   Large doses of thionamides,

   ii.  Iodides,

   iii. β-adrenergic blockade,

   iv.  Glucocorticoids,

   v.   Fluid and electrolyte (and nutrient) replenishment and support, and

   vi.  Uncover and treat the underlying cause!

g.  Graves' Ophthalmopathy is managed with:

   i.   Supportive measures – elevation of the head of the bed, dark glasses, methyl cellulose and other artificial eye lubricants, local antibiotics (as necessary),

ii. Avoidance of hypothyroidism – it appears to worsen the ophthalmopathy,

iii. Glucocorticoids – local and systemic,

iv. Orbital radiation – proptosis may persist, and

v. Orbital decompression – for severe disease.

vi. Total thyroid ablation does not appear to affect the natural course of the disease.

# 11

# NEOPLASTIC DISEASE OF THE THYROID

## THE CLINICAL PARADOX OF THE NODULAR THYROID

1. Thyroid nodules are common and are estimated to affect at least 4% of the US population. The incidence increases with age. Also, careful clinical examination is likely to reveal an even greater likelihood of thyroid nodules in any given patient. Ultrasonography is a still more sensitive diagnostic modality capable of diagnosing nodules that are beyond the range of reasonable clinical dexterity. As the ultimate 'gold standard', pathologic section of the gland in otherwise normal, asymptomatic individuals, without abnormal physical examination, may reveal nodules in as many as 50% of specimens.

2. Yet, thyroid cancer is uncommon – 36 new cases per million population per year; nine deaths from thyroid cancer per million population per year.

## WHY IS THERE AN APPARENT DISPROPORTIONATE PREOCCUPATION WITH THYROID CANCER?

1. Although not all thyroid nodules are cancer, virtually all thyroid cancers present as nodular growths – hence, cure is possible.

2. The thyroid gland (unlike other endocrine structures) is easily palpated so 'lumps and bumps' are more readily brought to attention. (Although not palpable, a comparable situation has arisen in the case of the pituitary and adrenal glands where newer imaging technologies have uncovered a significant incidence of 'serendipitous' nodules.)

3. There are well-defined risk factors and clinical features associated with thyroid cancer.

4. There are a wide range of laboratory and imaging studies that have increased the database and have provided discriminating information. Included are thyroid function studies, conventional radiography, CT, MRI, thyroid scan, thyroid ultrasound and needle aspiration and biopsy.

5. A dilemma is that many benign conditions may present as nodules.

   a. Structural irregularities – incomplete genesis, thyroglossal duct cyst, focal hyperplasia (spontaneous or following surgery or radioactive iodine).

b. Inflammatory disease – Hashimoto's thyroiditis, 'silent thyroiditis', subacute thyroiditis.

c. 'True' neoplastic disease: microfollicular, macrofollicular, fetal, embryonal, papillary and Hürthle cell adenoma.

## TYPES OF THYROID CANCER (Table 11-1)

With the exception of medullary carcinoma, all primary thyroid cancers are of follicular origin.

1. Papillary Carcinoma

   a. Accounts for most cases of thyroid cancer (up to 75%) and has the best prognosis (death rate with this disease: 6.5%) – the course, if there is metastatic disease, is also long and protracted.

   b. Predominance in younger ages and in women.

   c. Younger ages have a better prognosis (perhaps because cancer later in life arises from *in situ* or small foci of 'controlled' thyroid cancer) – very young, however, have a poorer prognosis.

   d. Even if follicular elements are present, as long as some papillary components exist, the tumor is considered papillary and behaves as such. Psammoma (calcium-containing) bodies may be present, as well as Hürthle cells.

   e. Growth is primarily by direct extension and the lymphatic route – nodal involvement may be even more predominant than the primary lesions or may be the only obvious lesion ('lateral aberrant thyroid').

### TABLE 11-1.   TYPES OF THYROID CANCER

Papillary Carcinoma
Follicular Carcinoma
Anaplastic Carcinoma
Medullary Carcinoma
Other Causes

    f.  Nodal involvement is not a prognostic factor for either recurrence or death – documented prognostic factors are presence of distant metastases, size (greater than 4 cm), extension beyond the capsule, older age and cancer not associated with Hashimoto's thyroiditis.

    g.  May be responsive to thyroid stimulating hormone (TSH) (but generally not to the same extent as benign nodules) and take up iodide less avidly than surrounding normal tissue (hence, 'cold' lesions).

2.  Follicular Carcinoma

    a.  Affects women predominantly, but in a statistically older age group than papillary.

    b.  Accounts for only about 15% of thyroid cancers.

    c.  Metastases tend to be blood borne – e.g. lung, bone (pathologic fracture) – the extent of metastases is prognostic.

    d.  Although less able to take up iodide than surrounding tissue, iodide avidity after ablation of normal thyroid tissue forms the rationale for radioactive iodine therapy.

    e.  Extensive metastatic disease may give rise to an autonomous thyrotoxic state (but rather uncommon and usually not profound).

3.  Anaplastic Carcinoma

    a.  Approximately 5% of thyroid cancer.

    b.  Somewhat more common in women, may arise in a pre-existing goiter and has an aggressive, rapidly progressive and inexorable course.

    c.  Produces local (and distant) symptoms and signs – poorly responsive to therapy.

4.  Medullary Carcinoma

    a.  Arises from parafollicular cells (C cells) of 'last' (ultimo) branchial body originating in the 5th pharyngeal pouch.

    b.  Endocrinologically active – produces calcitonin (useful as a marker but its excess does not cause a distinct endocrinologic syndrome).

c. Can also produce serotonin, ACTH, histamine, prostaglandins and kinins and these may be responsible for additional clinical manifestations (e.g. watery diarrhea).

d. Sporadic (generally in older patients) and familial (commonly in younger patients) – somewhat more common in women. May be seen as part of multiple endocrine neoplasia (MEN) Type IIa (Sipple's Syndrome – hyperparathyroidism commonly secondary to parathyroid hyperplasia, and pheochromocytoma) or IIb (distinguished from IIa by the general absence of hyperparathyroidism and the presence of mucosal neuromas).

e. Familial cases may be multifocal and begin initially with C-cell hyperplasia (detectable by screening those at risk for stimulated calcitonin levels – pentagastrin and calcium stimulation test).

5. Other cancers of the thyroid – includes lymphoma (develops most often in association with Hashimoto's thyroiditis, although as a rare complication), metastatic disease (breast, lung, melanoma, etc.).

## DISCRIMINATING CLINICAL CLUES

1. History – the following features increase the index of suspicion:

a. Radiation – all varieties (for acne, tonsillitis, 'mantle' radiation, nuclear 'fallout'). The incidence of benign nodules following radiation is as high as one in three, but the likelihood of cancer development in a nodular situation is one in six – papillary is the most common histology. The paradox that therapeutic $^{131}$I for thyrotoxicosis does not appreciably increase the likelihood of thyroid cancer is probably best explained because thyroid cells are 'too destroyed' (initially or later) to become neoplastic.

b. Appearance of the nodule prior to the age of 14 or after the age of 65.

c. Local symptoms – hoarseness, dysphagia, discovery of a 'new' neck mass, change in size of a pre-existing goiter.

d. Family history of medullary carcinoma (alone or as part of a multiple endocrine neoplasia syndrome)

2. Physical Examination – the following features increase the index of suspicion:

   a. Solitary nodule (although cancer can certainly be found in a multinodular gland), lymphadenopathy (particularly ipsilateral), laryngeal stridor, vocal cord paralysis, 'hard' lesion, 'fixation'.

   b. Male; young individual.

3. Imaging Studies – solitary 'cold' nodule on thyroid scan; 'solid' on ultrasound (necessity for ultrasound as part of the screening process is somewhat controversial since 'cystic' lesions may be malignant, but the ultrasound is more sensitive in picking up multiple nodules). CT and MRI may be helpful in delineating the extent and in picking up distant metastases. Proton magnetic resonance spectroscopy may hold future potential in discriminating benign follicular lesions from follicular tumors.

4. Serum Parameters – Thyroid function studies including TSH (autonomous hyperfunctioning nodules are virtually never cancerous; metastatic follicular carcinoma can produce elevation of thyroid hormone levels including isolated elevation of serum triiodothyronine ($T_3$); thyroglobulin (not useful in initial discrimination, but high levels may be a helpful clue and levels are useful in following the course of the disease); calcitonin (basal and stimulated, when necessary; additional 'ectopic' parameters may also be of value if there is suspicion of medullary carcinoma – e.g. 5-hydroxyindoleacetic acid, cortisol, ACTH).

## MANAGEMENT

1. Fine Needle Aspiration – this has been an extremely important diagnostic adjunct; technical and cytopathologic expertise are imperative.

   a. It has to be used with selective discrimination to be an effective tool.

   b. Sampling adequacy may be problematic with multinodular glands. Performance under ultrasonography can improve localization and sampling, particularly in more complex nodular settings.

c. In cystic lesions, fluid may not be indicative of the nature of the 'solid' tissue portion. Such lesions are best treated with surgery if follow-up ultrasound shows interim growth of the 'solid' or septate portion.

d. Incidence of thyroid cancer is sufficient in patients with nodular disease who have had thyroid radiation to warrant surgery without prior aspiration. These patients also do better with postoperative radioactive iodine ablation and long-term thyroid hormone suppression.

e. If the aspirate reveals 'malignant' cells, surgery is warranted.

f. In situations where the aspirate is read as 'benign' or 'suspicious', there can be clinical follow up and the patient placed on thyroid hormone suppression. If re-examination reveals no regression, the lesion may be rebiopsied or excised. While lesion enlargement under suppressive therapy warrants surgical extirpation, the lesion that remains unchanged is more problematic. Such patients can continue to be maintained on suppressive hormone therapy (which decreases TSH) but this can result in diminished bone density, over time, and increase their vulnerability to atrial fibrillation. After several years of unchanged size, the thyroid hormone may be discontinued and the lesion followed clinically – repeat aspirations may be included in the follow-up process.

2. Surgery

a. Unilateral lobe resection for papillary carcinoma less than 2 cm; subtotal thyroidectomy for larger papillary and all follicular carcinomas. Removal of all affected nodes.

b. Total thyroidectomy with adjacent nodal and soft tissue dissection for medullary carcinoma.

c. As 'reasonably extensive' surgery as possible for undifferentiated carcinoma.

3. Postoperative Management

a. $^{131}$I radiation to the thyroid remnant for all papillary and follicular carcinomas except for lesions less than 2 cm. (Patients under 20 and perhaps over 50 are exceptions and should receive $^{131}$I irrespective of lesion size.)

b.  Metastatic ablation with $^{131}$I (metastases will 'light up' if normal thyroid tissue is previously fully ablated and cancer is capable of taking up iodide). All patients should be on suppressive doses of thyroid hormone, but the patient may benefit in particular from changing to Cytomel (T$_3$) prior to initiation of any isotopic body scan or the actual $^{131}$I therapy, itself. When the Cytomel is then discontinued prior to the isotopic procedure, a shorter period of time is required for the patient to be off the medication (because of its briefer half-life); thus, the patient experiences a hypothyroid state of shorter duration.

c.  It is not clear to what level the TSH must decrease to produce adequate suppression. Values of 0.1–0.2 mU/l seem reasonable – lower values might not render additional benefits and must be achieved at the price of iatrogenic hyperthyroxinemia.

d.  Repeat radioactive iodine isotopic body scan every 6–12 months with follow-up $^{131}$I, as necessary. Initial absence of metastatic lesions or cure of lesions with $^{131}$I warrant a significantly decreased frequency of scan – clinical judgement determines how often this will be required.

e.  The serum thyroglobulin level can be helpful in follow up, particularly in lieu of long-term total body scans, as its presence would indicate regrowth of thyroid tissue.

f.  Medullary carcinoma does not respond to $^{131}$I and (as with undifferentiated carcinoma) is resistant to chemotherapy.

# Section D

# DISORDERS OF THE ADRENAL GLAND

# 12

# THE ADRENAL CORTEX: OVERVIEW

**Embryology and Functional Anatomy**
**Steroidogenesis**
**Glucocorticoid Action**
**Measurement of Adrenal Function**

## EMBRYOLOGY AND FUNCTIONAL ANATOMY

1.  The adrenal cortex is of mesodermal origin; identifiable as a distinct organ at 2 months' gestation. Two zones evolve: a thin outer 'definitive' zone and a larger inner 'fetal zone'.

2.  The fetal zone lacks 3-β-hydroxysteroid dehydrogenase and thus cannot make either cortisol or certain androgens (e.g. androstenedione). It does make dehydroepiandrosterone (DHEA) and can sulfate it to form dehydroepiandrosterone sulfate (DHEA-S). The placenta can desulfate DHEA-S (by the action of steroid sulfatase) and aromatize it to form estradiol. If the fetal liver prior hydroxylates it to form 16 α-hydroxy DHEA, the placenta converts it to estriol. Most estriol and 50% of estradiol during pregnancy is ultimately of fetal adrenal origin.

3.  The fetal zone atrophies during the first 3 months of life during which time the 'definitive' zone takes on the three distinct layers of the adult gland: the zonae glomerulosa, fasciculata and reticularis.

4.  The zona glomerulosa, by lacking the 17-hydroxylase enzyme, cannot make cortisol or androgens. It can produce mineralocorticoids including deoxycorticosterone, corticosterone and aldosterone. As opposed to the zonae fasciculata and reticularis which are primarily ACTH driven, angiotensin II is the major driving force to aldosterone production.

    a.  Angiotensin II is formed when renin is produced by the juxtaglomerular apparatus. Major stimuli to renin formation are perfusion pressure of the afferent arterioles, perception of sodium concentration by the adjacent macula densa cells, and β-adrenergic stimulation. In clinical actuality, hypovolemia is probably the most significant influence.

    b.  Renin (MW – 40 000; derived from pro-renin) acts on renin substrate (also known as angiotensinogen; MW – 60 000) to produce angiotensin I (decapeptide) which is converted to angiotensin II (octapeptide) by angiotensin converting enzyme (ACE).

    c.  Hyperkalemia and hyponatremia are additional direct aldosterone stimuli; ACTH is a stimulus but its effect is more episodic than sustained.

5. The adrenal is a richly vascular gland supplied by branches from the inferior phrenic, aorta and renal arteries. The left adrenal vein drains into the left renal vein, the right adrenal vein drains directly into the inferior vena cava.

6. Each adrenal gland weighs 4–5 g. They may increase in weight by as much as four- to fivefold (as seen at autopsy) in non-adrenal disease – indicative of the trophic effect of stress on adrenal stimulation.

## STEROIDOGENESIS (Figure 12-1)

1. Adrenal steroids require cholesterol for synthesis – this may be taken up by the gland from circulating lipoproteins or be synthesized *de novo* from acetyl coenzyme A (as is a property of most bodily cells).

2. The cleavage of the cholesterol side chain to produce pregnenolone is both the major effect of ACTH and the rate limiting step to steroid production.

3. Cortisol production requires conversion of pregnenolone to progesterone (via 3 β-hydroxysteroid dehydrogenase) and the three consecutive hydroxylations at the 17, 21, and 11 positions, respectively. (The 3 β-hydroxysteroid dehydrogenase step can also take place after the 17-hydroxylation).

4. Androgens require 17-hydroxylation of pregnenolone (21 and 11 hydroxylation steps not required):

   a. Dehydroepiandrosterone (DHEA) and its sulfated derivative (DHEA-S) are derived directly from 17-hydroxy pregnenolone by action of a 17, 20 desmolase (side chain is split).

   b. Androstenedione formation requires an additional 3 β-hydroxysteroid dehydrogenase step.

   c. DHEA and DHEA-S are the most abundant adrenal androgens but androstenedione is more significant in its greater ability to be converted to testosterone (this is done primarily in peripheral tissues).

   d. Adrenal androgens can also be converted to estrogens but this is done primarily in peripheral (e.g. adipose) tissues.

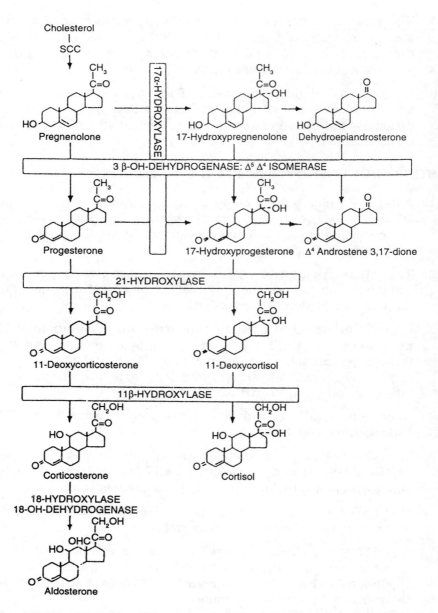

**Figure 12-1.** Pathway of Biosynthesis of Corticosteroids: Reproduced with kind permission from *Endocrinology*, DeGroot, L.J. (ed.) 1989, Philadelphia: W.B. Saunders Company, p. 1544

5. Cortisol (including its structural analogs) is the most potent inhibitor of adrenal androgen and glucocorticoid steroidogenesis.

   a. Inhibition by glucocorticoids occurs at both the hypothalamic (corticotropin releasing hormone (CRH)) and pituitary (pro-opiomelanocortin (POMC)-ACTH) level.

   b. ACTH, and hence cortisol, is additionally made in a circadian pattern (greater levels occurring between the 6th and 8th hours of sleep and the lowest sleep levels in the earliest part – but levels are already low in the hours before sleep). This is subject to alteration by time zone change and altered sleep–wake patterns but only after an 'adjustment phase'. (Interesting nuances: peak ACTH levels occur several hours earlier in the elderly; in blind individuals, the circadian periodicity is 24–25 hours).

   c. ACTH is also made episodically in response to stress and its associated physiologic provocateurs – CRH, vasopressin, hypoglycemia and immune modulators (interleukin-1,-2,-6, and cachectin).

   d. While adrenal androgen production is largely determined by ACTH stimulation and glucocorticoid-mediated feedback inhibition, other pituitary factors may be operant (although not clearly defined).

## GLUCOCORTICOID ACTION

1. Glucocorticoids are carried in the plasma primarily in the bound state (more than 95%: corticosteroid binding globulin (CBG) is the primary binding protein, albumin is less significant). Androgens and estrogens are primarily bound by sex hormone binding globulin (SHBG) rather than CBG. Like glucocorticoids, they are also carried by albumin (which binds the androgens and estrogens more tightly than it does glucocorticoids).

2. Glucocorticoids bind to specific cytosol receptor sites in responsive cells – these complexes are carried to specific receptors in the nucleus. This initiates the transcription process that will ultimately result in the production of specific DNA-mediated protein products.

3. Primary Physiologic Actions of Glucocorticoids

   a. Metabolic Effects

      i. Gluconeogenesis – a major effect of glucocorticoids (hence their name). Increased glucose production through activation of glucose 6 phosphatase and phosphoenolpyruvate carboxykinase (PEPCK). They additionally have a permissive role in the action of glucagon and epinephrine.

      ii. Decrease peripheral glucose uptake and insulin effectiveness.

      iii. Increase glycogen synthesis.

      iv. Increase lipolysis but in excess states also produce obesity through fat redistribution (both hyperinsulinemia and increased substrate intake may be operant).

   b. Immunologic and Hematologic Effects

      i. T lymphocytes are particularly affected (suppressed interleukin may play a role).

      ii. Inhibit monocytic activation and number.

      iii. Indirectly affect B-cell function through T-cell action.

      iv. Decreased inflammatory response (phospholipase inhibition).

      v. Leukocytosis (increased intravascular compartmentalization; increased half life).

      vi. Eosinopenia.

   c. Although necessary for normal growth enhancement and maturation, pathologic concentrations inhibit growth (gluconeogenesis; growth hormone and somatomedin inhibition).

   d. Maintenance of normal cardiovascular tone (permissive effect on catecholamines) and glomerular filtration rate (regulation of antidiuretic hormone (ADH) 'set point'?).

## MEASUREMENT OF ADRENAL FUNCTION

1. Steady State and Static Parameters

   a. Plasma Cortisol – has a diurnal variation with peak value at 08.00 (normal: 6–24 µg/dl) and nadir at 16.00 (normal: 3–12 µg/dl). Cortisol is produced in 'pulses' and this can result in variability in individual determinations. The values are also affected by physiologic stimuli that increase ACTH.

b.  Plasma ACTH – useful in distinguishing pituitary from adrenal disease. It is elevated in primary but decreased in secondary adrenal insufficiency. Conversely, it is elevated in ACTH-dependent but suppressed in ACTH-independent Cushing's syndrome. ACTH levels in the ectopic syndrome are generally higher than with pituitary adenomas in the standard assay, but they are also characteristically suppressed when an immunoradiometric ACTH assay is used. Hence, both types of ACTH assay can be useful.

c.  Urinary Cortisol and Metabolites

   i.  Urinary Free Cortisol – an excellent measure of daily production of cortisol and a very useful screening test for Cushing's syndrome (normal range: 20–90 mg/24 hours).

   ii.  17-Hydroxy Corticosteroids – Historically a useful test of daily cortisol production (Porter–Silber reaction) but there are many causes of false negatives and positives (e.g. can be elevated in obesity) (normal values: 3–15 mg/24 h (male); 3–12 mg/24 h (female)).

   iii. 17-Ketogenic Steroids – like the 17-hydroxy corticosteroids, a measure of the metabolites of cortisol, but it also measures non-glucocorticosteroid metabolites such as pregnanetriol. Historically, it has been adjunctively useful in the diagnosis of the 11-hydroxylase and 21-hydroxylase deficiency etiologies of congenital adrenal hyperplasia. Direct plasma measurements of specific corticoids, however, have supplanted its value. The assay is also affected by many drugs (e.g. penicillin, radiocontrast agents, meprobamate).

   iv.  17-Ketosteroids – a measure of androgenic metabolites, but rarely used because this test has been supplanted by direct serum measurements. Elevated in congenital adrenal hyperplasia associated with 11-hydroxylase or 21-hydroxylase deficiency states, and often disproportionately elevated in Cushing's Syndrome secondary to adrenocortical carcinoma (normal values: 10–20 mg/24 h (male); 5–15 mg/24 h (female)).

2. Dynamic Tests of Adrenal Function

   a. Dexamethasone Suppression Test – the rationale for this test is that normal suppressibility of the pituitary–adrenal axis occurs when the glucocorticoid level exceeds the hypothalamic–pituitary 'set point' for stimulation. The 08.00 plasma cortical level should be less than 5 µg/dl in normal individuals who take 1 mg of dexamethasone between 23.00 and midnight of the prior night.

   b. ACTH Stimulation Test – the rationale for this test is that the adrenal gland in primary Addison's disease is incapable of response to ACTH, whereas it can respond to ACTH if the deficiency is pituitary in origin. Because it can increase adrenal cortisol production in ACTH-dependent etiologies of Cushing's syndrome (but generally not in primary adrenal etiologies), it has been used as an ancillary test in the work-up of Cushing's disease – but it is of little additional benefit.

   c. Metyrapone Test – the rationale for this test is that 11-hydroxylase blockade by metyrapone results in ACTH stimulation and secondary adrenocortical activation. Although cortisol production is suppressed, its immediate precursor, 11-deoxycortisol should increase. The resultant increase would reflect adequacy of the hypothalamic–pituitary–adrenal axis. As with the ACTH stimulation test in Cushing's syndrome, this test has also been used to screen ACTH- from non-ACTH-mediated etiologies and to distinguish between pituitary and ectopic sources of ACTH. The rationale is that patients with non-ACTH-dependent Cushing's syndrome would not increase their cortisol production with metyrapone, but those who are ACTH dependent would. Further, those with pituitary-mediated Cushing's syndrome would have a greater response than those with an ectopic ACTH source.

   d. Insulin-mediated Hypoglycemia – hypoglycemia is an important stimulus to ACTH activation. The resultant ACTH and cortisol response tests the intactness of the hypothalamic–pituitary–adrenal axis.

   e. CRH Stimulation Test – the rationale is that in pituitary-mediated adrenal insufficiency, the ACTH (and secondarily, cortisol) responses to CRH administration are muted. In hypothalamic disease, the ACTH response is augmented, but because of 'chronic disease', the cortical response is blunted. In primary adrenal insufficiency, basal ACTH is high and even more augmented after CRH. In pituitary-mediated Cushing's Syndrome (Cushing's disease), ACTH levels are augmented. In all other etiologies of Cushing's syndrome, ACTH levels should not rise.

# 13

# HYPERFUNCTION OF THE ADRENAL CORTEX

General Features
Etiologies of Cushing's Syndrome
Laboratory Methods in Establishing the Diagnosis
Special Laboratory Tests
Imaging Tests
Treatment

## GENERAL FEATURES

1. The syndrome that is associated with the name of Harvey Cushing was first described in 1912 in a 23-year-old woman with 'painful obesity, hypertrichosis and amenorrhea' who had a 'polyglandular syndrome'. In 1932, Cushing attributed its causality to the trophic effect of pituitary basophils.

2. The clinical manifestations represent the cumulative effects of glucocorticoid excess on the body. Most striking are (Table 13-1):

   a. Obesity – this is centripetal or 'truncal' with involvement of the face, abdomen and 'scruff' of the neck. It is a 'grotesque' obesity, not to be confused with the obesity of overweight (indeed, the commonest clinical manifestation that generates a 'rule-out Cushings' referral is obesity). In children and adolescents, the weight gain is commonly associated with growth retardation.

   b. Weakness – this is primarily caused by a proximal myopathy and the weakness should be objectively evident. Loss of protein secondary to accelerated gluconeogenesis is the physiologic reason. Hypokalemia can be an aggravating factor.

   c. Ecchymoses and striae – secondary to loss of subcutaneous collagen matrix which renders vasculature unprotected to trauma, thus producing skin fragility. Striae are wide and red. Skin readily 'peels off' (Liddle's sign) and is subject to fungal infection.

## TABLE 13-1. CLINICAL FEATURES OF CUSHING'S SYNDROME

Obesity
Weakness
Ecchymoses and Striae
Androgen Excess
Osteoporosis
Hypertension
Psychiatric Manifestations
Glucose Intolerance
Depressed Immune Function
Increased Intraocular Pressure

d. Androgen excess – produces hirsutism (usually facial) in women along with increased sebum production, acne and some scalp hair regression. Irregular menses are very common. (In men, androgen excess is inconsequential when compared with testosterone levels, but impotence and decreased libido can occur as a direct effect of the glucocorticoid excess).

e. Osteoporosis – enhanced bone resorption (loss of matrix, negative calcium balance) with increased fracture diathesis. Increased outflow resisitance in the intraosseous circulation by hyperplastic and hypertrophic lipocytes can also lead to osteonecrosis (e.g. femoral head).

f. Hypertension – a common accompaniment; patients with Cushing's syndrome are also subject to dependent edema and congestive heart failure.

g. Additional clinical manifestations include a wide spectrum of psychiatric features (e.g. agitation, depression, frank psychoses), polydipsia and polyuria (glucose intolerance and hypokalemia can be operant), depressed immune function and increased intraocular pressure.

h. It is important to note that while the sensitivity for the findings of obesity, hypertension, irregular menses and glucose intolerance is high, they are so exceedingly common in many other guises that their specificity for Cushing's syndrome is low.

3. Ancillary but non-specific laboratory findings include: polycythemia, relative leukocytosis and neutrophilia ('demargination' of polymorphonuclear neutrophil leukocytes), lymphopenia and eosinopenia, increased very low-, low-, and high-density lipoprotein concentrations, hypercalciuria (rarely hypercalcemia), and hypokalemia. Rarely, factors V and VIII may be elevated (increased tendency to thrombophlebitis).

## ETIOLOGIES OF CUSHING'S SYNDROME (Table 13-2)

Although the common denominator in all causes is glucocorticoid excess, there are multiple etiologies that can produce this. They can be divided into ACTH-dependent and ACTH-independent categories. Cushing's syndrome, as may be caused by exogenous sources (e.g. pharmacotherapeutic agents) will be excluded from discussion.

## TABLE 13-2. ETIOLOGIES OF CUSHING'S SYNDROME

| | |
|---|---|
| ACTH-Dependent | Pituitary-Mediated |
| | Ectopic ACTH |
| ACTH-Independent | Adrenal Adenoma |
| | Adrenal Carcinoma |
| | Micronodular Adrenal Hyperplasia |

1.  ACTH-Dependent – can result from exaggerated pituitary ACTH production or from an ectopic source of the ACTH.

    a.  Pituitary-mediated (by definition, Cushing's Disease)

        i.   Accounts for 60% of all cases of Cushing's syndrome.

        ii.  Bilateral adrenal hyperplasia; proportional production of cortisol and its precursors.

        iii. Persistent secretion of ACTH and associated peptides with higher amplitude of secretory bursts, but with unchanged frequency (diurnal variation, however, is lost).

        iv.  Evidence strongly suggests a primary pituitary rather than a hypothalamic etiology (e.g. abnormalities of other pituitary trophic hormones reverse after surgical extirpation, recovery of normal ACTH rhythm and responsiveness occurs after surgery and there is a low incidence of recurrence in cured patients).

        v.   Although most cases are associated with a microadenoma, production of ACTH is not totally autonomous but rather capable of cortisol-mediated suppression, albeit at a higher 'set point'.

    b.  Ectopic ACTH Production

        i.   Fifteen per cent of all cases of Cushing's Syndrome.

        ii.  Most frequently associated with malignant tumors (small cell carcinoma of the lung accounts for 50% but noted in other tumors of foregut origin – e.g. bronchial carcinoid; also seen in thymoma, medullary carcinoma of the thyroid and islet cell tumor).

iii. May be associated with ectopic production of other hormones (e.g. syndrome of inappropriate antidiuretic hormone).

iv. In many cases, the classical appearance of Cushing's syndrome may be subdued (e.g. because of rapid tumor growth and course as well as the catabolic effects of the underlying malignancy) – instead, profound electrolyte imbalance (notably hypokalemia) and gluconeogenic effects of the glucocorticoids (wasting, hyperglycemia) may predominate.

v. In cases of bronchial carcinoid, however, the classic features of Cushing's syndrome may be present and the tumor is often occult. These patients may not have the carcinoid syndrome (L-amino acid decarboxylase may be deficient). Furthermore, these tumors may show feedback inhibition with dexamethasone suppression and stimulation with metyrapone. Bilateral inferior petrosal sinus sampling for ACTH can be a useful, if not invaluable, tool for definitive diagnosis.

c. Ectopic corticotropin releasing hormone (CRH) production – very rare; usually non-suppressible (testing studies often similar to ectopic ACTH – in fact, some tumors make both CRH and ACTH).

2. ACTH-Independent (aggregate 25% of Cushing's Syndrome).

a. Adrenal Adenoma

i. Ten per cent of cases of Cushing's syndrome.

ii. Tend to be slow growing and usually feature 'pure' hypercortisolism (this phenomenon is paralleled by complementary laboratory studies which demonstrate high levels of cortisol metabolites compared with precursor metabolites).

iii. Remainder of normal adrenal tissue on both sides develops secondary atrophy.

b. Adrenal Carcinoma

i. Fifteen per cent of cases of Cushing's syndrome.

ii. In contrast to the adenoma, these masses are larger in size (may even be palpable or demonstrate renal distortion or displacement on imaging studies). They may also produce abdominal and flank symptoms.

iii. Carcinomas also tend to elaborate more cortisol precursors and adrenal androgens than do adenomas. Concomitant laboratory studies should demonstrate high levels of cortisol precursors and androgen products.

c. Micronodular Adrenal Hyperplasia

i. A rare disorder usually seen in younger individuals.

ii. When familial, it is autosomal dominant and associated with a variety of other structural lesions: multiple pigmented lentigines, atrial myxomas and other tumors (e.g. pituitary, testicular).

iii. Hyperplastic micronodules are interspersed between regions of atrophic but otherwise seemingly normal adrenal tissue (why some foci of adrenal tissue become autonomous and others do not is not clear).

iv. This entity should not be confused with a variant of Cushing's disease which produces macronodules (in lieu of diffuse hyperplasia). Some of these macronodules may even remain autonomous after treatment of the primary pituitary disorder but they ultimately regress when their trophic stimulation is lifted.

v. This entity may be food-dependent as a result of increased adrenal cell sensitivity to gastric inhibitory polypeptide (GIP).

## LABORATORY METHODS IN ESTABLISHING THE DIAGNOSIS

1. Overnight Dexamethasone Suppression Test

a. The simplest and most cost-effective screening test. If the test is normal, the patient does not have Cushing's syndrome.

b. The patient is given 1 mg of dexamethasone between 23.00 and midnight and a plasma cortisol is drawn the following morning between 08.00 and 09.00. The $t_{1/2}$ of the dexamethasone is such that its sustained effect prevents the morning cortisol burst. Plasma levels in normal individuals should be less than 5 µg/dl (and are often substantially less).

c.  Although comparison of morning and afternoon plasma cortisol levels in patients with Cushing's syndrome would reveal lack of diurnal variation, there is sufficient episodic variability in normal bursts to make this an ineffective screening test. Certainly, random cortisol levels are of no value (especially in the context of physiologic stress).

d.  False-positive tests (i.e. failure to demonstrate suppression) occur in obesity, psychiatric illness and alcoholism, stress, renal failure and with drugs that induce dexamethasone metabolism (e.g. anti-seizure drugs – phenobarbital, dilantin, primidone and tegretol; and rifampin).

e.  If there is a suspected false-positive result, using a 2 mg dose in a repeat study is often helpful.

2.  Urine Free Cortisol

a.  Normal range: 20–90 µg/24 h.

b.  An excellent screening test for Cushing's syndrome – can supplement the dexamethasone suppression test if a false-positive result is suspected.

c.  It has supplanted the classic 24-hour 17-hydroxysteroid urinary excretion test which is based on the Porter–Silber reaction and measures metabolites of cortisol and deoxycortisol (normal range: 3–15 mg/24 h in men, 3–12 mg/24 h in women).

d.  The 24-hour 17-ketosteroid urinary excretion test has not been supplanted but its role continues to remain that of an adjunctive measure of adrenal androgen production. (This test does not measure testosterone, the most potent androgen, yet it measures etiocholanolone which is not an androgen.) Normal range: 5–15 mg/24 h in women; 10–20 mg/24 h in men).

3.  Structured Prolonged Low- and High-Dose Dexamethasone Suppression Tests

a.  The classic testing sequence for distinguishing between Cushing's disease and other causes of Cushing's syndrome.

b. The Low-Dose Test – dexamethasone administration, 0.5 mg orally every 6 hours, for 2 days. Urine is collected on the second day and measured for 17-hydroxysteroids and creatinine. All patients with Cushing's syndrome will have 17-hydroxysteroid values greater than 4 mg/day (or 2.5 mg/g creatinine/day). Variations on this test can be done with urinary free cortisol or plasma cortisol levels.

c. The High-Dose Test – dexamethasone administration, 2.0 mg orally every 6 hours, for 2 days. Patients with Cushing's disease generally show 17-hydroxysteroid suppression – other etiologies generally do not (some patients with ectopic ACTH, however, may suppress). Use of urinary free cortisol as an adjunct has been additionally helpful. An intravenous test variant has also been used.

d. An additional distinction, more relevant for historical purposes, is the comparison of the urinary excretion of 17-hydroxysteroids and 17-ketosteroids. Adrenal adenomas would tend to be associated with a disproportionately higher 17-hydroxysteroid excretion while adrenal carcinoma would be associated with a higher 17-ketosteroid excretion.

4. Plasma ACTH Level

a. A helpful test in distingushing between ACTH-dependent and -independent Cushing's syndrome.

b. All ACTH-independent etiologies have very low or undetectable levels (normal: 20–100 pg/ml). Although both pituitary and ectopic etiologies have elevated levels, ectopic values are significantly higher, while values in true Cushing's disease can overlap the normal range.

c. If the immunoradiometric assay is used (this is a double antibody assay directed at both the N and C terminals of the ACTH molecule), values in the ectopic syndrome may be low or undetectable (this may be used advantageously in the differential diagnosis).

d. Plasma ACTH levels (with simultaneous plasma cortisol) after CRH administration can help to discriminate among etiologies of Cushing's syndrome.

i. In Cushing's disease, CRH produces an increase in both ACTH and cortisol levels.

ii. There is no response to CRH in pituitary-independent etiologies.

iii. Patients with ectopic ACTH generally do not respond to CRH but exceptions have occurred. These have demonstrated a disproportionate increase in ACTH (as opposed to cortisol) which is suggestive of a structurally different ACTH molecule ('Big' ACTH).

iv. Patients who have an abnormal low-dose or overnight dexamethasone suppression test and are felt to have 'non-Cushing's hypercortisolism' (e.g. depression) tend to have a blunted response to CRH.

## SPECIAL LABORATORY TESTS

Not generally necessary in establishing the diagnosis, but they may be of selectively useful adjunctive value.

1. Metyrapone Test

   a. Metyrapone blocks the synthesis of cortisol and thus stimulates endogenous ACTH. Deoxycortisol is measured in the 17-hydroxysteroid assay and would increase if ACTH were increased and the adrenal cortex capable of response.

   b. Patients with Cushing's disease are capable of an exuberant response while those with ACTH-independent Cushing's syndrome are not. Among patients with ACTH-dependent Cushing's syndrome, those with ectopic ACTH production do not generally have the same magnitude of response as patients who have pituitary-mediated Cushing's syndrome. Combining these test results with the high-dose dexamethasone suppression test could make the discrimination between pituitary-mediated and ectopic ACTH syndromes even greater.

2. ACTH Infusion Test – this test is not of practical value. Although it can generally distinguish between pituitary-dependent and -independent etiologies, it cannot distinguish between Cushing's disease and ectopic ACTH etiologies.

3. Insulin-Induced Hypoglycemia Test – this test is not of value because there is blunted ACTH and growth hormone response to chronic hypercortisolemia, irrespective of etiology. It may be helpful in distinguishing Cushing's syndrome from non-Cushing's hypercortisolism.

## IMAGING TESTS

1. Adrenal CT – important for structural confirmation of an adrenal lesion when ACTH-independent Cushing's syndrome is chemically diagnosed. False negatives are rare (although incidental adrenal masses serendipitously noted on abdominal CT can be seen in anyone).

2. Cranial MRI

   a. Important for structural confirmation of pituitary lesions when ACTH-dependent Cushing's syndrome is chemically diagnosed. In general, the MRI has a greater sensitivity than CT, especially when gadolinium enhancement is used. Unfortunately, false negatives occur.

   b. Because there can be overlap with the biochemical features of ectopic and pituitary-mediated Cushing's syndrome, a search should be done for ectopic lesions if cranial MRI is negative. A negative chest X-ray mandates chest CT with follow-up abdominal CT, as necessary.

   c. If the suspicion is compelling, the above studies should be done in the presence of a pituitary lesion on MRI because of the possibility that this lesion may be a 'true–true-unrelated' one (analogous to incidental adrenal lesions) that are seen in otherwise normal people.

3. The problem can be resolved using bilateral inferior petrosal sinus sampling for ACTH levels.

   a. This test is a powerful tool when utilized for substantiation of a pituitary etiology of Cushing's syndrome – it is reserved for those clinical situations in which there is some elevation of ACTH.

   b. The rationale is that there should be some pituitary : peripheral gradient if ACTH secretion is pituitary in origin whereas there should not be one if the ACTH source is ectopic.

c . Indeed, the ratio is never less than 2.0 if pituitary or greater than 2.0 if ectopic. If this test is modified with CRH stimulation, a pituitary lesion would never have a ratio less than 3.0. (In actuality, the gradients are generally more discriminating but lower ranges can be approached because of the pulsatile nature of ACTH release.)

d. An added benefit of sampling is that lateralization of a pituitary lesion can be determined. There is independence of left and right pituitary venous drainage into their respective ipsilateral inferior petrosal sinuses.

e. Logistically, catheters are fed up both femoral veins and placement confirmed by fluoroscopy – the pulsatile nature of ACTH release mandates that blood samples be simultaneously obtained from both sides.

f. An ACTH ratio between the two sides of greater than 1.4 indicates lateralization to the higher side.

g. Sources of potential error include unavoidable technical problems, aberrancy of venous drainage, prior surgery, presence of a midline lesion or ectopic CRH production.

4. The increased affinity of ectopic ACTH-producing lesions for somatostatin makes somatostatin receptor scintigraphy a potentially valuable tool.

## TREATMENT

1. For pituitary-mediated Cushing's syndrome, pituitary surgery is the treatment of choice.

   a. The above-noted tests result in a success rate up to 90% following ipsilateral surgery.

   b. If no isolated adenoma is noted on ipsilateral exploration of the side showing inferior petrosal sinus lateralization, a hemihypophysectomy is usually performed.

   c. If a second procedure is required, the success rate is in the 50–75% range.

   d. Because of chronic suppression of CRH and ACTH in normal pituitary tissue, patients successfully operated on may need long-term steroid therapy with gradual tapering (for up to a year or more).

e. Follow up is mandatory as recurrence rate is 5%.

f. Although used as a primary modality in the past, bilateral adrenalectomy remains a second-line therapy for persistent Cushing's syndrome following pituitary surgery. Complications include a higher mortality than with pituitary surgery, permanent Addison's disease, the risk of recurrence from ectopic embryologic 'adrenal rest' tissue and Nelson's syndrome (symptomatic enlargement of the pituitary adenoma).

g. Pituitary radiation can control the disease when used in concert with o'p' DDD (Mitotane, Lysodren) – the long-term effect may be curative but medical therapy may have to be sustained in some patients. Delayed hypopituitarism and non-pituitary radiation damage are potential complications.

2. Adrenalectomy is the treatment of choice for primary adrenal lesions; long-term antecedent suppression requires glucocorticoid replacement therapy with gradual tapering.

3. If resectable, surgery is the treatment of choice for ectopic ACTH-producing lesions.

4. Medical therapy is indicated for:

a. Ectopic ACTH- or CRH-producing lesions that are non-identifiable, non-resectable or metastatic.

b. Metastatic adrenal carcinoma.

c. Persistent pituitary-mediated Cushing's syndrome in patients post-bilateral adrenalectomy whose source of excessive glucocorticoid is still unclear.

d. As a preoperative adjunct in some patients.

e. As an adjunct to radiation therapy of the pituitary gland.

f. Available medications include:

i. Agents which inhibit the synthesis or action of glucocorticoids:

(a) o'p' DDD (Mitotane, Lysodren): adrenalytic agent and inhibitor of cholesterol desmolase and 11-hydroxylase.

(b) Aminoglutethimide (Cytadren): inhibitor of cholesterol desmolase.

(c) Metyrapone: inhibitor of 11-hydroxylase.

(d) Ketoconazone (Nizoral): inhibitor of cholesterol and 17, 20-desmolase and 11-hydroxylase. It also inhibits the peripheral effects of glucocorticoids and androgen synthesis.

(e) Additional drugs include: Etomidate (originally used as an anesthetic and limited in its treatment of hyperglucocortisolism by the side-effect of drowsiness), Trilostane and RU 486 (Mifepristone). Mifepristone is both a glucocorticoid and a progesterone antagonist. It is best known (and has received world-wide attention) for that latter effect and its resultant abortifacient action. When used as an abortifacient, it is generally combined with a prostaglandin.

ii. Neuromodulatory agents:

(a) Bromocriptine – a dopamine agonist.

(b) Cyproheptidine – antiserotonergic, anticholinergic and antihistamine.

(c) Octreotide – a somatostatin analog. It may also serve as a helpful tool in distinguishing between pituitary and ectopic ACTH production in that the ectopic, but not pituitary-mediated Cushing's syndrome, is more likely to suppress with octreotide.

(d) Valproic Acid – a $\gamma$-aminobutyric acid receptor blocker.

# 14

# ADRENAL CORTICAL INSUFFICIENCY

## GENERAL CONSIDERATIONS

1. Can be classified according to primary and secondary (includes pituitary and hypothalamic) etiologies. Primary etiologies invariably involve all three layers (in physically extensive disease, the medulla is involved as well). Thus, mineralocorticoid deficiency is an integral part of the syndrome complex. In addition, compensatory pituitary production of ACTH (as part of the pro-opiomelanocortin (POMC) 'package') contributes to clinical findings. Secondary adrenal insufficiency is associated with normal or near-normal mineralocorticoid function and does not have any findings associated with increased ACTH.

2. Can be classified according to the acuteness or chronicity of onset – these categories have their own unique presentations, etiologies, clinical course and gravity of illness.

## CHRONIC PRIMARY ADRENAL INSUFFICIENCY

**Etiologies** (Table 14-1)
1. Idiopathic

   a. The most common etiology today, comprising about 80% of all cases.

   b. An autoimmune disease with corresponding histopathology of lymphocytic infiltration and fibrous stroma and loss of functioning adrenal cells.

### TABLE 14-1.   ETIOLOGIES OF CHRONIC PRIMARY ADRENOCORTICAL INSUFFICIENCY

Idiopathic (Autoimmune)
Tuberculosis and Fungal Disease
HIV-Associated
Metastatic Disease
Sarcoidosis
Iatrogenic
Congenital
Drugs
Lipid Storage Disease

c.  The autoimmunity is both cell-mediated and humoral. A number of anti-adrenal antibodies have been identified. While these antibodies may be shown to attach to the ACTH receptor site, none has been shown to have the stimulating effect of that seen with the thyroid-binding immunoglobulins of Graves' disease. Antibody appearance may antedate the clinical disease, but the titers wane over the duration of the process.

d.  Associated with other autoimmune diseases – gonadal failure, immune thyroid disease (goitrous, hypothyroidism, and Graves' disease), Type I diabetes mellitus, vitiligo, hypoparathyroidism and pernicious anemia. Can also occur without these other clinical disorders although immunologic evidence of disease potential may exist (e.g. parietal cell and intrinsic factor antibodies). Conversely, related disorders (most notably hypoparathyroidism) may independently be associated with anti-adrenal antibodies. Linkage to other endocrine deficiencies (especially diabetes mellitus and hypothyroidism) is often referred to as Schmidt's syndrome.

e.  Distinct polyglandular syndromes, whose spectrum include primary adrenal insufficiency, have been codified. Type I Syndrome additionally includes mucocutaneous candidiasis, hypoparathyroidism, chronic active hepatitis and hypophysitis, and has no HLA-DR association. Type II Syndrome does not include candidiasis, hypoparathyroidism is unusual and there is association with HLA-DR3 and DR4. Isolated adrenal insufficiency is also linked to DR3, DR4, and B-8.

2.  Adrenal Tuberculosis

a.  The most common etiology in the past – noted in Addison's original cases.

b.  Results from hematogenous spread of the organism from other sites. The organism 'thrives' in the steroid-rich environment – although the medulla is preferentially destroyed.

c.  Adrenal glands may be initially large, then atrophic and calcify about 50% of the time.

d.  Fungal diseases (e.g. histoplasmosis and paracoccidioidomycosis) can produce a comparable effect (coccidiomycosis is a rare cause).

3. HIV-Associated Disease

   a. Adrenal insufficiency may occur as a primary process or secondary to opportunistic infection.

   b. The overt clinical state may be enhanced when rifampin (accelerated cortisol metabolism) and ketoconazole (decreased steroidogenesis) are used in a setting of decreased adrenal reserve.

4. Metastatic Disease

   a. While metastatic disease to the adrenal glands is common, adrenal insufficiency is rare, as 90% of the gland has to be functionally replaced for overt disease to develop.

   b. Common primary tumors are breast, lung and melanoma.

5. Miscellaneous (and uncommon)

   a. Sarcoidosis, hemochromatosis, syphilis.

   b. Iatrogenic (surgery).

   c. Congenital – enzyme deficiency states, ACTH receptor insensitivity (mineralocorticoid production is not affected), profound cholesterol deficiency (abetalipoproteinemia; impaired response to ACTH but not overt deficiency may be seen in patients with cholesterol receptor defect – familial hypercholesterolemia), congenital hypoplasia.

   d. Drugs – ketoconazole, o'p'-DDD (Mitotane, Lysodren), metyrapone (these drugs can be used to treat glucocorticoid excess). Drugs which accelerate glucocorticoid metabolism can 'unmask' an insufficient state.

   e. Adrenoleukodystrophy and adrenomyeloneuropathy – pathologic accumulation of lipids (e.g. cholesterol esters, gangliosides) in multiple tissues (including adrenal glands) secondary to failure to metabolize long-chain fatty acids. Inheritance is X-linked recessive. Neurologic deterioration is a hallmark of this disease. The Hollywood-generated publicity notwithstanding, there is no evidence that dietary treatment with oleic and erucic acids ('Lorenzo's oil') is beneficial.

### TABLE 14-2.   CLINICAL MANIFESTATIONS OF ADRENOCORTICAL INSUFFICIENCY

Weakness, Fatigue, Anorexia, Weight Loss
Hyperpigmentation
Clinical Manifestations of Hyponatremia
Gastrointestinal Symptoms
Hypoglycemia
Androgen Deficiency
Myalgia, Arthralgia
Ear Calcification
Costovertebral Angle Tenderness
Psychiatric Manifestations

---

f.  Glucocorticoid Resistance States – Receptor dysfunction with variability of clinical expression based on different sensitivities of target tissues. It may theoretically appear surreptitiously and be difficult to diagnose.

**Clinical Manifestations** (Table 14-2)

1.  Weakness, fatigue, anorexia and weight loss are invariably present.

2.  Hyperpigmentation

a.  Both ACTH and related Pro-opiomelanocortin (POMC)-derived melanocyte stimulators are purported factors.

b.  As opposed to the hyperpigmentation of 'suntan', Addisonian hyperpigmentation can occur in non-solar exposed areas (skin creases and folds). Hands may have a 'dirty' appearance. Buccal mucosa and gingiva are involved. Solar-exposed areas, however, do become more deeply pigmented.

c.  Scars and traumatized areas occurring after the onset of Addison's disease are more intensely pigmented than those which have existed previously.

d.  Hyperpigmentation can occur superimposed on any racial background.

e.  Vitiligo, if present, can be all the more profound (by contrast).

157

3. Manifestations of Hyponatremia – hypotension (often orthostatic); inexplicable improvement in pre-existing hypertension; 'small quiet heart'; salt craving.

4. Gastrointestinal Symptoms – nausea, vomiting, abdominal pain, bowel dysfunction.

5. Hypoglycemic Manifestations

   a. Fasting (as opposed to reactive) hypoglycemia, although Addisonian patients can 'adapt' to chronically low levels.

   b. Caused by failure of gluconeogenesis and increased insulin sensitivity (glucocorticoid absence prevents insulin antagonism).

   c. May be brought out by acute precipitating events (e.g. infection); alcohol, by inhibiting gluconeogenesis, is also a provocateur.

   d. Improved glycemic control in a previously diagnosed diabetic may be an early clue.

6. Androgen Deficiency

   a. Clinically manifest in women as loss of bodily hair and decreased libido; amenorrhea may, independently, occur in women.

   b. Although testicular androgens are still operant in men, generalized lassitude and ill health contribute to sexual dysfunction.

   c. Hypogonadism may be an independent immune-mediated finding.

7. Other Clinical Aspects

   a. Myalgias and arthralgias,

   b. Auricular (ear) calcification (Thorn's sign),

   c. Costovertebral angle tenderness (Rogoff's sign),

   d. Psychiatric manifestations.

**Diagnostic Studies**
1. General Laboratory Studies

   a. Hyponatremia and hyperkalemia; non-anion gap metabolic

acidosis; paradoxical urine sodium wasting in the presence of hyponatremia and hypovolemia.

b. Complete blood count – normocytic, normochromic anemia (may become more obvious after fluid replacement); if there is macrocytosis, it may suggest early pernicious anemia; lymphocytosis; eosinophilia. As opposed to the demargination and leukocytosis of glucocorticoid excess, there may be a mild leukopenia.

c. Hypoglycemia (fasting).

d. Azotemia secondary to dehydration (loss of gluconeogenesis actually results in decreased urea production).

e. Tendency to mild hypercalcemia.

f. Increased ADH (stimulated by hypovolemia) with impaired free water clearance contributing to the hyponatremia.

g. Non-specific EKG changes, or the more specific T-wave changes seen with hyperkalemia.

h. The chest X-ray would show a relative decrease in heart size. If studied radiographically, ear calcification might be noted (Thorn's sign).

2. Definitive Laboratory Studies

a. ACTH and associated POMC derivatives are elevated but maintain their normal diurnal variation; 'random' cortisol and other adrenal steroid levels (e.g. dehydroepiandrosterone, aldosterone) are low – but this is not definitive (it is useful, however, if an 'inappropriately' low cortisol level is obtained in the context of physiologic stress).

b. The definitive test measures adrenal response to ACTH:

i. A simplified procedure involves the use of an intravenous injection of synthetic ACTH (cosyntropin; ACTH 1-24; Cortrosyn), 250 µg; 1 hour plasma levels greater than 20 µg/dl rules out adrenal insufficiency (in a test modification, salivary cortisol levels have been used). In reality, patients with Addison's disease have substantially lower values.

ii. More prolonged testing protocols ranging from 8 hours to 5 days have been employed but are generally not necessary. They are of value in distinguishing between primary and secondary disease because long-term ACTH deficiency renders the adrenals unable to respond to exogenous ACTH without further 'priming'.

   iii. Additional tests that measure the competence of the pituitary gland to stimulate the adrenals may be necessary if the diagnosis of primary adrenal insufficiency is not clear (see below).

  c. Mineralocorticoid deficiency is demonstrated by showing an appropriate increase in plasma renin (values may be initially high because of the dehydration) with upright posture, but the absence of a concomitant rise in plasma aldosterone.

## ACUTE ADRENAL INSUFFICIENCY

### Etiologies

1. Can occur in the setting of borderline compensated chronic adrenal insufficiency with an acute superimposed event – e.g. surgery, myocardial infarction, trauma.

2. Can occur in a person with known Addison's disease and already on replacement therapy who does not receive adequate 'stress' doses of glucocorticoid at times of physiologic need. The need for mineralocorticoid (and NaCl and volume replacement) may be particularly important.

3. Associated with acute adrenal hemorrhage – secondary to multisystem failure; anticoagulant therapy; circulating 'procoagulants' (e.g. lupus 'anticoagulant').

4. Associated with fulminant septicemia (Waterhouse–Friderichsen Syndrome) which is a special form of adrenal hemorrhage. The pathologic state is a result of disseminated intravascular coagulation, referred to in the past as a 'Schwartzman phenomenon' (classically described with meningococcemia but seen with other septic etiologies).

### Clinical Presentation

1. Unlike chronic adrenal insufficiency in which many clinical findings have had the opportunity to evolve, the major manifestations in acute adrenal insufficiency are hypotension and shock, dehydration, altered mental status, gastrointestinal and

abdominal symptoms (nausea, vomiting, pain) and signs (rebound, rigidity), and fever.

2. Classic electrolyte patterns may be mild or absent, and hyperpigmentation would not have had the opportunity to evolve. Metabolic acidosis (peripheral hypoperfusion) and azotemia (dehydration) can be seen. Other studies may suggest etiology (e.g. elevated prothrombin time (PT) and partial thromboplastin time (PTT), fibrin split products, positive blood cultures); eosinophilia may be present.

**Management**
1. Definitive diagnosis using previously described protocols can be made at a subsequent time when the acute crisis has abated and the patient is more stable.

2. Presumptive clinical diagnosis warrants immediate intervention even without a definitive diagnosis. Included in initial blood work are plasma cortisol and ACTH levels – they can be helpful in that profound physiologic stress should result in significant elevations. Other laboratory studies such as complete blood count, electrolytes and basic chemistries would undoubtedly be done anyway in an acute care setting.

3. Volume repletion with glucose/isotonic saline solutions.

4. The average amount of saline infusion will be 3–6 liters for the initial 4–6 hours with the actual amount a function of both the clinical need and patient tolerance – central blood pressure monitoring may be necessary.

5. Hydrocortisone, 100 mg, is given as an intravenous bolus and every 6 hours thereafter. If the underlying cause of the Addisonian crisis abates, this may be tapered over 3–4 days with maintenance therapy thereafter (oral medication may be substituted if the patient is tolerant of oral intake).

6. As long as saline infusion persists (the high-dose hydrocortisone will also have mineralocorticoid activity), there is no need for oral mineralocorticoid therapy. When saline is discontinued, Fludrocortisone (Florinef), 0.1 mg by mouth daily should be started – the final dose to be determined later.

7. When able to tolerate oral glucocorticoids, the patient may be changed to maintenance therapy (with initial high doses if

tapering is still in progress). Testing for adrenal responsiveness to ACTH stimulation will require the patient to be on dexamethasone so that laboratory results can be interpreted.

8. Intramuscular cortisone acetate has no role in acute management because of the unpredictability of absorption and the need for hepatic conversion (reduction) of cortisone to hydrocortisone.

9. Simultaneous with the management of adrenal insufficiency, precipitating and coincident disease must be managed.

## MAINTENANCE THERAPY OF ADRENAL INSUFFICIENCY

1. Although glucocorticoid is given to parallel the normal diurnal variation, it is often difficult to mimic the morning surge (because ACTH levels are highest prior to waking) – this may result in both the tendency to sustained hyperpigmentation and morning constitutional symptoms that are not abated until after a significant blood level of steroid is achieved.

2. The shorter acting preparations (cortisol and cortisone acetate) may also produce supraphysiologic levels of glucocorticoid in the late morning which could give rise to chronic Cushingoid manifestations.

3. Dosing Schedules

   a. Longer acting preparations (dexamethasone and prednisone) could provide a smoother course and may also be taken at bedtime in doses of 2.5–7.5 mg of prednisone or 0.25–0.75 mg of dexamethasone. This could reduce the morning ACTH surge, but some patients have insomnia and may become 'hyperactive and charged' with this dosing pattern. Further, the steroid 'effect' may wear off prematurely during the day when compared with the 'natural endogenous fall off'.

   b. A more traditional approach would be two-thirds of the daily dose in the early morning and one-third in the late afternoon (although some patients may not require the second dose because normal afternoon cortisol production is very low).

   c. Patients who have an inverse day/night schedule (on a continuous basis) should alter their pattern of administration according to their sleep–wakefulness cycle and not the time of day.

4. Morning ACTH levels may be a helpful guide to dosimetry but must be interpreted in the appropriate clinical context.

5. Concomitant medication use which can increase glucocorticoid metabolism (e.g. phenobarbital, dilantin, rifampin) may result in the need for an upward dosing change in glucocorticoids (medications that block steroidogenesis – e.g. ketoconazole, are of no relevance).

6. Mineralocorticoid dosage range is 0.05–0.2 mg, of fludrocortisone (Florinef) daily – blood pressure (basal and postural), weight, presence of edema, and electrolyte concentrations are important guidelines for dosimetry.

7. Acute physiologic stress such as trauma, infection, or surgery, warrants dose augmentation (usually four to six times the normal dose during the first day of the event) with progressive tapering (as the inciting event abates).

    a. Surgery requires intravenous supplementation.

    b. An appropriate regime following major trauma would be hydrocortisone, 100 mg intravenous every 8 hours, for the first 24 hours.

    c. The patient should always carry an 'emergency syringe' (dexamethasone, 4 mg) for acute events until professional medical care can supervene. The patient should also wear an appropriate identification tag.

## SECONDARY ADRENAL INSUFFICIENCY

1. Occurs as a result of pituitary or hypothalamic insufficiency – it is often one aspect of a larger syndrome in which manifestations may be caused by multiple endocrine deficiencies, the mass effect of the lesion or even hormonal excess states (e.g. prolactin, growth hormone (HGH)).

2. Major distinctions from primary adrenal insufficiency are the absence of hyperpigmentation (indeed, hypopigmentation may occur) and classic electrolyte patterns. While hyperkalemia is rare, some degree of hyponatremia often occurs because of the effect of ACTH (albeit mild) on mineralocorticoid production and because of excessive water retention (decreased free water

clearance). Hypoglycemia may be more pronounced (although rarely severe without other underlying conditions) because of concomitant HGH deficiency.

3. Baseline hormonal measurements may be of general screening value (urinary hydroxycorticoids and free cortisol are low), but dynamic tests are required for determining the type of insufficiency.

   a. The ACTH stimulation test may be abnormal if an 'abbreviated' version is used. Given sufficient 'priming' with a more prolonged test, there should be an adequate (if not exuberant) adrenal response.

   b. Insulin-induced hypoglycemia – a very potent test that can additionally measure HGH. It is potentially dangerous in that those most likely to show a positive response (absent activation of the pituitary–adrenal axis) and hence, the most likely to be tested, are also at greatest risk to the effects of the hypoglycemia. For that reason, the usual dose of 0.15 U/kg of insulin, given intravenously, can be decreased to 0.1 U/kg because it is not the insulin *per se* but its hypoglycemic effect that is the test stimulus. Ideally, the ACTH response should be the discriminant (cortisol levels can be low because of either a primary or secondary deficiency) but values for ACTH have not been well standardized.

   c. Metyrapone Stimulation Test – acts by blocking cortisol synthesis and thus preventing cortisol-mediated ACTH suppression. Because cortisol deficiency is more potent a provocateur than hypoglycemia, a patient may have a 'normal' hypoglycemic test yet have 'early' or 'partial' ACTH deficiency as manifest by an abnormal metyrapone test. Both an overnight (abbreviated) and 3-day test protocol are available.

   d. CRH (Corticotropin-Releasing Hormone) Stimulation Test – the rationale is that pituitary deficiency will result in no ACTH production after CRH stimulation but the pituitary can still respond to CRH if only the hypothalamus is affected. ACTH response can be high and sustained, thus serving as a discriminant between hypothalamic and pituitary etiologies. Although not a necessary test for the diagnosis of primary adrenal insufficiency, basal ACTH levels in this condition are elevated and have an augmented response to CRH. (CRH is sometimes administered as part of a pituitary work-up 'cocktail' along with thyrotropin-releasing hormone, growth hormone-releasing hormone and gonadotropin-releasing hormone.)

4. Glucocorticoid Replacement Therapy – the dosage and patterns are the same as with primary disease. Although some patients with chronic ACTH deficiency may develop decreased aldosterone production, mineralocorticoid therapy is rarely necessary. Other hormonal replacement therapy is based on the presence or absence of other deficiency states.

# 15

# CONGENITAL ADRENAL HYPERPLASIA

CLINICAL HANDBOOK OF ENDOCRINOLOGY AND METABOLIC DISEASE

## GENERAL CONSIDERATIONS

1. A family of autosomal recessive syndromes all having the common denominator of inadequate cortisol synthesis. As cortisol is the most potent feedback inhibitor of ACTH, ACTH production increases in compensation and the adrenal is 'overdriven'. To sustain life, the increased stimulation to cortisol production must result in sufficient circulating levels.

2. Although basal cortisol levels may be adequate, 'stressed' levels may not be and a cortisol deficiency state could occur when there is an acute illness. If the defect affects mineralocorticoid synthesis as well (as most do), a salt-wasting hypovolemic presentation is superimposed.

3. The clinical syndromes also reflect the accumulation of excessive metabolites proximal to the enzymatic defect (e.g. resulting in hirsutism, virilization, or precocious puberty) or sex hormone deficiency states (because of impaired synthesis of sex steroids) contribute to the clinical presentation.

## ETIOLOGIES OF CONGENITAL ADRENAL HYPERPLASIA
(Table 15-1)

### 21-Hydroxylase Deficiency
1. Depending on the severity of the defect, varying degrees of hyperandrogenism and salt-losing states characterize this disorder. In males, hyperandrogenic states are most relevant prepubertally as adrenal androgens are not consequential when compared with testicular androgens (testosterone) postpuberty. Nonetheless, there is an increased risk of infertility and embryologic 'adrenal rest' tissue tumors arising in men with this

### TABLE 15-1. ETIOLOGIES OF CONGENITAL ADRENAL HYPERPLASIA

21-Hydroxylase Deficiency
11-Hydroxylase Deficiency
17-Hydroxylase Deficiency
3β-Hydroxysteroid Dehydrogenase Deficiency
Cholesterol Side-Chain Cleavage Enzyme Deficiency

disorder. Excessive prepubertal androgens can give rise to accelerated growth and precocious puberty (with ultimate stunting of stature). The spectrum of disease in males may vary and the clinical scenario can range from a 'subtle' one (e.g. a 'shorter' male with earlier puberty) to the 'Infantile Hercules' syndrome. Ironically, because they might not have come to medical attention, males with the least overt clinical manifestations may be at greatest risk for consequences of mineralocorticoid deficiency when subject to dehydration.

2. The spectrum in women can range from neonatal female pseudohermaphroditism to manifestations only of hirsutism and perhaps irregular menses later in life.

3. This disorder is sometimes divided into Type I (minimal mineralocorticoid defect) and Type II (salt-wasting).

4. Incidence is 1 in 14 000 births. The coding gene locus is on the short arm of chromosome 6 (close to C4 and between HLA-B and HLA-D). Several types of gene disorders have been associated with the syndrome (e.g. mutations, deletions).

5. Elevated plasma 17-hydroxyprogesterone is characteristic (this can be incorporated into a neonatal screening protocol) – this has supplanted urinary 17-ketosteroid and pregnanetriol determinations. In 'subtle' cases, the 17-hydroxyprogesterone determination may be elevated only in the early morning (in response to the 'natural' ACTH peak) or following an actual ACTH stimulation test. Other elevated androgens include dehydroepiandrosterone sulfate and androstenedione. The mineralocorticoid defect results in hyperkalemia, a relative hyponatremia and an inappropriately low plasma and urine aldosterone level (in comparison to an elevated plasma renin level).

6. Treatment requires glucocorticoid replacement as maintenance (with episodic 'stress' doses, as required). Unlike Addison's disease where all adrenal cortical function is shut down, the relative composition of adrenal products (indeed, magnified, because the glands are hyperplastic) is altered. Thus, even 'normal' ACTH levels lead to excessive androgen production. The following are important considerations:

a. Excessive glucocorticoid necessary to 'shut down' ACTH (and hence prevent excessive undesired adrenal 'by-products') will produce a Cushingoid state – thus, the tendency to short stature may be aggravated.

b. Accelerated sexual maturation has an augmenting effect on the timing of hypothalamic–pituitary–gonadal activation – the tendency to short stature may again be aggravated.

c. Although the renin–angiotensin–aldosterone axis is independent of the pituitary, aldosterone deficiency results in ACTH activation. To minimize compounding the effects of excessive ACTH, mineralocorticoid therapy must be administered as well.

d. Use of androgen-receptor blockade may have a role – e.g. spironolactone, flutamide. Since small amounts of estrogen (synthesized from the androgens) may also accelerate growth, aromatase inhibition (testolactone) may also have merit.

e. Additional considerations: gonadotropin-releasing hormone antagonists to turn off gonadotropins; timing of cortisol administration; is bilateral adrenalectomy ever justified ?; pregnancy (dexamethasone turns off maternal and fetal ACTH but it must be given early in pregnancy to prevent virilization of fetal female external genitalia; dexamethasone, itself, may alter genital development); reconstructive surgery to correct physical effects of masculinization.

## 11-Hydroxylase Deficiency

1. Virilization associated with hypertension – secondary to increased deoxycorticosterone production (this and deoxycortisol elevation are biochemical markers). Hypokalemia and hypernatremia may be concomitants.

2. One in 100 000 live births. The 11-hydroxylase gene is on the long arm of chromosome 8.

3. Aldosterone is suppressed because of increased deoxycorticosterone. (Mineralocorticoid therapy may be necessary in patients treated with a glucocorticoid who are on a reduced salt intake.)

## 17-Hydroxylase Deficiency

1.  Impaired 17-hydroxyprogesterone and 17-hydroxypregnenolone synthesis. Androgen and cortisol synthesis are impaired but corticosterone and deoxycorticosterone production is increased (because of excessive ACTH).

2.  Clinically, there is hypertension and hypokalemic metabolic alkalosis – elevated deoxycorticosterone with suppressed plasma renin and aldosterone. In women, there is female (but infantile) external genitalia because decreased androgen production results in decreased estrogen synthesis. In men, genitalia are usually ambiguous (male pseudohermaphroditism).

## 3β-Hydroxysteroid Dehydrogenase Deficiency

A disorder usually seen in early infancy; inadequate androgens result in male sexual ambiguity; in females, there may be sufficient ACTH-stimulated dehydroepiandrosterone for some of its conversion to testosterone to result in 'mild masculinization'.

## Cholesterol Side-Chain Cleavage Enzyme Deficiency

A rare neonatal disorder; there is female external genitalia in both sexes; it is fatal unless diagnosed early.

# 16

# PRIMARY HYPERALDOSTERONISM

General Considerations
General Screening
Diagnostic Confirmation
Identification of Subtype

## GENERAL CONSIDERATIONS

1. Accounts for less than 2% of the identified hypertensive population.

2. The clinical syndrome is that of hypertension (may be severe but rarely malignant) and hypokalemia.

3. Because the hypertension is 'volume dependent' and atrial natriuretic hormone (ANH) is elaborated in response to it, edema is rare.

4. Manifestations of hypokalemia include metabolic alkalosis (also a primary effect of excess aldosterone), impaired glucose tolerance and associated muscle weakness and cramping, polydipsia, polyuria and nocturia.

5. There are five identifiable subtypes – the issue being not merely academic because the genetics and therapy are different depending on etiology:

   a. Aldosterone-producing adenoma,

   b. Aldosterone-producing carcinoma,

   c. Bilateral adrenal hyperplasia,

   d. Unilateral adrenal hyperplasia, and

   e. Glucocorticoid suppressible hyperaldosteronism.

6. In addition to primary hyperaldosteronism, there are other causes of adrenal hypertension.

   a. Syndromes in which deoxycorticosterone is the major mineralocorticoid include enzymatic defects in cortisol synthesis (17α-hydroxylase deficiency and 11β-hydroxylase deficiency) as well as in carcinoma of the adrenal gland or adrenal hyperstimulation in ectopic ACTH syndromes.

   b. Recently understood are the rare disorders of 11β-hydroxysteroid dehydrogenase deficiency in which congenitally or acquired (e.g. licorice and its active alkaloid, glycyrrhetinic acid; carbenoxolone – an anti-ulcer drug) inhibition of the enzyme results in impaired cortisol conversion to cortisone. Cortisol (prevented from local conversion to cortisone) is more tenaciously bound to mineralocorticoid type I receptors and thus is able to exhibit a significant mineralocorticoid effect.

c. A syndrome first described by Grant Liddle and originally felt to be secondary to overproduction of a non-aldosterone glucocorticoid, resulting in a clinical syndrome similar to that of primary hyperaldosteronism. It is now believed to be caused by enhanced distal tubule sodium reabsorption (hence its clinical response to potassium-sparing diuretics).

7. The clinical approach is in three phases: general screening, diagnostic confirmation, and identification of subtype.

## GENERAL SCREENING

1. Do not screen all hypertensives for hyperaldosteronism; it is wasteful and inappropriate. Only screen hypertensives who have spontaneous or easily induced (e.g. diuretic) hypokalemia.

2. If the patient has spontaneous hypokalemia, do a 24-hour urine for potassium and an upright plasma renin and plasma aldosterone level (the patient must be on a diet of at least 100 mEq of sodium/day). Look for kaliuresis greater than 30 mEq/day with a suppressed plasma renin (less than 3 ng/ml/h) or an increased aldosterone : renin ratio (greater than 20–25 when aldosterone is expressed as ng/dl and renin is expressed as ng/ml/h).

3. If the patient is on a diuretic, demonstration of an inappropriately suppressed upright plasma renin in the presence of an increased aldosterone : renin ratio is still a useful screening test. The patient need not stop the diuretic, but the urine potassium level is not going to be of value.

4. If the diuretic can be safely discontinued, the patient should be given oral potassium replenishment and an added salt diet. If the serum potassium corrects after 2 weeks, primary hyperaldosteronism is unlikely.

5. An alternative test is the administration of 25–50 mg of captopril (this can be done on an outpatient basis) and demonstrating persistence of an elevated plasma aldosterone : renin ratio greater than 50 or a plasma aldosterone value greater than 15 ng/dl, 60–120 minutes after drug administration.

## DIAGNOSTIC CONFIRMATION

1. Whereas initial screening is to see if the renin–angiotensin–aldosterone axis could be activated by physiologic stimulation, the rationale of diagnostic confirmation is to demonstrate failure of axis suppression.

2. If possible, the patient should be off antihypertensive therapy. If not, the following drugs, used in moderation, will probably not adversely affect the results: prazosin, terazosin, doxazosin, guanadrel and guanethidine.

3. The suppression test is effected by a sodium challenge. Normal saline, 2 liters, intravenously over 4 hours is administered to a recumbent patient after an overnight fast. A plasma aldosterone greater than 10 ng/dl is highly likely to be indicative of primary hyperaldosteronism. If less than 5 ng/dl, the diagnosis is unlikely.

4. Alternatively, a high salt diet (greater than 200 mEq of sodium daily) for 3 days (with KCl supplementation) can be used. If urine sodium is greater than 200 mEq/day but urine aldosterone is greater than 10–14 µg, the diagnosis of primary hyperaldosteronism is highly likely.

5. Urine free cortisol may be obtained if glucocorticoid excess is felt to be a possibility.

## IDENTIFICATION OF SUBTYPE (Table 16-1)

1. Aldosterone-Producing Adenoma – this comprises about 60% of cases of primary hyperaldosteronism.

   a. Statistically, these patients tend to be younger and have higher aldosterone levels and as a result have generally more severe hypertension, hypokalemia and inappropriate kalliuresis.

## TABLE 16-1.  SUBTYPES OF PRIMARY HYPERALDOSTERONISM

Aldosterone-Producing Adenoma
Aldosterone-Producing Carcinoma
Bilateral Adrenal Hyperplasia
Unilateral Adrenal Hyperplasia
Glucocorticoid Suppressible Hyperaldosteronism

b.  When changing from a recumbent to upright posture, plasma renin and aldosterone levels do not change – indeed, aldosterone levels may paradoxically decrease. The patients also tend to have higher 18-hydroxycorticosterone levels than those with bilateral adrenal hyperplasia.

c.  CT is necessary for anatomic delineation. MRI or iodo-cholesterol isotopic study may be of supplementary value. In addition, selective adrenal vein sampling may be necessary. To allow for episodic ACTH stimulation of the adrenal glands, intravenous Cortrosyn is continuously infused and aldosterone : cortisol ratios, on both sides, evaluated and compared.

d.  Hypertension (as well as the associated electrolyte imbalance) is usually cured by surgical extirpation. Adrenal carcinoma, if removed intact, could have the same favorable response. Further, the remaining contralateral adrenal gland can assume all normal adrenal function.

e.  If an aldosterone-producing adrenal carcinoma is not cured with surgery, additional therapies will be required. These include potassium-sparing agents (spironolactone and potassium-sparing diuretics), adrenolytic agents (e.g. o'p'-DDD (Mitotane, Lysodren)) and other antineoplastic agents and adrenal enzyme inhibitors (e.g. ketoconazole).

f.  A spironolactone trial may be a helpful clue as to etiology since it will usually cure the hypertension without changing urinary aldosterone excretion in both aldosterone-producing adenoma and unilateral hyperplasia. Indeed, from a functional and therapeutic point of view, unilateral hyperplasia can be treated like an adenoma.

2.  Bilateral Adrenal Hyperplasia – this comprises nearly 40% of cases of primary hyperaldosteronism.

a.  Etiology is unknown, but there may be excessive production of a pituitary intermediary lobe trophic hormone.

b.  Syndrome is generally less severe than that of an aldosterone-producing adenoma.

c.  Bilateral adrenalectomy is not only generally ineffective but also renders the patient Addisonian.

d. Spironolactone will correct the aldosterone-mediated electrolyte imbalance but will generally not correct the hypertension. It may also have significant estrogenic side-effects (especially in males). Amiloride and triamterene are also effective (and avoid the estrogenic side-effects). Additional secondary agents include angiotensin-converting enzyme inhibitors, nifedipine and hydrochlorthiazide.

e. A rare subset of patients are glucocorticoid suppressible. They produce excessive abnormal steroids (18-oxocortisol and 18-hydroxycortisol) in addition to aldosterone. The disease is autosomal dominant, has been associated with a mutation on chromosome 8 and may be related to the persistence of fetal 'hybrid' cortical cells.

# 17

# PHEOCHROMOCYTOMA

**General Considerations**
**Clinical Presentation**
**Diagnostic Work-up**
**Therapy**

## GENERAL CONSIDERATIONS

1. Accounts for less than 0.1% of the identified hypertensive population.

2. It is talked about far more often than clinically seen. Yet, most cases of pheochromocytoma are serendipitously found at post-mortem examination. Indeed, the name is Greek for its gross description (dusky-colored tumor).

3. Equal prevalence in both sexes (third to fifth decades).

4. The 'Rule of Tens' – the 'approximate' likelihood of associated presentations.

   10% – Familial
   10% – Children
   10% – Multiple
   10% – Bilateral
   10% – Malignant
   10% – Recur after Surgical Extirpation
   10% – Extra-adrenal

5. Differential diagnosis includes endocrine (e.g. hypoglycemia, estrogen withdrawal, thyrotoxicosis), cardiac (other causes of hypertension and tachycardia) and neuropsychiatric disease.

## CLINICAL PRESENTATION (Table 17-1)

1. Hypertension

   a. May be sustained or paroxysmal.

### TABLE 17-1.    CLINICAL PRESENTATION OF PHEOCHROMOCYTOMA

Hypertension
Cardiac Manifestations
Metabolic Aspects
Neuropsychiatric Aspects
Association With Multiple Endocrine Neoplasia Syndromes
Association With Other Syndromes
Renal Artery Stenosis
Cholelithiasis

b.  May be spontaneous or precipitated by diagnostic procedures, drugs (e.g. opiates, histamine), emotional or physiologic stress or increased intra-abdominal pressure. In the very rare instances of a bladder wall pheochromocytoma, micturition may be a provocateur.

c.  May occur in the setting of the '5-Ps': Pressure (hypertension), Pain (headache), Perspiration (diaphoresis), Pallor (intense vasoconstriction), Palpitations (tachyarrhythmias).

d.  Episodes are of variable duration (minutes to hours).

e.  Orthostatic hypotension may be an accompaniment because of loss of the physiologic response to peripheral pooling of blood in the context of a patient who is already maximally vasoconstricted and hypovolemic.

2.  Cardiac Manifestations

a.  Tachycardia and arrhythmias.

b.  Symptomatic coronary insufficiency.

c.  Cardiomyopathy.

3.  Metabolic Aspects

a.  Hypermetabolism, hyperthermia, weight loss.

b.  Tendency to glucose intolerance (increased glucose production, decreased insulin release).

c.  May have symptoms related to other accompanying endocrinopathies (e.g. hypercalcemia, watery diarrhea with hypokalemia).

d.  Relative polycythemia.

4.  Neuropsychiatric Aspects

a.  Anxiety, tremulousness, fear of impending doom, headache.

b.  Manifestations mimic that which normal individuals would perceive in extreme 'fright or flight' (piloerection, however, does not occur; although this process is dispatched through the sympathetic nervous system, acetylcholine is the effector neurotransmitter).

5. Associated Clinical Entities

   a. Multiple Endocrine Neoplasia Type II a – (also known as Sipple's Syndrome): pheochromocytoma, hyperpara-thyroidism and medullary carcinoma of the thyroid.

   b. Multiple Endocrine Neoplasia Type II b – pheochromocytoma with increased tendency to bilaterality, medullary carcinoma of the thyroid, mucosal neuromas, Marfanoid habitus, intestinal ganglioneuromatosis and thickened corneal nerves.

   c. Von Hippel–Lindau Disease – cerebellar hemangioblastoma and retinal angiomata.

   d. Von Recklinghausen's Disease (neurofibromatosis).

   e. Sturge–Weber Syndrome.

   f. Ataxia Telangiectasia.

   g. Tuberous Sclerosis.

   h. Carney's Triad – gastric leiomyosarcoma, pulmonary chondroma, extra-adrenal pheochromocytoma.

   i. Renal Artery Stenosis – may contribute to ambiguity of the etiology of the hypertension.

   j. Cholelithiasis.

## DIAGNOSTIC WORK-UP

1. General Considerations

   a. Catecholamines are synthesized *de novo* as follows: (Figure 17-1):

      Phenylalanine → Tyrosine → DOPA → Dopamine → Norepinephrine

      (Phenylethanolamine *n*-methyl transferase, an enzyme enriched by high cortisol levels, catalyzes the conversion of norepinephrine to epinephrine)

   b. There are four mechanisms by which catecholamines are disposed:

      i. Neuronal reuptake,

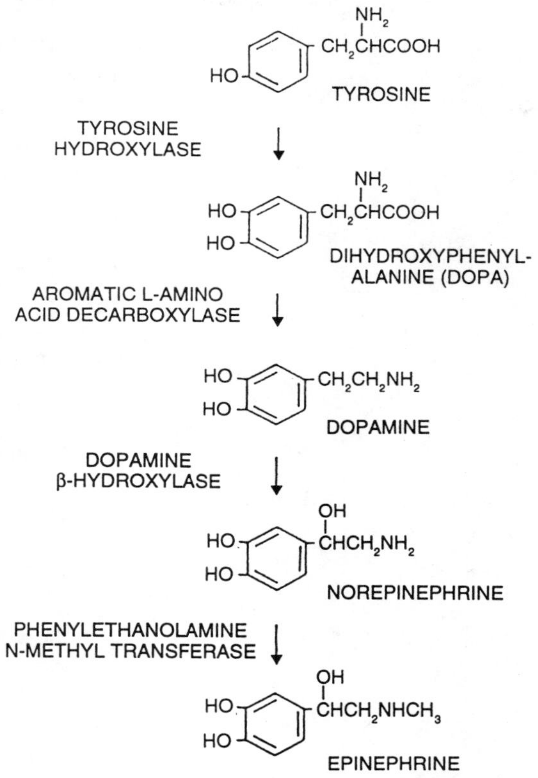

NH$_2$
|
CH$_2$CHCOOH

HO —

TYROSINE

TYROSINE
HYDROXYLASE

NH$_2$
|
CH$_2$CHCOOH

HO —
HO —

DIHYDROXYPHENYL-
ALANINE (DOPA)

AROMATIC L-AMINO
ACID DECARBOXYLASE

HO —
HO —  CH$_2$CH$_2$NH$_2$

DOPAMINE

DOPAMINE
β-HYDROXYLASE

OH
|
HO —  CHCH$_2$NH$_2$
HO —

NOREPINEPHRINE

PHENYLETHANOLAMINE
N-METHYL TRANSFERASE

OH
|
HO —  CHCH$_2$NHCH$_3$
HO —

EPINEPHRINE

**Figure 17-1.** Catecholamine biosynthesis. Reproduced with kind permission from *Endocrinology and Metabolism,* 2nd edn., Felig, P., Baxter, J.D., Broadus, A.E. and Frohman, L.A. (eds.), New York: McGraw-Hill Book Company, p.653

    ii. Unchanged excretion in the urine,

    iii. Degradation by monoamine oxidase – production of dihydroxymandelic acid, and

    iv. Degradation by catecholamine ortho-methyl transferase – production of metanephrine and normetanephrine

  c. When the last two mechanisms are operant, the end product is 3-methoxy, 4-hydroxy-mandelic acid, commonly known as VMA (Figure 17-2).

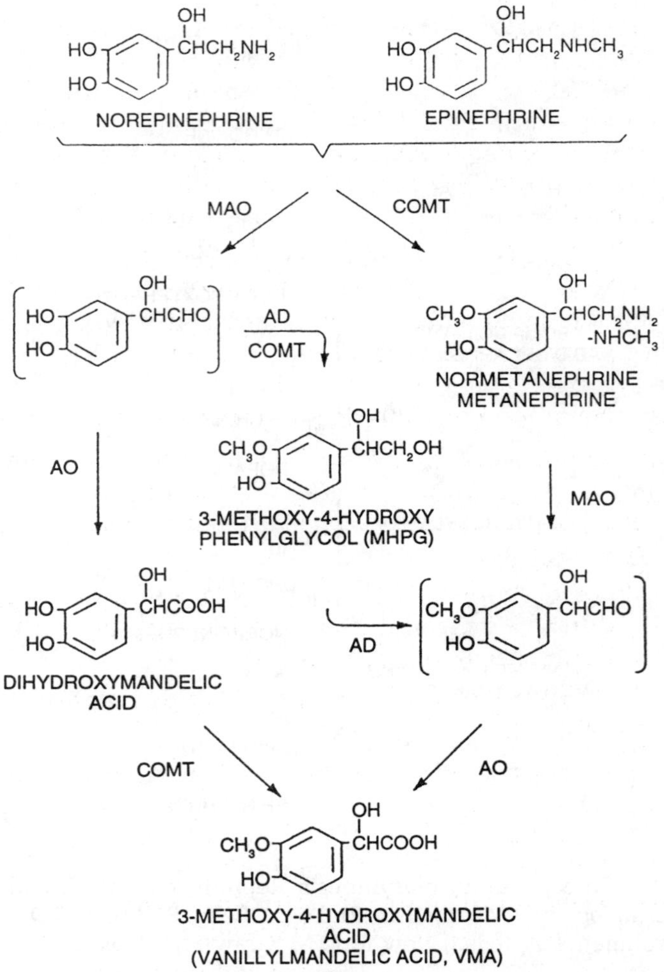

**Figure 17-2.** Catecholamine Degradation: MAO, Monoamine oxidase; COMT, catecholamine ortho-methyl transferase; AD, alcohol dehydrogenase; AO, aldehyde oxidase. Reproduced with kind permission from *Endocrinology and Metabolism,* 2nd edn., Felig, P., Baxter, J.D., Broadus, A.E. and Frohman, L.A. (eds.), New York: McGraw-Hill Book Company, p. 654

2. Chemical Analysis

   a. Urinary metabolites – urinary metanephrines and free catecholamines are the most sensitive tests (close to 100%), but the specificity is less. While values for 24-hour collections in pheochromocytoma are generally and substantially elevated (often greater than twice normal) in sustained hypertension, values may be normal in the setting of hypertension occurring only in paroxysms. In such cases, a shorter urine collection that encompasses the period of time of the paroxysm (with comparison with the urine creatinine in that same specimen) can be very helpful.

Be mindful of the assay procedures used by your laboratory, as false positives and negatives occur and vary according to laboratory methodology. Newer tests using high-pressure liquid chromatography, radioimmunoassay, and radioenzymatic assays avoid many of the pitfalls incumbent in the older assays which use colorimetric or fluorimetric procedures.

    i. Common causes of false–positive VMA, metanephrines and free catecholamines: amphetamines, labetalol, ethanol, major stress, α-methyl DOPA, and clonidine (or related drug) withdrawal.

    ii. Common causes of false-negative VMA, metanephrines and free catecholamines: reserpine, guanethidine, central α-2 agonists, and metatyrosine.

    iii. Phenothiazines and tricyclic antidepressants have a variable effect.

b. Plasma catecholamines are elevated in pheochromocytoma, but unfortunately, there is also a high frequency of false positives. However, markedly elevated values (especially during paroxysms) are meaningful. Plasma metanephrines may also be a more sensitive assay than plasma catecholamines (or urinary metanephrines).

c. Clonidine Test – rationale is the failure to suppress ectopic catecholamine production that normally would be suppressed if centrally mediated. Thus, failure of catecholamine suppression after clonidine administration supports the diagnosis.

d. Provocative (and Suppressive) Tests – (e.g. phentolamine, glucagon, histamine, tyramine and metoclopramide) – potentially dangerous and not generally recommended.

3. Tumor Localization

a. Statistical odds, clinical nuances and chemical fractionation are important clues.

b.  Computed imaging of the abdomen (MRI preferred over CT) is the preferred initial imaging procedure.

c.  Pending above results, additional studies include computed imaging of other areas of the body, meta-iodobenzylguanidine (MIBG) isotopic study (this can be selectively taken up by tumor) and selective venous sampling.

## THERAPY

1.  Surgery is the only definitive initial approach.

2.  It is imperative that patients be appropriately managed pre-operatively.

3.  α-Adrenergic blockade must be initiated first to control hypertension and to prevent paradoxical increases in blood pressure. Phenoxybenzamine is the preferred drug in initial doses of 10 mg, twice daily, with incremental increases of 10–20 mg, every 2 days as necessary. Liberalization of salt and water intake will counteract the tendency to orthostatic hypotension mediated by increased vascular capacitance. α-1 blocking agents may also be considered for long-term symptomatic treatment of metastatic disease.

4.  When blood pressure is controlled, a β-adrenergic blocking drug should be added – in theory, a non-selective β antagonist is preferred; in actuality, it does not really matter.

5.  Labetalol (combined α and β antagonism) is an 'all purpose' agent. If used as initial therapy, however, it may acutely provoke a worsening of the blood pressure.

6.  Metastatic disease is treated with symptomatic control of catecholamine excess, biochemical suppression of catecholamine synthesis (e.g. α-methyl para-tyrosine) and tumoricidal therapy.

# Section E

# DISORDERS OF GLUCOSE METABOLISM

# 18

# GLUCOSE METABOLISM: NORMAL PHYSIOLOGY AND OVERVIEW

Normal Glucose Homeostasis
Insulin
Glucagon

## NORMAL GLUCOSE HOMEOSTASIS

1. From a teleologic point of view, normalcy of the blood glucose level has to be maintained because neuronal tissue cannot acutely utilize any other alternative fuel.

   a. Obviously, this is not a problem if eating were a continuous process (assuming adequate intestinal digestion and conversion of more complex fuel sources to glucose).

   b. Since such is not the case (as certainly ancestrally in the human species when food availability was unpredictable), mechanisms had to evolve whereby glucose could be formed from endogenous sources – implicit in such an infrastructure would be mechanisms of storage in the fed state (serving as 'glucose-producing factories') and 'switches' which could activate glucose production from these storage sites and deactivate the process when glucose production was no longer necessary.

   c. Not only must there be assurance that 'too low' a glucose level never occurred but that hyperglycemia would be avoided as well.

      i. Hyperglycemia would be indicative of either a wasteful inability to store fuel or an inappropriate breakdown of storage resources – or both.

      ii. Hyperglycemia could lead to a clinical syndrome of its own.

2. One cannot talk of glucose metabolism without discussing its interrelationship with protein and fat metabolism.

   a. Overlapping pathways allow for interconversion of moieties because 'building blocks' of one component can be utilized for another.

   b. Postprandial anabolism of glucose is paralleled by the synthesis of fat and protein. Conversely, euglycemia is maintained in the postabsorptive (fasted) state by the ability of fat and protein to make products that augment glucose production.

3. In the normal postprandial state, glucose is taken up by cells and

a glycolytic sequence is activated where the glucose is converted to glucose 6-phosphate, fructose 6-phosphate, fructose 1,6-biphosphate, glyceraldehyde 3-phosphate (and dihydroxyacetone phosphate) and ultimately to pyruvic acid (Figure 18-1).

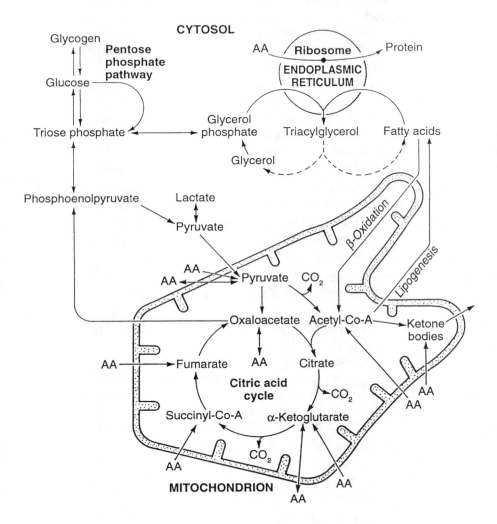

**Figure 18-1.** Overview of Metabolic Pathways: AA, amino acid; Acetyl CoA, acetyl coenzyme A. Reproduced with kind permission from *Harper's Biochemistry*, 23rd edn., Norwalk, CT: Appleton and Lange, 1993, p. 159

a.  If oxygen is available, the pyruvate can be converted to acetyl coenzyme A (acetyl CoA) which then becomes 'completely consumed' after one complete passage through the citric acid or Krebs (tricarboxylic acid; TCA) cycle. It is initially taken up by oxaloacetate to form citric acid but this ultimately 'regenerates' oxaloacetic acid after one complete revolution of the cycle. This overall process of aerobic metabolism is very 'energy giving' with one mole of glucose ultimately able to form 38 moles of ATP.

b   If oxygen is not available, the pyruvate can be converted to lactate – it is not very 'energy giving' (only 2 moles of ATP per mole of glucose) but it may still meet limited energy requirements. If the hypoxic state continues, then the energy produced may be marginal or inadequate, and the lactate generated in such excess as to result in lactic acidosis.

c.  With plentiful glucose and no bodily energy demands in excess of the calorific value of the glucose (the 'fed state'):

   i.  The glucose can be stored as glycogen – the glucose 6-phosphate is converted to glucose 1-phosphate which is then acted upon by glycogen synthetase.

   ii. Fat can be synthesized as well from products of glucose metabolism (even if no dietary fat is consumed).

      (a) The acetyl CoA can be carboxylated to form malonyl CoA (subsequent acetyl CoA moieties can be added to 'lengthen' the chain until the desired 16, 18, etc. carbon lengths are achieved). (This process initially requires production within the mitochondria of citric acid from oxaloacetate and acetyl CoA; after the formed citric acid leaves the mitochondria, it can be cleaved back to its respective components.)

      (b) Ample energy is available from glycolysis to achieve this process - it has already been noted that any acetyl CoA directed through the TCA cycle will ultimately generate 38 ATP per mole from its precursor glucose.

      (c) Glyceraldehyde 3-phosphate, an above noted component of glycolysis, serves as the 'backbone' onto which fatty acids can attach (via glycerol phosphate acyltransferase) to form triglycerides.

(d) Cholesterol synthesis is also enhanced by the conversion of acetyl CoA to 3-hydroxy-3-methyl-glutaryl (HMG) CoA and the activation of HMG CoA reductase to produce mevalonic acid, the next step.

  iii. Amino acids can be synthesized because of the following (unlike the synthesis of fats from glucose, however, an amino group must be available):

(a) The available energy from glycolysis,

(b) The availability of pyruvate (as the corresponding keto-acid to several amino acids, especially alanine), and

(c) The availability of other keto acids (e.g. oxaloacetate, α-ketoglutarate) to form their corresponding amino acids.

4. When glucose is not plentiful, however, (the postabsorptive or fasted state) and glucose must be endogenously formed to normalize the circulating glucose concentration (a process known as gluconeogenesis), the following sequences occur (Figure 18-2).

a. Glycogen is broken down from its storage sources.

  i. There are limits to the amount of glucose to be generated in this fashion – only 100 g of glycogen are stored in the liver and less than 1000 g in skeletal muscle (even in a physically well-developed individual).

  ii. The production of glucose is facilitated by a parallel decrease in the synthesis of glycogen.

b. Fat synthesis is curtailed and replaced by catabolism – glycerol can be 'recycled' as a substrate to generate glucose.

c. Amino acids are catabolized and the corresponding keto acids that enter the glycolytic and TCA cycles are available for 'reversal' and 'recycling' – this process of gluconeogenesis is augmented by the 'switching off' of enzymes that favor forward glycolysis and aerobic metabolism and the 'switching on' of 'reverse enzymes'.

  i. Pyruvate carboxylase 'shunts' pyruvate directly into oxaloacetate – by preventing acetyl CoA formation from pyruvate, lipogenesis is curtailed.

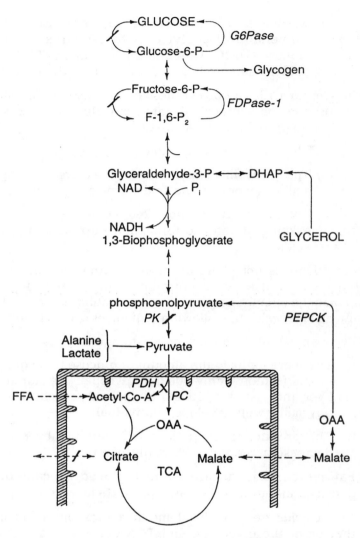

**Figure 18-2.** Regulatory Steps in Hepatic Gluconeogenesis under the Conditions of Fasting and Insulin Deficiency: P, phosphate; G6Pase, glucose-6-phosphatase; FDPase, fructose bisphosphatase; DHAP, dihydroxy acetone phosphate; PK, pyruvate kinase; PEPCK, phosphoenolpyruvate-carboxykinase; PDH, pyruvate dehydrogenase; PC, pyruvate carboxylase; OAA, oxaloacetic acid; FFA, free fatty acids; TCA, tricarboxylic acid. Reproduced with kind permission from *Endocrinology and Metabolism*, 2nd edn., Felig, P., Baxter, J.D., Broadus, A.E. and Frohman, L.A. (eds.), McGraw-Hill Book Company

    ii.  Phosphoenolpyruvate carboxykinase converts oxaloacetate to the precursor of pyruvate, phosphoenol pyruvate.

    iii. Fructose 1-6-bisphosphatase and glucose 6-phosphatase are the 'reversal counterparts' to glucokinase and phosphofructokinase and thus move the reaction in a reverse fashion to the direction of glucose synthesis.

  d.  While striated muscle cannot reverse the process all the way back to glucose (it lacks glucose-6-phosphatase), any lactate generated on route can be taken up by the liver (which has glucose 6-phosphatase), and there, it can be converted to glucose (Cori Cycle). Alternatively, as muscle has aminotransferases, alanine can be synthesized from pyruvate within the muscle and then released into the circulation where the liver can take it up and convert it to glucose through gluconeogenesis.

5.  That this process succeeds so elegantly is a a tribute to the role of regulatory hormones. A corollary is that hormonal dysfunction can result in serious derangement of the process.

## INSULIN

1.  Made by specialized pancreatic $\beta$ cells (directed by a gene on the short arm of chromosome 11) – initially made as a preproinsulin (analogous to other protein hormones such as growth hormone and parathyroid hormone). Proinsulin consists of the two-chain insulin product (A chain of 21 amino acids and B chain of 30 amino acids) connected in a 'number 9' configuration by a 35-amino acid peptide – 31 of those amino acids ultimately form the C-peptide which is released into the circulation (along with two dipeptides) whenever insulin is released.

2.  The two chains of insulin are connected by two disulfide linkages (the A chain also has one 'intra-chain' disulfide linkage) at cysteine sites.

3.  Insulin release is a calcium-dependent process. Although glucose is the most significant secretagogue, insulin is also stimulated by direct vagal stimulation, leucine and sulfonylurea oral

hypoglycemic agents (hence, the therapeutic value of the latter). Release is augmented by gastrointestinal hormones (e.g. gastric inhibitory polypeptide, GIP), arginine, and β-adrenergic stimulation. Release is diminished by β-adrenergic blockade, α-adrenergic stimulation and somatostatin. Certain drugs can decrease stimulation (e.g. diazoxide – it is used therapeutically when this effect is desired; dilantin; pentamidine – this initially enhances release, then it is β-destructive).

4. Insulin acts on a specific two-component receptor site setting off a sequence of post-receptor 'messenger' responses (although several 'second messengers' are purported including diacylglycerol, cyclic AMP is not one of them and is actually inhibited by insulin). Receptor activity is enhanced by fasting, exercise and hypoinsulinemic states – conversely, eating, a sedentary state, obesity and hyperinsulinemia decrease insulin receptivity.

   a. The propensity for Type II diabetes mellitus (or at least its clinical expression) may be explained by decreased insulin receptivity.

   b. Altered receptivity is usually 'postreceptor'.

5. Insulin in the most anabolic hormone and promotes glycogen synthesis (liver and muscle), protein synthesis (liver and muscle) and fat synthesis (adipose tissue and liver – this helps explain the fatty liver of overeating and obesity).

6. Insulin acts by stimulating specific enzymes – glucokinase and phosphofructokinase (this results in fructose 1,6-bisphosphate production – insulin promotes this by increasing the amount of fructose 2,6-bisphosphate through enhanced synthesis and diminished degradation).

7. Insulin also stimulates pyruvate kinase and 'diverts' acetyl CoA to fat synthesis by stimulating citrate 'cleavage enzyme' and acetyl CoA carboxylase.

8. Conversely, the gluconeogenic enzymes of pyruvate carboxylase, phosphoenolpyruvate-carboxykinase, fructose 1,6-bisphosphatase and glucose 6-phosphatase are inhibited in the presence of insulin.

## GLUCAGON

1.  Like insulin, it is derived from a larger precursor protein molecule – glucagon is a single 29-amino acid polypeptide chain (the directing gene is on chromosome 2).

2.  A wide range of provocateurs stimulate glucagon – amino acids, many gastrointestinal hormones and catecholamines. Hypoglycemia is a very important stimulant of glucagon. Conversely, hyperglycemia is a suppressant (somatostatin suppresses as well).

3.  The actions of glucagon and insulin are antagonistic.

    a.  Although there are many shared enzyme systems in which insulin and glucagon are operant, direction of the path of reaction is dependent on the glucagon–insulin balance. The phosphorylation by glucagon or the dephosphorylation by insulin of shared enzymes are crucial to enzymatic activity and thus to the direction of reaction.

    b.  The anatomic juxtaposition of α and β cells in islet tissue allows for additional facets of the insulin–glucagon relationship. Insulin is locally inhibitory to α cell function.

        i.  Somatostatin (a 14-amino acid peptide made from a larger precursor molecule and produced in D cells of islet tissue) is inhibitory to both α and β cells and is also anatomically close to both. Somatostatin is stimulated by the same provocateurs that stimulate insulin release and is also the same hypothalamic peptide that inhibits growth hormone (HGH) production.

        ii.  Pancreatic peptide, made by a fourth cell type, the F cell (located mainly in the posterior lobe of the head of the pancreas) is not operant in glucose homeostasis. Major physiologic actions are to decrease pancreatic protein and bicarbonate secretion and to decrease hepatic bile secretion and gall bladder contraction.

4.  Glucagon promotes catabolism – those enzymatic systems which are catabolic are activated and those which are anabolic are inhibited. (The actions of glucagon are felt to be directed solely at hepatic tissue.)

a. Glycogen is broken down to glucose by activation of phosphorylase b (which activates phosphorylase a) ultimately leading to a sequence of events that leads to glucose 1-phosphate which can then be converted to glucose 6-phosphate.

b. Activation of glucose-6-phosphatase to act on glucose-6-phosphate produces glucose.

c. Glucose-6-phosphate is also generated by 'reversal' of the glycolytic scheme. Pyruvate is diverted from formation of acetyl CoA to form oxaloacetic acid (by action of pyruvate carboxylase). The oxaloacetic acid can be shunted to phosphoenolpyruvate, the step before pyruvate, by phosphoenolpyruvate-carboxykinase. Fructose 1,6-bisphosphate generation can be reversed by activation of a phosphatase.

d. Lipid synthesis is reversed. Although acetyl CoA generation from pyruvate is decreased, acetyl CoA is amply generated from lipolysis. Glucagon further inhibits lipogenesis by inhibiting acetyl CoA carboxylase.

   i. The resultant decrease in malonic acid (as malonyl CoA) allows fatty acids to be converted to ketone bodies by creating a 'transport bridge' across the mitochondrial membrane where ketogenesis occurs. The enzyme operant in this is carnitine palmitotransferase I, which is activated when malonic acid decreases.

   ii. Ketone production (acetoacetate and $\beta$-hydroxybutyrate) is also enhanced by glucagon-mediated synthesis of carnitine (this is the actual 'carrier' of fatty acids to the mitochondria where ketones are generated).

# 19

# HYPOGLYCEMIA

**General Considerations**
**The Two Major Divisions of Hypoglycemia**

## GENERAL CONSIDERATIONS

1. Hypoglycemia occurs when any of the previously discussed components (substrate or hormone), single or multiple, fail in their responsibility to maintain an adequate circulating concentration of blood glucose.

2. Although the role of glucagon was discussed in depth and glucagon is the most critical counterregulatory hormone, there are other counterregulatory hormones:

    a. Growth hormone (HGH) – activates lipolysis and antagonizes the peripheral effect of insulin.

    b. ACTH – acting directly, it is lipolytic; through adrenal stimulation, it generates cortisol which is catabolic, gluconeogenic and lipolytic (at responsive adipose sites).

    c. Catecholamines – very important counterregulatory hormones; glycogenolytic and lipolytic; the $\alpha$-adrenergic effect is stimulatory to glucagon and inhibitory to insulin.

3. The clinical syndrome of hypoglycemia has two physiologic effects (Table 19-1).

### TABLE 19-1. THE CLINICAL SYNDROME OF HYPOGLYCEMIA

Sympathetic Nervous System Activation
      Tachycardia
      Hypertension
      Tremulousness
      Anxiety
      'Cold' Diaphoresis

Neuroglycopenic Manifestations
      Mental Status Changes
      Behavioral Abnormalities
      Altered Consciousness
      Focal Deficits
      Coma
      Death

a.  Sympathetic Nervous System Effect – includes elaboration of catecholamines with resultant tachycardia, hypertension, tremulousness and anxiety ('flight and fight' response). Sympathetic nervous system activation of cholinergic effectors also produces diaphoresis (but it is 'cold' because of associated vasoconstriction) and pilo-erection.

b.  Neuroglycopenic Effect – manifest because of vulnerability of the nervous system to lack of glucose. There is a wide spectrum of clinical manifestations depending upon presence of any underlying central nervous system (CNS) disease (e.g. atherosclerosis), magnitude and abruptness of fall in blood glucose and absolute level of severity. The clinical scenario can range from alteration in alertness and mental concentration to focal neurologic defects, coma and death. The duration of hypoglycemia is an important determinant of irreversibility.

c.  The catecholamine response can be attenuated.

    i.   β-blocking agents may diminish the clinical response to hypoglycemia that is produced by heightened adrenergic activity (this can occur even with 'cardioselective' agents). On the other hand, by inhibiting β-adrenergic-mediated stimulation of pancreatic β cells, β blocking agents can also decrease the tendency to hypoglycemia insofar as the hypoglycemia is mediated through endogenous insulin production. Caffeine, conversely, can augment the catecholamine mediated manifestations of hypoglycemia, for any given level of blood sugar.

    ii.  In tightly controlled diabetes mellitus, the adrenergic response to hypoglycemia is less intense than in less well-controlled diabetes. Curiously, as demonstrated in patients with insulinoma whose 'unawareness' of hypoglycemia abates after surgical extirpation and 'normalization' of blood glucose, hypoglycemia (as appears to be an almost inevitable consequence of tightly controlled diabetes) can induce neuroglycopenic and autonomic 'unawareness' as well as decreased hormonal counterregulatory response. The hypoglycemic episodes, themselves, may be operant in promoting this 'unawareness'.

    iii. Autonomic neuropathy (as may occur in diabetes) diminishes the sympathetic nervous system mediated catecholamine response.

## THE TWO MAJOR DIVISIONS OF HYPOGLYCEMIA

The two major divisions of hypoglycemia are based on the state of alimentation: fasting hypoglycemia and postprandial hypoglycemia

1. Fasting (Post-absorptive) Hypoglycemia (Table 19-2)

### TABLE 19-2. ETIOLOGIES OF FASTING HYPOGLYCEMIA

Major Organ System Failure
Starvation and Malnutrition
Endocrine Deficiency States
Drugs
Inborn Errors of Metabolism
Treated Diabetes Mellitus
Non-Pancreatic Tumors
Autoimmune
Islet Cell Tumors
Factitious

---

a. Major Organ System Failure

   i. Liver Disease – a combination of glycogen depletion and impairment of gluconeogenesis. Usually indicative of severe organ damage (e.g. fulminant hepatitis, hepatic coma) with loss of other hepatic functions (e.g. synthetic abilities, metabolism of bilirubin).

   ii. Severe heart failure, renal failure or septicemia.

b. Profound Starvation and Protein-Energy Malnutrition – hypoglycemia results from the loss of 'substrate reservoir' to provide 'resource fuel' for gluconeogenesis. Seen also in severe muscle wasting states.

c. Endocrine Deficiency States – ACTH, Cortisol, or HGH deficiency (loss of hormonal counterregulation). Very rarely seen in hypothyroidism.

d. Drugs

   i. Ethanol – inhibits gluconeogenesis because the obligatory metabolism of ethanol to acetaldehyde and acetyl coenzyme A 'consumes' NAD (vital for gluconeogenesis) and generates NADH. Particularly vulnerable are diabetics on hypoglycemic medication (insulin, oral hypoglycemic agents) and those with superimposed endocrine deficiency states (e.g. Addison's disease) or poor nutritional intake (glycogen depletion); hypoglycemia should always be in the differential diagnosis of the seemingly 'confused', 'inebriated' patient, even if the blood alcohol level is not very elevated.

ii. Pentamidine – β-cell toxin (initially, however, it is a stimulator).

iii. Quinine – insulin secretagogue, originally noted as a consequence of quinine treatment of malaria (although hypoglycemia can be seen in malaria not treated with quinine). Hypoglycemia has also been reported with quinine treatment of leg cramps.

iv. Ritodrine – $\beta_2$ agonist, used as a tocolytic agent.

v. Salicylates (high dose) – unclear mechanism (children are vulnerable).

vi. Disopyramide (Norpace) – unknown mechanism.

vii. Sulfonylureas – usually seen in the context of a treated diabetic whose ability to metabolize the drug is impaired by organ failure, or who is rendered hypoglycemic by the concomitant administration of drugs which prolong the metabolism of sulfonylureas.

   (a) Sulfonamides, phenylbutazone and coumadin impair hepatic sulfonylurea metabolism.

   (b) Liver disease will prolong the half-life of all sulfonylureas except chlorpropramide.

   (c) Chlorpropramide is excreted by the kidney unchanged – renal disease can severely prolong the half-life.

e. Inborn Errors of Metabolism – rare disorders most often seen in the pediatric age group. Von Gierke's Disease (glucose 6-phosphatase deficiency), gluconeogenic enzyme deficiencies (fructose 1,6-bisphosphatase, phosphoenolpyruvate carboxykinase, pyruvate carboxylase). Galactosemia and fructose 1-phosphate aldolase deficiency are disorders in which glycogenolysis is inhibited and are thus not 'pure fasting' disorders – i.e. ingestion of the offending substrate, galactose or fructose, precipitates the hypoglycemia.

f.  Treated Diabetes Mellitus

   i.   A basic problem (and this can amplify the severity of the hypoglycemia) is that gluconeogenesis is impaired if there is a hyperinsulinemic state – whether due to insulin itself or secondary to sulfonylurea stimulation. Thus, the hypoglycemic state may not readily 'right itself'.

   ii.  Diabetics are always vulnerable because their food intake has to match their anticipated insulin surges (not the other way around as exists in normals).

   iii. Factors that contribute to the vulnerability of the diabetic patient include:

      (a) Autonomic neuropathy – leading to erratic food transit time, absorption and diminished sympathetic counterregulatory response.

      (b) Visual problems – errors in dosage and mixtures.

      (c) Renal Disease – decreases insulin requirements in the insulin-dependent diabetic, as the kidney metabolizes insulin.

      (d) Variability of absorption of insulin depending on the site and regional blood flow (e.g. the effect of exercise).

      (e) Increased (albeit uncommon) incidence of other endocrine deficiency states in Type I Diabetes Mellitus (e.g. Schmidt's Syndrome).

g.  Non-Pancreatic Tumors

   i.   Associated with a wide range of tumors – most common are mesenchymal (e.g. fibrosarcoma, mesothelioma) with abdominal and retroperitoneal predominance (less commonly located in the chest); other tumors known to be associated with this syndrome include hepatocellular carcinoma, carcinoid and adrenocortical carcinoma.

ii. Mechanisms appear to be increased glucose consumption and elaboration of insulin-like growth factor (IGF-II). These two mechanisms are not mutually exclusive as IGF-II acts to increase peripheral utilization of glucose. It is also inhibitory to HGH. Variability of the IGF-II molecule renders its assay unreliable.

h. Autoimmune-Mediated Hypoglycemia – may be mediated by an antibody to insulin or the insulin receptor; may be associated with acanthosis nigricans and androgenic features (depending on the predominance of the 'blocking' or 'stimulating' effect of the antibody on the insulin receptor, this syndrome can also be associated with diabetes mellitus).

i. Islet Cell Tumor of the Pancreas

   i. May be an isolated tumor or as a part of Multiple Endocrine Neoplasia Type I syndrome (10% are malignant, but the clinical course and not the histology is the best determinant of malignancy).

   ii. Because the course is generally insidious and rather chronic, the neuroglycopenic (as opposed to the sympathetic) symptoms predominate. Thus, psychiatric manifestations (at times even leading to psychiatric referral and treatment) and neurologic features (e.g. seizures, syncope, transient ischemic attack) may be the mode of clinical presentation.

   iii. Symptoms are made worse by exercise and food abstinence (patients, however, tend to have excessive hunger and a particular craving for sweets and there is a tendency to weight gain as a result).

   iv. The inappropriateness of persistent hyperinsulinemia in the presence of hypoglycemia may be explained by an abnormal glucose transporter protein. Because of its low $K_m$, that protein requires a lesser concentration of glucose for activation of insulin synthesis.

   v. Although stimulation tests using leucine, glucagon and tolbutamide have been used, the prolonged fast with determination of the glucose : insulin ratio remains the best test (the 72-hour fast is a 'gold standard' but such a protracted fast is rarely necessary – and may be poorly tolerated).

vi. Curiously, the oral glucose tolerance test is not a good screening test – it is not only not 'flat' but because insulinoma tissue is associated with decreased insulin reserve, it is less responsive to glucose than normal islet tissue. In addition, normal islet tissue is suppressed in insulinoma and the oral glucose tolerance test curve is often 'diabetic'.

vii. Proinsulin and C-peptide measurements may be helpful. They are inappropriately elevated in insulinoma.

viii. Because many tumors are small and 14% are multiple (nesidioblastosis, or diffuse foci of islet cell tissue, is rare, except when part of Multiple Endocrine Neoplasia Type I syndrome), MRI, CT and ultrasound are often not helpful – angiography remains a useful diagnostic procedure.

ix. Surgery is the therapy of choice – at times, distal pancreatectomy must be performed.

    (a) Depending on surgical success, and even as a general part of preoperative management, adjunctive therapy (e.g. glucose infusion, diazoxide) is necessary.

    (b) Carcinoma may be additionally responsive to glucagon, dilantin, streptozotocin, octreotide, diazoxide and verapamil.

2. Reactive Hypoglycemia (Table 19-3)

a. Untreated Diabetes Mellitus – occurs late after eating and is related to the 'dysinsulinism' of diabetes (caused by a delayed insulin release produced when the hyperglycemia is waning). Associated with obesity and a family history of diabetes.

**TABLE 19-3. ETIOLOGIES OF REACTIVE HYPOGLYCEMIA**

Untreated Diabetes Mellitus
Alimentary Hypoglycemia
'Functional' Hypoglycemia
Factitious Hypoglycemia

b. Alimentary Hypoglycemia – associated with a structural process (e.g. postpeptic ulcer surgery) or with physiologic 'overshoot' (in response to a glucose load). Usually occurs within 1–2 hours of eating. Symptoms are primarily autonomic (as opposed to neuroglycopenic). The mechanism appears to be augmentation by gastrointestinal hormones of an exaggerated insulin response.

c. 'Functional' Hypoglycemia – so named because of autonomic symptoms associated with hypoglycemia but without clear-cut documentation.

   i. At times, there is a disparity between the nadir of blood glucose and symptoms, even though an oral glucose tolerance test may show some 'low readings'. (A 'mixed' meal often does not reveal hypoglycemia.)

   ii. Otherwise normal people can be asymptomatic with a low blood glucose level (e.g. normal women after a fast).

   iii. Patients with 'functional' hypoglycemia often have associated problems of 'somatization' – e.g. fatigue, headache, irritability.

   iv. Nonetheless, it is arrogant and condescending to dismiss these patients' symptoms without being supportive and understanding. Little is known about intracellular glucose (and associated metabolite) concentrations in these situations. If a 'hypoglycemic diet' (frequent small feedings; avoidance of simple sugars) is of benefit, there is no harm in recommending it as long as the patient is not 'labelled' with an inappropriate diagnosis.

3. Factitious Hypoglycemia

   a. Can occur as a 'postabsorptive' or 'reactive' phenomenon – the 'randomness' of hypoglycemia may be a clue.

   b. Often difficult to diagnose as patients may resort to elaborate schemes. Disproportionately seen in health-care workers.

   c. Insulin antibodies may be positive from repeated injections, even if human insulin is used (it is not a helpful test in a diabetic previously treated with insulin).

   d. C peptide is suppressed with exogenous insulin (but not if oral agents are used); oral agents may be measured directly in serum or urine.

# 20

# DIABETES MELLITUS

## GENERAL CONSIDERATIONS

1. Defined as the clinical syndrome of hyperglycemia secondary to a deficiency of, or resistance to insulin. For empiric categorization, it is diagnosed by a fasting plasma glucose concentration greater than 140 mg/dl on at least two separate occasions. If an oral glucose tolerance test is used, the plasma glucose has to be greater than 200 mg/dl at 2 hours and at least one other time during the test. (A minimum of 150 g/day of carbohydrate must be taken for the 3 days prior to the test.)

2. Impaired glucose tolerance is defined as a 2-hour plasma glucose value less than 200 mg/dl but with a value between 0 and 2 hours greater than 200 mg/dl.

3. The plasma glucose (rather than whole blood glucose) value is used because it is better standardized (not subject to changes in hematocrit) and it lends itself to analysis by the automatic analyzer. Blood glucose values (because of the admixture of cellular elements) would be 10–15% lower – this relationship has to be appreciated in light of the frequent use of finger stick glucose determinations.

4. Diabetes Mellitus is empirically classified according to etiology:

   a. Type I ('Insulin-Dependent'),

   b. Type II ('Non-Insulin-Dependent'),

   c. Impaired Glucose Tolerance,

   d. Gestational Diabetes,

   e. Secondary Etiologies

      i. Secondary etiologies are capable of producing the same type of diabetic syndromes that are seen with primary etiologies.

      ii. Additional manifestations will depend on other features of the secondary cause (e.g. hemochromatosis, chronic pancreatitis), whether glucagon is present or absent (e.g. in pancreatectomized patients, the diabetic state is easier to control but more subject to hypoglycemia), and the potentially reversible nature if drug-induced (e.g. thiazide diuretics, glucocorticoids, β-adrenergic blockade).

## TYPE I DIABETES MELLITUS

1. Etiologic in 10–15% of all diabetics (about 20 000 new cases per year in the USA; more frequent in whites than blacks); associated with well-defined genetic markers of the major histocompatibility complex (genetically directed within the short arm of chromosome 6). Class II antigen associations are DR3 and DR4 (DR2 is 'protective'); class I antigens include B8, B15, and B18. The proximity to immune response genes is felt to be the basis for such linkage.

   a. Having genetic linkage represents increased risk but additional factor(s) have to be operant, because the concordance rate for Type I diabetes mellitus in identical twins is only 50%. Such factors may be viral (e.g. mumps, cytomegalovirus, coxsackie-viruses B4 and B5, etc.), environmental 'toxins' and allergens (e.g. bovine albumin in cow's milk).

   b. Type I diabetes is associated with antibodies to insulin, islet cells and glutamic acid decarboxylase (GAD). The latter can be an early predictive marker of the diabetes. The corresponding pathology is islet cell inflammation and ultimate destruction.

   c. It is possible that pre-emptive treatment with immunosuppressive agents (e.g. cyclosporine) may retard or thwart the development of diabetes – the major problem is finding a safe drug whose benefit outweighs risk. At present, lifelong therapy is necessary.

   d. The most current theory regarding pathophysiology is that the pathogenesis resides not in the T cell but in the antigen-presenting cell and that the process is a systemic one.

   e. There is statistical linkage with other autoimmune diseases – Hashimoto's thyroiditis, Graves' disease, pernicious anemia, rheumatoid arthritis, vitiligo.

2. The clinical syndrome is generally acute and almost always affects younger individuals – included are the classic polyuria, polydipsia, weight loss, nausea, vomiting, dehydration and weakness. In the very young, subtle manifestations such as enuresis with a 'peculiar' breath odor (ketosis) may be observed by the parent. There may be history of an antecedent 'viral illness'.

3. Physical examination will be confirmatory of dehydration with hypotension (with or without orthostasis) and varying degrees of fat and muscle wasting (Type I diabetics are generally already of thin habitus); with acidosis, there may be Kussmaul respiration. On occasion, there may be physical evidence of hyperlipidemia (e.g. lipemia retinalis).

4. Laboratory studies will demonstrate hyperglycemia and glycosuria. Electrolytes will generally show hyponatremia unless the total body water loss is disproportionately profound (because of the osmotic effect of glucose in 'drawing water' out of cells). While total body potassium is depleted, this may not be reflected in serum levels; as ketoacidosis is a frequent mode of presentation, serum bicarbonate is low and chloride is decreased disproportionate to the fall in serum sodium because of the 'anion gap' acidosis. Arterial blood gases will demonstrate a decreased pH, decreased $pCO_2$ (because of hyperventilation) and increased $pO_2$ (because of $pCO_2$ depression). Complete blood count (CBC) may demonstrate hemoconcentration, leukocytosis and relative thrombocytosis. There may be 'mild' liver function abnormalities (usually secondary to 'fatty infiltration'), hyperlipidemia (may be seen as lactescent serum), elevated blood urea nitrogen (BUN) because of prerenal azotemia (creatinine should be normal as long as glomerular filtration rate (GFR) is normal) and hyperamylasemia (salivary and pancreatic in origin – elevation in uncontrolled diabetes is thus not a predictor of inflammatory disease of those organs).

5. Type I diabetics will invariably require insulin therapy and this will be necessary in the acute management. Because of the 'inflammatory' nature of the lesion, however, there may be a subsequent clinical 'honeymoon' period (en route to ultimate islet cell 'exhaustion') when either a decrease in the insulin dose or oral hypoglycemic agents will suffice.

## TYPE II DIABETES MELLITUS

1. The most common type of diabetes mellitus – accounts for about 85% of all diabetics and affects over 6% of the American population (about half a million new cases a year); the incidence appears to be increasing.

2. More common in older people – the incidence increases with age (infrequently seen in young, the so-called maturity-onset diabetes of youth (MODY), which is rarely caused by an abnormal insulin molecule); seen more often in blacks than in whites; among certain cultures, it is highly endemic (e.g. South-west native Americans, Nauru).

3. There is a high association with obesity (85% of Type II diabetics). While there are no known immunologic markers, there can be association both with polymorphism of the glycogen synthase gene, with mutations of glucokinase, and with increased intracellular calcium levels in most tissues. Further abnormalities in the sensitivity of the $\beta_3$-adrenergic receptor of adipocytes is associated with increased insulin resistance. Genetic predilection is strong (virtual 100% concordance in identical twins). A subtype of both Type I and Type II diabetes is associated with a mutation of mitochondrial DNA.

4. A major pathophysiologic mechanism is peripheral insulin resistance (obesity without overt diabetes does this as well) – this appears to result from 'down regulation' of the 'receptor process' (postreceptor defect). This resistance can be observed before there is chemical or clinical evidence of diabetes mellitus. Increased hepatic gluconeogenesis results in fasting hyperglycemia. Postprandial hyperglycemia occurs secondary to decreased glucose uptake. There may be compensatory islet cell hyperplasia (this explains the possibility of elevated insulin levels early in the pathogenesis) – ultimately, there may be relative or absolute pancreatic 'exhaustion'. Always, the insulin output is inadequate relative to the degree of hyperglycemia.

5. Because of the loss of insulin-mediated suppression of glucagon, there is an inappropriate hyperglucagonemia (also seen in Type I diabetes but not necessarily early in its course). Thus, hyperglycemia does not suppress glucagon (there may even be a paradoxical increase) and amino acid stimulation of glucagon may be augmented. Restoration of normal insulin balance may be corrective.

6. Unlike the 'explosive' way in which Type I diabetes may present, Type II presentations tend to be more insidious. By example:

   a. Inappropriate hyperglycemia may be noted on 'routine' screening (e.g. chemical screening prior to elective surgery).

b. There may be a tendency to increased thirst and urination (compensated; nocturia may be a clue); blurriness of vision (refraction impairment because of hyperosmolality of the lens), candidal infection (e.g. vulvovaginitis); peripheral paresthesias (these are reversible and not the neuropathy of long-term diabetes).

c. Physiologic stress (e.g. pregnancy) or the use of medications which impair glucose tolerance (e.g. thiazide diuretics, glucocorticoids, oral contraceptives) may 'unmask' diabetes.

d. While Type II diabetics generally do not present with ketoacidosis and do not usually require insulin (initially), a major medical event may make insulin therapy necessary (e.g. myocardial infarction, sepsis, surgical abdomen). As a corollary, an otherwise stable diabetic can decompensate when acute medical crises supervene.

## ADDITIONAL MARKERS OF DIABETES MELLITUS

1. Glycosylated Hemoglobin ('Glycohemoglobin') – the result of an irreversible bond between the $NH_2$ group of the hemoglobin $\beta$ chain and the aldehyde group of glucose. This forms a Schiff base (and a secondary Amadori rearrangement). As this lasts the life of the red blood cell, measurement can provide an integrated picture of the glycemic state over the last 3 months.

a. Hemoglobin $A_{1c}$ is the specific moiety used in clinical measurement; it is non-phosphorylated. The other components of 'glycohemoglobin' are hemoglobin $A_{1a}$ and $A_{1b}$.

b. Non-diabetics do not have a hemoglobin $A_{1c}$ of zero. Normals have a 'normal' blood glucose and this results in a hemoglobin $A_{1c}$ range of 6-8% (normal ranges may vary among laboratories). There is little value in using a 'low' value of hemoglobin $A_{1c}$ to diagnose hypoglycemia.

c. Hemoglobinopathies and anemia can affect the hemoglobin $A_{1c}$ value – glycosylated albumin (fructosamine) is not affected by these. Fructosamine is additionally advantageous in providing an 'overview' of the glycemic state over a shorter time span.

2. Glycosuria – useful only as a general screening technique. Not valuable in ongoing monitoring (even the 'double voiding technique' is not clinically useful). Affected by certain proximal tubular disorders and pregnancy (decreased tubular absorption of glucose) and renal failure (increased renal threshold for glycosuria). When glucose oxidase strips are used, sugars other than glucose (e.g. pentosuria, lactosuria) will not be measured.

3. Urine and Serum Ketone Determinations – adjunctive; utilizes nitroprusside reaction; useful for screening for ketosis (helpful for diabetics self-monitoring their blood sugar); β-hydroxybutyrate is not measured by this technique.

4. Intravenous Glucose Tolerance Test (IVGTT) – not a very good screening test because it is 'inconvenient' (as a result of the need to administer glucose intravenously and take multiple samples – albeit over only 30 minutes); a more significant problem is its relative insensitivity because it does not mimic the natural state of gastrointestinal hormone-mediated augmentation of the insulin response. The actual calculation is in solving for $K$ (the rate constant of the disappearance of glucose) where $K = 0.693/t \times 100$ and $t =$ the time (in minutes) for the peak glucose level (this is determined by extrapolation to 0 time using a semilogarithmic plot) to be reduced by 50%. Normal $K$ values should be greater than 1.2.

## ACUTE COMPLICATIONS OF DIABETES MELLITUS

### Diabetic Ketoacidosis (DKA)

1. In Type I diabetes, it may occur without an obvious precipitating cause; in Type II diabetes, there is usually some antecedent reason – even if it is an issue of compliance (not infrequently the case).

2. Additionally, the brittle nature of Type I diabetes makes these diabetics vulnerable to DKA.

3. High on the list of precipitating etiologies is infection. This may be overt (e.g. pneumonia, septicemia) or subtle (e.g. a 'cryptic' soft tissue or urinary tract infection). DKA can also be precipitated by a cardiovascular event such as an overt (or 'silent') myocardial infarction or cerebrovascular accident – or these may also follow an event of DKA (in the appropriate risk setting). The greater the

insulin dependency, the more likely a given inciting factor will bring about DKA.

4. Once the process is initiated, a chain of events takes place which amplifies the sequence. These include:

   a. Dehydration secondary to the obligatory loss of water and electrolytes with the osmotic diuresis. This may be compounded by gastrointestinal distress (nausea, vomiting, diarrhea – whether or not these were initial provocateurs) and inability of the patient to keep up with fluid replacement.

   b. Other organ systems may falter – e.g. renal insufficiency, decreased myocardial contractility.

   c. The limits of endogenous utilization of ketones, buffering of excessive keto-acids, renal excretion of acids and hyperventilation. When these limits are exceeded, metabolic acidosis ensues.

5. The clinical manifestations include overt dehydration, hypotension, abdominal pain, nausea and vomiting, hyperventilation (Kussmaul respiration), warm dry skin, ketotic breath and urine, and varying levels of confusion or obtundation.

6. The pertinent laboratory studies include hyperglycemia, hyponatremia (a frequent concomitant, but dependent on the extent of water loss in excess of electrolytes – also depending on hyperlipidemia); a variable potassium concentration; a variable serum chloride and a significant absolute decrease in serum bicarbonate (although a non-anion gap acidosis could be additionally operant). There is increased serum osmolality (it can be calculated by $2 \times Na + Glucose/18 + BUN/2.8$) and decreased pH and $pCO_2$. As noted earlier, there may be abnormalities of renal and hepatic function as well as hemoconcentration, leukocytosis and hyperamylasemia (but lipase will be normal in the absence of pancreatic disease). Other clinical and laboratory features may reflect superimposed disease (e.g. myocardial infarction, nitrite-positive urine with pyuria).

7. It is clear at this point that although insulin inadequacy may have been the initial event in the cascade, the process has gone well beyond that point ('For the want of a nail, the shoe was lost; for the want of a shoe, the horse was lost . . .') and merely replacing

the insulin without correcting the secondary events will be woefully inadequate. Indeed, insulin therapy alone without fluid and electrolyte replenishment can worsen the hypovolemia by 'driving' glucose into cells. Specific measurements of management include:

a.  Appropriate work-up of the precipitating causes and careful documentation of laboratory parameters (electrolytes, blood glucose, ketones, arterial blood gases as well as supplementary laboratory studies such as calcium, phosphorus and magnesium) along with documentation of therapeutic measures (fluid and electrolyte administration, insulin, other therapeutic measures). Flow sheets are extremely helpful in organizing data and in charting the clinical course.

b.  All patients require fluid replacement – as the average deficit is usually 5 liters (clinical dehydration is apparent at 6% and profound at 10% of total body weight), isotonic saline should be given up to the rate of 500–1000 ml/hour over the first 2–3 hours. Tapering can occur thereafter depending on patient response and tolerance (if there is underlying cardiovascular disease, the rate may have to be tempered – some patients may require coronary care unit monitoring and Swann–Ganz catheterization). Some advocate Ringer's lactate solution (more 'alkaline' than NaCl as NaCl has a pH of 7.0 – on the other hand, DKA is associated with hyperlactic acidemia and Ringer's solution will increase the serum lactate concentration). Ultimately, adequate restoration of cellular metabolism and circulation will correct acid–base imbalance. Half-normal saline may be administered after the first 1–2 liters and 5% dextrose/0.45% normal saline should be given once the blood glucose falls to 250 mg/dl.

c.  Insulin is administered as an intravenous 'loading dose' first (generally 25–50 units) and then as a separate insulin 'drip' (generally 5–10 units/hour based on the approximate need of 0.15 U of insulin per kilogram of body weight per hour). This should be administered through an access line independent of fluid replacement; 1 unit/10 ml of normal saline is a recommended dilution – the intravenous tubing should be 'flushed' adequately with this solution prior to administration to prevent future insulin adherence. Although higher doses of insulin are used by some (and were the standard of therapy in the past), they are rarely necessary.

d.  Unless there is evidence of renal failure (even with renal insufficiency, however, some potassium deficit is common) and urine output is not adequate, potassium should be replaced (the rate is generally up to 10 mEq/hour – rarely is a higher rate necessary, even though insulin administration and correction of acidosis will 'drive' potassium into cells).

e.  Bicarbonate administration is not indicated unless pH is less than 7.1 (some utilize pH of 7.0 and serum bicarbonate of 5 mEq/l as cutoff levels) – 50 ml of sodium bicarbonate (44 mEq) can be added to each liter of half normal saline solution.

f.  Although DKA is associated with phosphate depletion (which theoretically decreases buffering capacity of the blood and diminishes tissue oxygenation because of decreased levels of 2,3 diphosphoglycerate (DPG), it is rarely necessary – if given, the rate should be no greater than 3–4 mmol/hour (if all of potassium replenishment is given as potassium phosphate, too much phosphorus is given too soon with the resultant danger of calcium phosphate deposition and hypocalcemia).

g.  Once clinically stabilized, a 'sliding scale' regime of regular insulin can be instituted – do not stop the insulin drip until the effect of the first subcutaneous regular insulin can be realized (about 1 hour).

## Hyperglycemic Hyperosmolar Non-ketotic Syndrome

1.  Generally seen in older patients with underlying medical problems (e.g. cardiovascular, renal disease); fluid intake often decreased (e.g. situational circumstances, altered mental status); aggravated by superimposed clinical events (e.g. hip fracture, pneumonia) or medication (e.g. thiazide diuretics, glucocorticoids).

2.  Levels of hyperosmolality greater than that seen in DKA. Acidosis is prevented by the presence of some insulin and the continued ability to carboxylate acetyl coenzyme A (rather than conversion to ketone bodies – there is no obvious difference in counterregulatory hormone concentration between this condition and DKA).

3. Dehydration is generally severe (with associated finding of 'skin tenting', orthostatic hypotension, decreased 'eyeball resilience' and dry mucous membranes). There is often evidence of other underlying medical problems. No ketosis on breath; no Kussmaul respirations, but obtundation may be severe (with other neurologic findings).

4. Laboratory studies reveal hemoconcentration, leukocytosis, hyponatremia (with corresponding decreases in other electrolytes secondary to 'osmotic correction') – if serum sodium is 'normal', this is indicative of a profoundly hyperosmolal state. Serum bicarbonate is not inappropriately depressed (except there may be associated lactic acidosis secondary to peripheral hypoperfusion).

5. The mainstay of therapy is fluid replenishment – isotonic saline may be given initially (because of the need to maintain intravascular integrity) but half normal saline is generally given earlier in this condition than in DKA. The rate of administration (generally 500–1000 ml/hour) depends upon the clinical response and tolerance but overall fluid deficit is often 5 liters or more. As the serum glucose falls, 5% dextrose/half normal saline will be the replacement fluid. Caution: as long as the patient is 'on the right path' and there is clinical restitution, do not attempt too rapid normalization of laboratory values!

6. Bicarbonate therapy is not indicated; potassium replacement is generally less than in DKA (no more than 10 mEq/hour). Insulin drip may not be necessary (there is no contraindication to its use except that patients with non-ketotic hyperglycemia generally respond more rapidly and the initial bolus of intravenous insulin (10 to 20 Units) can be followed by hourly injections of 5 to 10 Units, as needed.

### Lactic Acidosis

1. Can occur for metabolic (increased generation or decreased metabolism) or cardiovascular–pulmonary reasons – can be independent of, or an integral part of other acute diabetic crises.

2. In its 'pure' state, it is a non-ketotic, anion gap, metabolic acidosis – the clinical syndrome often takes the 'scenario' of the primary precipitating disorder. Laboratory studies include those that may

219

be relevant to the primary problem(s) as well as abnormal arterial blood gases (decreased bicarbonate and $pCO_2$) and a calculated 'anion gap'. Direct measurement of serum lactate would demonstrate a significant elevation (normal: 1 mEq/l).

3. As lactic acidosis is usually the consequence of a more primary process, therapy is directed against that particular disorder (e.g. DKA, sepsis, peripheral hypoperfusion). Ancillary fluid and electrolyte administration are given as indicated and tolerated – sodium bicarbonate is given for severe metabolic acidosis. While the therapeutic use of dichloroacetate improves the blood lactate and pH, it has no beneficial effect on hemodynamic status or outcome.

**Hypoglycemia**
Reviewed in Chapter 19.

## CHRONIC COMPLICATIONS OF DIABETES MELLITUS

1. Postulated Mechanisms (Table 20-1)

   a. Formation of polyols – polymerization of reduced glucose (sorbitol); activated by aldose reductase.

      i. May contribute to neuropathy, retinopathy, cataracts and nephropathy.

      ii. Associated with secondary myoinositol deficiency – this has been demonstrated in nerve tissue of diabetic rats, but its role in human disease is less clear. On the other hand, uridine, which increases phosphoinoside synthase, can improve neurophysiologic parameters in patients with diabetic neuropathy.

### TABLE 20-1. POSTULATED MECHANISMS OF CHRONIC COMPLICATIONS OF DIABETES MELLITUS

Formation of Polyols
Post-Translational Protein Glycosylation
Hyperlipidemia
Increased Platelet Aggregation
Increased Capillary Filtration ('Hyperfiltration')

iii. May be reversible with aldose reductase inhibition (sorbinil, and more recently, Tolrestat).

b. Post-Translational Protein Glycosylation

i. Associated with a virtually irreversible bond between aldose (of glucose) and amine (of protein) producing an aldimine (Schiff base) made stronger by an Amadori rearrangement.

ii. Concept of that type of bonding has multiple applications beyond diabetology (although its empiric utility in the role of glycemic surveillance using glycohemoglobin determinations has already been discussed). Other applications include the mechanism of the effect of aspirin, activation of glycoprotein hormones, post-translational modification of glutamic acid (to form $\gamma$-carboxyglutamic acid – relevant in the action of vitamin K), and binding of direct bilirubin to albumin.

iii. May contribute to multiple abnormalities seen in the diabetic – including nephropathy, retinopathy and connective tissue abnormalities.

iv. Preventive agents (e.g. aminoguanidine, which prevents advanced glycosylated end products) are actively being sought and developed.

c. Hyperlipidemia – decreased lipoprotein lipases produce hypertriglyceridemia; increased free fatty acid delivery to the liver results in increased very low-density lipoprotein (VLDL) synthesis; increased low-density lipoprotein (LDL) can result either from increased VLDL availability or decreased LDL receptors; high-density lipoprotein (HDL) is decreased.

d. Increased Platelet Aggregation – increased thromboxane $A_2$ and Von Willebrand factor; decreased prostacyclin.

e. Increased capillary filtration secondary to decreased arteriolar resistance (not reflected in blood pressure) – 'hyperperfusion'.

2. Specific Chronic Complications

a. Nephropathy

i. Affects 20–30% or more of all diabetics. The incidence has been declining (presumably secondary to improved glycemic control).

ii. Rare before 5 years and evident (in those who will be affected) after 15–20 years of diabetes.

iii. Evolutionary progression – initial hyperfiltration, microalbuminuria (normal, less than 10 μg/minute; in this stage of nephropathy, 20–200 μg/minute are usually seen), and then overt renal disease.

iv. Although histologic correlates include glomerular basement membrane thickening, the degree of mesangial expansion is the most closely correlated structural analog.

v. Tight diabetic control (if possible) appears to prevent or mitigate the severity but it must be initiated early – tight control 'after the fact' is not apparently beneficial. Restricted protein intake (0.6 g/kg of body weight/day) and use of angiotensin converting enzyme (ACE) inhibitors (even without overt hypertension) also appear beneficial. Control of overt hypertension appears important, but β blockers and diuretic therapy are associated with a greater deterioration of GFR when compared with ACE inhibitors, despite blood pressure equivalency.

vi. Other renal complications include:

   (a) Proclivity to pyelonephritis and necrotizing papillitis. The increased likelihood of a neurogenic bladder and impaired neutrophil function with hyperglycemia are predisposing factors to urinary tract infection.

   (b) Acute tubular necrosis (ATN) following radiographic contrast (but unlikely when newer 'reduced ionic contrast agents' are used as they are less hyperosmolal). Antecedent dehydration is an associated risk factor.

   (c) Accelerated atherosclerosis affecting the renal vasculature.

   (d) Hyperkalemia as a consequence of chronic renal failure or of hyporeninemic hypoaldosteronism.

b. Neuropathy

   i. Motor – isolated mononeuropathy; isolated cranial nerve palsies (III, IV, VI and VII most likely to be affected); mononeuritis multiplex; amyotrophy (pain, weakness, wasting, and fasciculations).

ii. Sensory – peripheral sensory loss (distal – 'stocking' more common than 'glove'); parasthesias, pain (may be radicular or tabetic) and dysesthesias; neuropathic arthropathy (Charcot joint); absent deep tendon reflexes (DTRs). Treatment of painful episodes include anti-seizure medication and tricyclic antidepressants (even though they are not used here for their 'antidepressant properties').

iii. Autonomic – includes postural hypotension, gastrointestinal dysmotility (gastroparesis, diarrhea, 'blind loop'), altered sexual function, bladder atony, failure of adrenergic hypoglycemic counterregulation. Diagnosed by clinical appraisal, failure of the Valsalva maneuver to produce expected changes in heart rate, cold pressor test (failure of anticipated blood pressure response to cold – e.g. immersion of hands in ice water). Treatment options include fludrocortisone (Florinef) and support hose for hypotension, antibiotic therapy for 'blind loop' and loperamide, diphenoxylate and atropine (Lomotil) for gastrointestinal hypermotility, and metclopramide (Reglan) and cisapride (Propulsid) for gastroparesis. A promising treatment for diabetic diarrhea is the somatostatin analog, octreotide. It is important to rule out vascular causes of impotence. Intracavernous papaverine (alone or with phentolamine) will be therapeutically effective for impotence if the penile circulation is intact (prosthetic implant is an additional consideration).

c. Eye Complications

i. Retinopathy

(a) 'Background' – caused by vascular dysfunction: 'leaky capillaries' ('waxy exudates', 'dot and blot' hemorrhages), venoendothelial 'bulge' (micro-aneurysms); 'cotton wool' exudates.

(b) Proliferative – the response by the retina to focal hypoxia with neovascularization (vascular endothelial growth factor (VEGF) appears to be a major mediator). Pre-emptive treatment with laser photocoagulation has been an effective modality.

    ii. Cataracts – 'Snowflake' variety seen primarily in Type I diabetes; all diabetics are more likely to develop 'senile' cataracts (and at an earlier age).

d. Dermatologic Changes – 'Shin spots', necrobiosis lipoidica diabeticorum, propensity to *Candida* infection and ischemic ulcers.

e. Cardiovascular Disease – accelerated atherosclerosis, congestive cardiomyopathy and peripheral vascular disease. The association of Type II diabetes mellitus, hypertension, obesity, atherosclerosis, hyperlipidemia (usually hypertriglyceridemia with increased LDL-cholesterol and decreased HDL-cholesterol), and (often) hyperuricemia is sometimes referred to as 'Syndrome X'. Risk factors for amputation include decreased peripheral circulation, unfavorable arm : leg blood pressure, decreased vibratory sensation, decreased HDL-cholesterol and lack of ambulatory diabetes education.

f. Miscellaneous – soft tissue thickening and contractures (Dupuytren's contracture, 'cheirarthropathy'); propensity to soft tissue infections; hyporeninemic hypoaldosteronism.

g. Although there is now strong evidence to suggest that tight glycemic control can ward off complications, there is no solid evidence to support the notion that tight control will reverse disease once it has occurred. In one study, retinopathy even worsened; in another study, microalbuminuria could be retarded but not overt renal disease. What constitutes 'tight control' is an additional dilemma because the body's response to hyperglycemia comprises a 'continuum'. Even if the 'clinical numbers are good', the ambient glucose concentration that tissues are chronically exposed to may be 'physiologically too high' and may be beyond their 'set point of tolerance'.

h. On the other hand:

    i. A Swedish study of 102 insulin-dependent diabetics studied prospectively and evaluated after 18 months, 3, 5 and 7.5 years, showed that intensified (versus standard) therapy significantly retarded the development of microvascular complications. Intense therapy required patient education, individual responsibility, and generally at least three insulin injections per day.

ii. In a widely publicized, expensive ($165 million), comprehensive (1441 volunteers; 35 280 clinic visits) and long-term (9 years, overall) study, the Diabetes Control and Complications Trial (DCCT) presented clear and convincing evidence in insulin-dependent diabetes mellitus that intensive therapy that normalizes the blood sugar as much as possible can improve the chronic consequences of insulin-dependent diabetes mellitus in the following manner: reduction of retinopathy by as much as 76%, reduction of nephropathy by as much as 56%, and reduction of neuropathy by as much as 64%.

iii. A 'trade-off' to tight diabetic control is the increased frequency of hypoglycemic episodes. The tighter the control, the less effective is counterregulatory activation, as well as the additional consequence of hypoglycemia unawareness. The avoidance of hypoglycemia (as possible) can play an important role in maintenance of cognitive awareness of hypoglycemia.

**MANAGEMENT OF DIABETES MELLITUS** (Table 20-2)

1. Diet – The American Diabetes Association (ADA)-recommended diet includes principles of weight reduction (if there is obesity), 50–60% of calories as carbohydrate (complex carbohydrates are recommended) and fat intake of less than of 35% of calories (two-thirds as unsaturated fat). Cholesterol intake should be less than 300 mg/day. A high fiber diet delays glucose absorption (thus preventing surges of hyperglycemia) and will decrease the serum cholesterol concentration. The daily caloric intake should be 'balanced' – three meals and mid-morning and mid-afternoon and

### TABLE 20-2.   MANAGEMENT OF DIABETES MELLITUS

Diet
Exercise
Oral Hypoglycemic Agents
Insulin

bedtime snacks to 'balance' the insulin action (by convention, the greatest caloric intake is usually at dinner). The principles behind this are:

a.  In a diabetic patient taking insulin, the food intake must 'match' the anticipated times of effect of the insulin and it makes sense to co-ordinate this process.

b.  Even if the diabetic patient is not taking insulin (or even an oral hypoglycemic agent), that patient's diminished insulin reserve should dictate avoidance of any glycemic 'bolus' that might 'overwhelm' β-cell capacity. A more 'evenly distributed' caloric intake should make euglycemia easier to maintain.

2.  Exercise – enhances glucose utilization. Consistency is important because episodic hypoglycemia can arise from exercise and thus augment the insulin effectiveness. Moreover, there is increased insulin absorption from the 'exercised site' (one might alternatively choose an injection site not generally exercised, e.g. the abdomen, although it is difficult to divorce any specific anatomical area from the improved circulatory effects of generalized exercise). Exercise also improves cardiovascular fitness and lipid profile. It helps maintain weight control and promotes a sense of well-being.

3.  Oral Hypoglycemic Agents – Sulfonylureas are presently the largest class of oral agents in use. Their primary mechanism of action is β-cell stimulation – hence, they are only useful in patients who have endogenous insulin reserve. There is some evidence that they also increase peripheral sensitivity to insulin (but this is debatable) – this forms the rationale for 'combined' (oral hypoglycemic agent and insulin) therapy which some physicians support. Most physicians, however, would opt for 'upward' insulin dosage, as necessary, and thus limit the patient to only one type of medication. Some evidence demonstrates, however, improved glycemic control with lower insulin levels and less tendency to weight gain if nocturnal insulin is administered as a supplement to oral hypoglycemic agents.

a.  The majority of Type II diabetics will respond to oral agents alone – about 75% of those will remain responsive in the long term. (Note: weight reduction, if applicable, should always be an important goal).

b.  Drugs should be chosen based upon duration of action and mode of excretion (e.g. the effect of chlorpropramide or acetohexamide can be potentiated in renal failure). Second-generation agents may be selectively more effective in some cases of first-generation failure.

c.  Side-Effects – Skin rash (occasionally erythema multiforme), abnormal liver function tests (LFTs), hematopoietic toxicity; syndrome of inappropriate antidiuretic hormone (Chlorpropramide).

d.  Tolbutamide has the briefest duration of action; chlorpropramide (up to 60 hours), the longest.

e.  Biguanides, until recently, were not available for use in the USA. Phenformin (phenylethylbiguanide) was taken off the market because of the increased incidence of associated lactic acidosis and the results of the University Group Diabetes Program study which showed a higher incidence of cardiovascular death among its users. A related compound, metformin (long available outside the USA), does not appear to have the same toxicity as phenformin because it does not inhibit the mitochondrial oxidation of lactate.

Biguanides work primarily by increasing peripheral sensitivity to insulin and by inhibiting hepatic gluconeogenesis. They may also produce weight loss, particularly in adipose tissue. Metformin should not be used in the presence of renal disease or hepatic dysfunction, or in hypoxic states.

f.  Summary of Currently Available Oral Hypoglycemic Agents:

i.  'First Generation' Sulfonylureas

(a) Tolbutamide (Orinase) – short duration of action (6–12 hours); daily dose range: 500–3000 mg (divided doses).

(b) Chlorpropramide (Diabenese) – long duration of action (60 hours); daily dose range: 100–500 mg (single dose).

(c) Tolazamide (Tolinase) – intermediate duration of action (60 hours); daily dose range: 100–1000 mg (single or divided doses).

(d) Acetohexamide (Dymelor) – intermediate duration (12–24 hours); daily dose range: 250–1500 mg (single or divided doses).

ii. 'Second Generation' Sulfonylureas – (less bound to circulating proteins; fewer drug interactions; less dose of medication is needed, but action is similar to that of first-generation agents and second-generation drugs, except in selected cases, are probably not more effective).

(a) Glyburide (Micronase, Diabeta) – intermediate duration of action (10–30 hours); daily dose range: 2.5–20 mg (single or divided doses). Glynase is a glyburide product that is more 'bioavailable'. Its effectiveness is comparable, however. Daily dosage range is 3–12 mg.

(b) Glipizide (Glucatrol) – intermediate to long duration of action (13–30 hours); daily dosage range: 5–40 mg (single or divided doses – although doses greater than 10 mg/day produce little or no added benefit and may even reduce β-cell function). A long-acting product is also available.

iii Metformin (Glucophage) – a biguanide that appears to be efficacious in the management of non-insulin dependent diabetes mellitus. It may be particularly useful in the obese diabetic. The usual starting dose is 500 mg twice daily (with the morning and evening meals) to minimize gastro-intestinal side-effects. The dose is increased in the second week by adding 500 mg to the morning dose and in the third week by adding 500 mg to the evening dose as well. Metformin may also be considered in combination therapy with sulfonylurea.

4. Other Therapeutic Modalities

a. While increased dietary fiber can improve glucose tolerance, guar, a soluble fiber, can decrease intestinal glucose absorption. Unpleasant gastrointestinal side-effects may limit its use.

b. Acarbose and miglitol (presently under investigation) are α-glucosidase inhibitors and thus produce a 'maldigestion syndrome' that inhibits intestinal glucose production from more complex dietary precursors. These agents can also produce gastrointestinal discomfort, bloating, flatulence and diarrhea.

c. Glucagon-like Peptide, a 37-amino acid peptide made in the terminal ileum, is a potent insulin secretagogue that may have future promise. Likewise, the growth hormone-dependent somatomedin or insulin-like growth factor-I (IGF-I) may be useful as an adjunct or even as a singular drug. A particular use may be in insulin resistant states.

d. D-Fenfluramine, a serotonin agonist used adjunctively in the management of obesity, increases insulin sensitivity and glucose uptake.

e. Troglitazone, a thiazolidinedione, by decreasing insulin resistance, has been shown to improve glucose tolerance in the obese state.

## INSULIN THERAPY

1. The 'definitive' hormone therapy for all diabetics, and the only long-term therapy for Type I diabetes. In other diabetics, it is always a potential consideration, even though oral agents (in concert with diet) may suffice.

2. The goals of therapy are to sustain normal growth and development, to maintain the euglycemic state, to prevent catabolism, to normalize pregnancy (when applicable) and to avoid the complications of diabetes. These goals are noble in intent and an ideal for which to strive.

3. Types of Insulin

   a. Short-Acting Preparations

      i. Crystalline Zinc Insulin (Regular, CZI) – onset within 30 minutes, peak within 4 hours, duration up to 8 hours.

      ii. Semilente – onset within 60 minutes, peak within 6 hours, duration up to 10–16 hours.

   b. Intermediate-Acting Preparations

      i. Neutral Protamine Hagedorn (NPH) – onset within 2–4 hours, peak within 10–12 hours, duration up to 24 hours.

      ii. Lente – onset within 2–4 hours, peak within 10–12 hours, duration up to 24 hours.

c. Long–Acting Preparations

    i. Ultralente – onset within 5 hours, peak within 14–24 hours, duration up to 36 hours.

    ii. Protamine Zinc Insulin – onset within 5 hours, peak within 14–24 hours, duration up to 36 hours.

d. The relative solubilities of insulin (and thus their absorption from tissue sites) are affected by the addition of protamine/phosphate buffer (NPH) or zinc in acetate buffer (Lente system). It is important to remember that the delivery of insulin to the body from an injected site is thus based upon physical and chemical realities – and not upon the biologic needs of the patient.

    i. NPH is also 'Isophane' (equal parts insulin and protamine) – it can be admixed with regular insulin with each retaining their identity.

    ii. Identity of regular insulin is lost when added to Lente. Lente is, in actuality, a 30:70 mixture of semilente: ultralente.

    iii. Regular insulin also loses its identity if added to protamine zinc insulin.

e. Insulins can also be characterized by source and purity.

    i. Most commercial insulins in the past were a beef–pork mixture (because it was economical to produce them that way), but their role diminished with the advent of recombinant genetic technology. Pork insulin more closely resembles human insulin (only one amino acid difference versus three for beef) and is less antigenic. This has some (but limited) clinical relevance.

    ii. 'Purified' is the 'highest standard' of animal insulin available (less than 10 parts per million (ppm) of proinsulin); 'single peak' insulin (of historical interest) has between 10 and 25 ppm.

    iii. The availability of recombinant human insulins has made supplies plentiful and has supplanted much animal insulin use (especially in the initiation of insulin therapy).

(a) These insulins can be made without using any animal insulin substrate (Humulin) or through genetic alteration of the pork insulin molecule (Novolin, Velosulin).

(b) Despite its 'purity', human insulins can have some (but limited) antigenicity.

iv. Insulin is bottled in 10 ml vials with 100 U/ml. Syringes are available in 1 ml (and smaller) sizes to maximize the accuracy of the administered dose.

4. Strategies of Insulin Administration

a. All Type I diabetics (and a number of other insulin-dependent diabetics) will optimally require two injections per day. (Type II diabetics may be well controlled with a single daily injection.) A 'traditional' method of administration is approximately two-thirds of the daily dose before breakfast and one-third before dinner of an intermediate-acting insulin. Regular (or Semilente if the Lente system is used) may have to be added to each injection to 'smoothen' the course (generally, the regular to intermediate ratio is one-third to one-half but flexibility has to be used based on the pattern of food intake and the degree of hyperglycemia). The availability of insulin in a prepackaged NPH to Regular ratio of 70 : 30 can render the administration of these two types of insulin logistically easier in those patients in whom this ratio appears effective.

b. Alternative ('more intensive') therapies have included:

i. Regular insulin dosing before each meal based on an empiric sliding scale with a small dose of long-acting insulin at bedtime (to cover the 'basal' insulin needs throughout the night).

ii. Regular insulin dosing before lunch and dinner and NPH with Regular before breakfast and NPH alone at bedtime.

iii. The insulin pump has been used by some diabetics – its use is not as widespread as was once predicted, and it is of value only for selected diabetics. Patients must be highly motivated and capable of benefiting from pre-emptive tight control. Pumps are available both for subcutaneous and intraperitoneal insulin delivery.

c.  Remember: the knowledge of diabetic pathophysiology may be intellectual and precise but its management is empiric; there are no perfect schemes and no absolutes.

   i.  Insulin dosage (type and amount) will vary based upon glycemic patterns, which in turn, will be contingent upon diet, life style, exercise and ancillary issues.

   ii.  Consistency of daily life and anticipation of expected times of peak insulin action are crucial in maintaining normalcy.

   iii.  Three factors that promote early morning hyperglycemia have to be appreciated and 'sorted out' (if necessary), as their causes and treatments are different.

     (a)  The 'dawn' phenomenon – the tendency to early morning hyperglycemia, probably mediated by the nocturnal 'growth hormone burst'. It is best treated in an anticipatory manner with increased evening or nighttime insulin coverage of a type whose anticipated peak would reduce the 'dawn' impact.

     (b)  The waning of insulin effect is another cause of early morning hyperglycemia. In one sense, it can be looked upon as a corollary to the 'dawn' phenomenon and it is treated with increased pre-emptive insulin coverage.

     (c)  The Somogyi phenomenon is reactive hyperglycemia in the early morning (because of the effect of counterregulatory hormones in response to nocturnal hypoglycemia) – it is probably not as common as once believed but it has to be distinguished from other causes of early morning hyperglycemia. If there is doubt as to its presence (and concomitant concern about making the patient hypoglycemic during the night), finger stick blood glucose testing can be done at selected times during the night.

   iv.  Self-monitoring of blood glucose is very important – the data one obtains are not only valuable in regulation, but this process incorporates patients into the overall management plan. It also sensitizes patients to a high level of awareness of their problem. They must not be so preoccupied by it that it detracts them from a normal and functional existence; neither can they 'give up their guard' and deny the existence of a chronic problem that requires ongoing management.

5. Pancreas Transplantation

   a. Although of small magnitude compared with the absolute number of diabetics, over 4000 pancreas transplants have now been performed. Most have been done in concert with concomitant renal transplantation. The failure rate, however, is higher than renal or heart transplantations and added complications are the increased incidence of infection and cancer, and the side-effects from immunosuppressive therapy. While transplantation can remove insulin dependence, organ scarcity, cost and failure to prove that chronic complications are mitigated after transplantation make this approach of insulin restoration a very limited one.

   b. Islet cell transplantation may be more efficacious, especially if tissue encapsulation could insulate the cells from the surrounding hostile immune environment.

## ANCILLARY ISSUES RELEVANT TO THE DIABETIC

1. Personal Hygiene – With particular emphasis on proper foot care (regular podiatric evaluation as necessary) and awareness of predilection to infection. This is one aspect of care where preventive measures can be invaluable.

2. The need for proper education and resource availability – additional aspects include identification bracelet, support groups and active participation in organizations committed to education, public enlightenment and ongoing research.

3. Diabetes and Surgery

   a. Interrelationships include:

      i. The greater incidence of certain types of surgical problems in the diabetic – e.g. gall bladder disease, bypass graft surgery (coronary and peripheral), ischemic bowel disease.

      ii. The greater surgical risk of the diabetic patient (e.g. cardiovascular disease, cerebrovascular disease, obesity).

    iii. The worsening of diabetic control by surgical crises.

    iv. The 'mimicking' of surgical conditions by DKA (e.g. acute abdomen, hyperamylasemia).

    v. The higher incidence of postoperative problems in the diabetic, including those relating to circulation, cardiovascular status and wound healing.

  b. Elective Surgery in the Diabetic

    i. In patients managed with diet or oral hypoglycemic agents, careful monitoring of blood glucose intra- and postoperatively with a sliding scale regime of regular insulin responses is usually satisfactory.

    ii. Insulin-dependent diabetics are best managed with a combined glucose and insulin infusion on the day of surgery (10 to 20 Units of regular insulin added to 1000 ml of 5% glucose in water with an infusion rate of about 150 ml/hour). Alternatively, they can be managed with supplemental subcutaneous insulin given intraoperatively, based upon their finger stick glucose determination. Generally, one-third of their daily insulin dose is given preoperatively and they would also have an intravenous infusion of 5% glucose in water – this is a less preferred approach than the glucose and insulin infusion technique because there is not the same level of control.

      (a) Patients undergoing major surgery should have at least one prior preoperative day in the hospital for stabilization – they can be managed in their normal manner until the midnight prior to surgery (nil by mouth (NPO) after midnight).

      (b) Barring urgent contingencies, their surgery should be scheduled as early as possible that day.

      (c) They can be followed with a 'sliding scale' throughout the perioperative period and 'weaned' into their standard pattern of insulin replacement when diet is normalized.

      (d) Remember – there is bound to be some disruption in the optimization of their blood glucose – expect this, but work within reasoned limits.

4. Diabetes and Pregnancy

   a. Gestational diabetes occurs in 2–3% of all pregnancies. The diagnosis is empirically made if two of the following plasma glucose values are exceeded: fasting, 105 mg/dl; 1 hour, 190 mg/dl; 2 hour, 165 mg/dl; 3 hour; 145 mg/dl. These values are obtained during an oral glucose test in which 100 g of glucose are taken after an 8–14-hour overnight fast following ingestion for 3 days of at least 150 g of carbohydrate ingestion per day.

   b. Data have unequivocally associated the degree of hyperglycemia in the third trimester with increased perinatal mortality.

   c. Even if the hyperglycemia is very early in fetal development, it is associated with multiple congenital anomalies involving, in particular, the cardiovascular, neurologic, renal and gastrointestinal systems. Offspring of diabetic mothers are more prone to neonatal hypoglycemia, hypocalcemia and hyperbilirubinemia.

   d. Fetal macrosomia is a frequent concomitant of maternal hyperglycemia – while the fetal hyperinsulinemic response to maternal hyperglycemia is still felt to be the prevailing mechanism, the transport of maternal insulin to the fetus, via antibodies, may also be of relevance.

   e. Polyhydramnios, hypertension and toxemia are among the effects of diabetes on the pregnancy.

   f. Treatment goals (glycemic goals are comparable whether or not the diabetes is pre-existing or gestational):

      i. Intensive Insulin Therapy – ideal laboratory values are a fasting blood sugar (FBS) of 60–100 mg/dl, 1 hour postprandial glucose of less than 140 mg/dl and a normal glycosylated hemoglobin. This invariably requires multiple insulin injections and frequent self-monitoring of blood glucose.

      ii. Proper obstetric care also includes frequent ultrasound monitoring, regular fetal monitoring with a non-stress test (and stress testing as additionally necessary), maternal α-fetoprotein determination, amniocentesis (for fetal lung maturity – lecithin : sphingomyelin ratio or phosphatidyl glycerol are measured) and optimal timing of delivery.

# Section F

# DISORDERS OF
# MINERAL METABOLISM

# 21

# MINERAL METABOLISM: NORMAL PHYSIOLOGY AND PATHOPHYSIOLOGY

## OVERVIEW OF MINERAL METABOLISM – CALCIUM, PHOSPHORUS AND MAGNESIUM

1. Metabolism of these minerals involves a complex interrelationship of dietary intake, intestinal absorption, cellular and matrix accretion and excretion. These minerals have overlapping relevance, are subject to common regulators (e.g. parathyroid hormone (PTH), calcitonin, vitamin D), and are affected by disease processes that alter some aspect of their handling (e.g. intestinal disease, renal failure).

2. These minerals are sufficiently unique in their own bodily roles, have different dynamics of handling, and their treatment strategies have respective uniquenesses. Thus, they are best discussed alone (but without losing sight of the dynamics of their interdependence). Their regulators will also be reviewed in the context of normal physiology and pathologic derangement.

### CALCIUM

1. Normal calcium intake ranges from 0.5 to 1.5 g/day in most American diets (although the recommended daily adult dietary allowance is 800 mg, this amount is being reconsidered in terms of specific physiologic needs – e.g. greater amounts earlier in life to offset a later negative balance; greater amounts in estrogen-deficient women).

   a. Approximately one-third to one-half is absorbed – the duodenum is the predominant site of absorption (this can be increased in calcium deficiency states or diets through the stimulation of PTH and the activation of vitamin D). Net absorption must take into account a daily 0.1–0.2 g/day active intestinal (intraluminal) secretion of calcium. Thus, on average, about one-half to two-thirds of the total amount of ingested calcium ends up in the feces. Absorption is decreased when there is an excessive amount of intraluminal fatty acids (e.g. malabsorption) or with excessive dietary fiber, phytate, or oxalate or with increased intraluminal alkali. Estrogens enhance absorption (glucocorticoids decrease it) – apparently mediated through the effects of activated vitamin D.

   b. The calcium absorbed from the gut enters into an

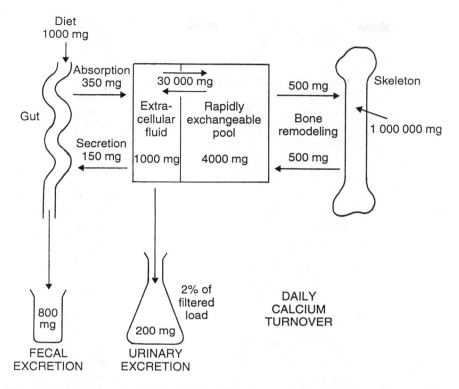

**Figure 21-1.** Average Daily Calcium Turnover in Humans. Reproduced with kind permission from *Physiology*, 2nd edn., Berne, R.M. and Levy, M.N. (eds.) St Louis: C.V. Mosby Company, 1988, p. 876

'exchangeable pool'. This pool is also in steady state with the bone. The overwhelming majority of calcium is stored in bone (1000–1400 g) – less than 0.1% is in the extracellular fluid and only 1% is within the cells (Figure 21-1).

c. Renal excretion of calcium in the stable adult in metabolic balance is equal to the amount absorbed.

    i. Losses in sweat are usually negligible but since sweat is a 'dilute ultrafiltrate' of plasma (i.e. the calcium concentration can be as high as 5 mg/dl), then up to 100 mg or more can be lost per day if perspiration is excessive.

    ii. Calcium undergoes complete glomerular filtration and thus 8000 to 10 000 mg/day are presented to the postglomerular portions of the nephron pool. Absorption is the singular process thereafter but it is usually so extensive that only 1–3% of the filtered load is ultimately excreted.

(a) About 60% of absorption takes place in the proximal tubule – this is associated with sodium absorption and explains the tendency to hypercalcemia in sodium avid states (it also explains the beneficial effect of saline infusion in the management of hypercalcemia, notwithstanding the independent ameliorative effect of reversal of dehydration).

(b) Twenty-five per cent of absorption occurs in the thick ascending limb of Henle's loop (this explains the beneficial effect of loop diuretics in promotion of a calciuresis).

(c) While only up to 8% of filtered calcium is absorbed in the distal tubule, it appears to be the site of PTH regulation of calcium absorption.

iii. PTH is the major hormonal regulator of calcium excretion.

(a) PTH increases calcium absorption.

(b) The paradox of hypercalciuria in hyperparathyroidism is readily explained by the increased filtered load of calcium in that disorder – no matter how effective PTH may be in enhancing absorption, it has only a small percentage of the filtered load to 'work with'.

(c) Hypercalcemic states associated with a depressed PTH (exclusive of the hypercalcemia of malignancy) thus results in a hypercalciuria (increased filtered load without compensatory increase in absorption) irrespective of the severity of the hypercalcemia.

(d) Other hormones that may produce hypercalciuria (e.g. growth hormone, vitamin D) do this primarily by indirect means. The effect of calcitonin in decreasing tubular calcium absorption is not significant (witness no characteristic pattern in medullary carcinoma). The effect of increased phosphate in decreasing urinary calcium is mediated through:

(1) Stimulation of PTH (increased phosphate

decreases the serum calcium because the solubility product [SP] of calcium × phosphate is a constant and 'has to be obeyed'),

(2) Decreased production of 'active' vitamin D (phosphate elevation inhibits 1-hydroxylation of vitamin D), and

(3) A direct effect of phosphate on the renal tubule.

(e) Hypermagnesemia and metabolic acidosis impair tubular calcium reabsorption. Metabolic acidosis also increases calcium mobilization from bone, thus turning off PTH.

2. Calcium is transported in the circulation in three forms: protein-bound (45–50%), complexed (about 5–10%; the complexing is to inorganic acids such as phosphate and sulfate and organic acids such as citrate and bicarbonate), and free (45–50%).

   a. The free is the 'metabolically active' form of calcium – its concentration is most closely correlated with calcium effect.

   b. The total protein concentration (whether 'true' as may be reflective of nutritional state, or 'artifactual' as may reflect the state of hydration) will affect the total serum calcium concentration. The degree to which a particular protein abnormality can affect this is best appreciated by noting that 80% of the normal binding of calcium is to albumin and 20% to globulin (by clinical corollary, note that the hypercalcemia of myeloma is rarely caused by enhanced calcium binding because an inordinate amount of globulin would have to be produced, or calcium-binding affinity would have to be enhanced by the abnormal globulin to result in overt hypercalcemia).

   c. The acid–base state can alter the compartmentalization (e.g. alkalosis, as in hyperventilation, can decrease the ionized – but not the total – calcium concentration).

3. Calcium has a variety of important extracellular and intracellular functions – clinical manifestations in hyper- and hypocalcemic states, by extrapolation, can help us to understand the role of calcium in normal physiology. Functions of calcium include: normal muscular contractility and nerve conduction (maintenance

## TABLE 21-1.   CLINICAL MANIFESTATIONS OF HYPOCALCEMIA

Parasthesias
Tetany
Seizures
Cardiac Arrhythmias
Miscellaneous:
    Fatigue
    Weakness
    Extrapyramidal Manifestations
    Intracranial Hypertension
    Psychiatric Manifestations
    Cataracts
    Bone and Dental Maldevelopment
    Malabsorption

of plasma membrane stability, a key component of normal electrophysiology, is operant here as is the direct effect of calcium in activating appropriate intracellular components), cellular secretion, regulation of enzymes, normal mineralization of calcified tissues, activation of prothrombin complex (factors VII, IX and X) and normal cellular growth and reproduction.

4.  The clinical syndrome of hypercalcemia is discussed in Chapter 22. Manifestations of hypocalcemia include: (Table 21-1):

    a.  Paresthesias – start in distal extremities in addition to the perioral region and the tip of the nose.

    b.  Tetany – usually heralded by antecedent paresthesias. May be spontaneous or elicited (e.g. Trousseau's and Chvostek's signs – Trousseau's sign is elicitation of carpal spasm, 'the sign of the Papal benediction' when the blood pressure cuff is inflated above systole; Chvostek's sign is facial twitching, brought on by tapping the facial nerve at its exit from the stylomastoid foramen). It may (ironically, when associated with paresthesias) also provoke hyperventilation and create a vicious cycle.

    c.  Seizures – also usually heralded by antecedent neuromuscular symptoms.

d. Cardiac Arrhythmias – initially may be only an 'EKG phenomenon' (prolonged QT interval), but it can lead to conduction abnormalities (e.g. atrioventricular block because prolongation of ventricular systole may make the ventricle unresponsive to the next atrial impulse) and decreased inotropy (e.g. refractory congestive heart failure).

e. More chronic changes may be fatigue and weakness, basal ganglia calcification (this may lead to extrapyramidal manifestations such as Parkinsonism or choreoathetosis), intracranial hypertension (with papilledema), psychiatric manifestations, posterior lenticular cataracts, maldevelopment of bones and teeth compounded by propensity to dental caries (if hypocalcemia occurs in childhood), abnormal skin and malabsorption (which can aggravate hypocalcemia by further decreasing calcium absorption). Despite the role of calcium in the coagulation cascade, clinically significant bleeding is not generally a feature of hypocalcemia.

## PHOSPHORUS

1. Normal dietary phosphate intake is about 1000–1500 mg/day (recommended daily adult dietary allowance = 800 mg/day).

   a. Phosphorus is ubiquitous in nature and it is therefore difficult not to have dietary adequacy, unless there are other nutritional issues (e.g. alcoholism). Meats and fish (e.g. flounder has 885 mg/100 g of edible fish) are the most concentrated source, but dairy products and vegetables are also significant.

   b. Absorption is about 80% (jejunum is the most significant site). Although 1,25-dihydroxycholecalciferol ($1,25-OH_2D$) is a potent stimulus to absorption, there are vitamin D-independent mechanisms. Further (unlike in the case of calcium) glucocorticosteroids increase absorption as does local environmental acidity. High calcium intake (2 g/day or more) may impair absorption. An active secretory mechanism for phosphorus in the gut has not been shown (Figure 21-2).

   c. In contrast to nearly all of the body's calcium being in bone, only 85% of phosphorus is 'stored' there (600–800 g) while 15% (100–150 g) is intracellular.

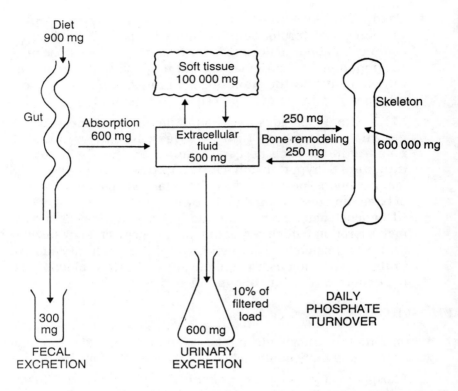

**Figure 21-2.** Average Daily Phosphate Turnover in Humans. Reproduced with kind permission from *Physiology*, 2nd edn., Berne, R.M. and Levy, M.N. (eds.), St Louis: C.V. Mosby Company, 1988, p. 877

   d. The major regulator of phosphate balance is the kidney (notwithstanding that significant fluctuations in serum levels can occur with cellular–extracellular shifts).

   i. Unlike the case of calcium, renal excretion of absorbed phosphorus is the major method of maintaining balance – the efficiency of intestinal phosphorus absorption cannot really be 'improved upon' except in states of significant phosphorus depletion.

   ii. Impairment of reabsorption is the major renal mechanism of phosphaturia.

   (a) PTH inhibits phosphate absorption primarily by its action on the proximal tubule.

## TABLE 21-2. ETIOLOGIES OF HYPOPHOSPHATEMIA

**Acute**

Respiratory Alkalosis
Active Cellular Glucose Uptake
Catecholamine Surges
Rapid Tissue Proliferation

**Chronic**

Phosphate-Binding Antacids
Primary Hyperparathyroidism
Renal Tubular Acidosis
Tumor-Mediated Hypophosphatemia

---

(b) Phosphate concentration, itself, independent of hormonal factors, regulates its own renal absorption.

(c) Increased calcium intake decreases urinary phosphate – multiple mechanisms appear to be operant (including decreased PTH and decreased serum phosphate).

(d) Metabolic acidosis, starvation, glucocorticoids, estrogen, many diuretics, hypokalemia and magnesium deficiency decrease renal phosphate reabsorption.

(e) Growth hormone and dehydration increase renal phosphate reabsorption.

e. Phosphorus circulates as phosphate bound to lipids and proteins (70%) and inorganic phosphate (30%). Based on the dissociation of phosphoric acid at physiologic pH, the ratio of $HPO_4^{-2}$ to $H_2PO_4^{-1}$ is usually 4:1 A normal serum phosphorus concentration is 2.5–4.5 mg/dl. Moderate hypophosphatemia is empirically defined at a value between 1.0 and 2.0 mg/dl, severe hypophosphatemia as less than 1.0 mg/dl.

**Hypophosphatemia** (Table 21-2)

1. Acutely seen in situations where there is rapid cellular uptake of phosphate and stimulation of glycolysis. Examples include:

    a. Acute respiratory alkalosis – initially described by Haldane and may be contributory to the hypophosphatemia seen in salicylate intoxication, gram-negative sepsis and toxic shock syndrome.

   b. Intravenous glucose administration and treatment of diabetic ketoacidosis, but it can also be seen with active nutritional repletion in a previously deprived person (e.g. a chronic alcoholic).

   c. Clinical situations associated with 'surges' of catecholamines which enhance cellular phosphate uptake.

   d. Rapid proliferation in tissue (e.g. rapidly growing neoplasms such as lymphoma) with a resultant increased capacitance of the intracellular phosphate pool.

2. Chronically seen in:

   a. Dietary inadequacy,

   b. Long-term use of phosphate-binding (e.g. non-absorbable) antacids,

   c. Primary hyperparathyroidism,

   d. Primary renal tubular disease – congenital (e.g. Fanconi syndrome, which is also associated with uricosuria, aminoaciduria and glycosuria) or acquired (e.g. toluene toxicity),

   e. Phosphate-wasting (renal) syndrome associated with some tumors – rare.

3. Manifestations of hypophosphatemia include:

   a. Impaired muscular and neuronal function (expressed in a wide range of clinical ways – felt to be related to impaired cellular energetics). Muscular dysfunction could progress to overt rhabdomyolysis.

   b. Impaired peripheral oxygenation (failure to generate adequate 2,3-diphosphoglycerate to 'unload' oxygen), with a wide range of clinical expressions. Other hematologic effects include decreased neutrophil chemotaxis and bactericidal action and impaired platelet function. 'Stiffening' of the red blood cell membrane could lead to hemolysis.

   c. Abnormal bone mineralization (chronic) – may produce clinical osteomalacia with overt bone deformity and pain.

d. Hypophosphatemia, itself, can decrease renal reabsorption of sodium, calcium and glucose, as well as cause renal tubular acidosis.

## Hyperphosphatemia

1. Most often seen in renal disease because of the significant role of the kidney in regulating phosphate balance. Also seen if a large amount of phosphate is 'delivered' to the body (e.g. tumor lysis) and 'overwhelms' normal excretory mechanisms. A rare disorder of hyperphosphatemia is associated with ectopic calcification ('tumor calcinosis' – failure of normal feedback inhibition by the hyperphosphatemia on vitamin D activation; conversely, ectopic calcification can be a consequence of hyperphosphatemia, *per se*).

2. The clinical syndrome in tumor lysis is related not only to the release of intracellular phosphate but to hyperkalemia (because of its high intracellular concentration) and to hyperuricemia secondary to degradation of pre-formed nucleic acids.

3. The major clinical effects of hyperphosphatemia are related to the secondary hypocalcemia.

## MAGNESIUM (Figure 21-3)

1. At 25 g, the fourth most plentiful cation in the body (after sodium, potassium and calcium). Somewhat more than half is in bone. Normal serum range is 1.4–2.1 mEq/l.

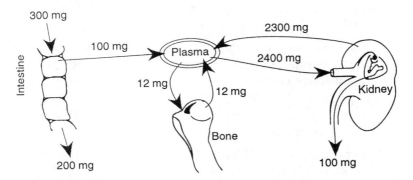

**Figure 21-3.** Metabolism of Magnesium. Reproduced with kind permission of S. Karger AG, Basel from Rude R.K. Physiology of magnesium metabolism and the important role of magnesium in potassium deficiency. *Am. J. Cardiol.* 1989, 63: 31 b–34 b

2. Although daily requirement is 200–400 mg, most Americans take in about 500 mg/day and unless there are dietary abnormalities, it is difficult to avoid access to it (plentiful in plant and animal food – an indispensable constituent of chlorophyll).

3. About one-third of ingested magnesium is absorbed (enhanced by 'active' vitamin D).

4. Approximately one-third of circulating magnesium is protein-bound. The unbound magnesium is completely filtered and about 95% of filtered magnesium is absorbed. Renal excretion is variable, but is an important determinant of serum concentration.

## Hypomagnesemia

1. Acute hypomagnesemia can be seen with enhanced tissue uptake (e.g. treatment of ketoacidosis or nutritional replenishment) – analogous to its effect in producing hypophosphatemia, but the magnitude of change is less. In pancreatitis, magnesium (like calcium) may be saponified. Following surgical remediation of hyperparathyroidism, the 'depleted' bones can become magnesium avid.

2. Chronic hypomagnesemia can be secondary to:

   a. Decreased dietary consumption – e.g. alcoholism (may also be associated with renal wastage), starvation, total parenteral nutrition without added magnesium.

   b. Impaired gastrointestinal absorption – e.g. chronic diarrhea, malabsorption syndromes, laxative abuse.

   c. Renal wasting – drugs associated with renal wasting of magnesium include loop and thiazide diuretics, aminoglycosides, carbenicillin, pentamidine, digoxin, cyclosporine, cisplatin and amphotericin B. 'Structural' (congenital or acquired) and tubulo-interstitial disease can also augment renal excretion.

   d. Endocrine disease – includes thyrotoxicosis, uncontrolled diabetes mellitus, vitamin D overdose and primary hyperaldosteronism.

3. The clinical syndrome includes a wide range of neuromuscular manifestations (e.g. muscle weakness, cramps and twitching),

mental status changes, insulin resistance, secondary hypocalcemia (from decreased PTH synthesis and activity) and cardiac consequences (e.g. arrhythmias, ST and T wave changes, coronary artery spasm, increased sensitivity to digitalis glycosides, and an increase in the size of an acute myocardial infarction).

**Hypermagnesemia**
1. Seen with tumor lysis syndrome and renal failure (augmented if oral intake is increased – e.g. magnesium-containing antacids). Less severe elevations seen in hypothyroidism, familial hypocalciuric hypercalcemia and mineralocorticoid deficiency. (Rarely seen in hyperparathyroidism – a normal or somewhat reduced serum magnesium level is more the rule.)

2. Clinical manifestations (e.g. neurologic and muscular depression) are secondary to impaired function; hypocalcemia may be seen here because of impaired PTH production (it ironically produces the same effect on PTH production as hypomagnesemia). Whether or not there is concomitant hypocalcemia, calcium administration can be an effective therapeutic antidote to symptomatic hypermagnesemia.

**PARATHYROID HORMONE (PTH)**

1. Chemical Structure

   a. Contains 84 amino acids; MW: 9500. Precursor molecules include a 'pre-pro' and a 'pro-PTH'.

   b. PTH elaboration is regulated primarily by serum calcium concentration which has an affect on parathyroid cell number, PTH synthesis and PTH secretion.

      i. Lesser stimuli to secretion include β-adrenergic agonists, histamine and prostaglandins (these are not clinically consequential, however, because drugs that antagonize their effects are neither useful adjuncts nor medical remedies for hyperparathyroidism).

      ii. $1,25\,(OH)_2\,D_3$ can impair PTH synthesis – hence an added benefit to its use in the hypocalcemia of renal disease.

    c. PTH circulates as an intact molecule and as multiple fragments.

        i. Until recently, PTH assays could not give 'reliable' information because they were directed against different parts of the molecule.

            (a) The '$NH_2$-site' is biologically active but is subject to greatest fluctuation and has a short half-life.

            (b) The 'mid-range' and 'COOH-site' have longer half-lives (but they are biologically inactive and their presence in blood can only imply prior PTH activity. Further, they are subject to elevations in renal failure which can be a complication of hypercalcemia, irrespective of etiology).

            (c) The use of a 'dual antibody' ($NH_2$ and mid-range or COOH) in a single assay appears to obviate the problem (this technology uses an immunoradiometric (IRMA) or chemoluminescence technology).

            (d) Bioassays have also been refined, but not to the point of generalized clinical utility.

2. PTH Action (binds to target cells with subsequent G protein activation)

    a. The effect on the kidney is to:

        i. Increase calcium absorption – PTH acts on distal tubule cells.

        ii. Decrease phosphate reabsorption.

        iii. Enhance 1-hydroxylation of vitamin D.

    b. The effect on bone is to increase osteoclast-mediated reabsorption.

        i. It appears to do this via production of an osteoblast-stimulated 'mediator'. Cortical bone is more affected than trabecular.

        ii. Ironically, acute (but not chronic) PTH can be primarily anabolic to bone (and PTH may have some role in the management of osteoporosis).

c. The action on the gut is indirect (mediated through vitamin D).

## VITAMIN D

1. It is a hormone – synthesized by the skin (from precursor 7-dehydrocholesterol made in the liver) upon action of ultraviolet light. In animals, it is $D_3$ (cholecalciferol). In plants, it is $D_2$ (ergocalciferol, which is derived from irradiated ergosterol).

2. It is 25-hydroxylated in the liver – this process is inhibited by dilantin and phenobarbital. Measured 25-OH D in the circulation is an index of its stores.

3. It is 1-hydroxylated in the kidney – the $1,25(OH)_2$ vitamin D is the most active form. This hydroxylation step is enhanced by PTH, low phosphate and (autoregulated, to some extent) by $1,25(OH)_2$ vitamin D, itself. The latter directs production of precursor vitamin D to the inactive $24,25(OH)_2$ D. (1-Hydroxylation may also occur ectopically in activated macrophages (e.g. sarcoidosis) or in lymphomas and lead to overt hypercalcemia.)

4. The major role of vitamin D is intestinal activation of a nuclear synthetic sequence that produces a calcium transport protein. A rare disorder of receptor inadequacy is Type II 'Vitamin D-Dependent Rickets'. Its given name is a misnomer because vitamin D is an ineffective therapy (calcium infusions, however, can be ameliorative by 'bypassing' the defect).

## CALCITONIN

1. It is a 32-amino acid protein (MW: 3700) – made from a larger precursor molecule and circulates with two other known peptide fragments from that precursor (katacalcin and calcitonin gene-related peptide).

2. Although its concentration inversely correlates with serum calcium levels, its physiologic role is not clear – its major effect is on osteoclasts (inhibitory). Gastrin is a secretagogue (but this is not of physiologic relevance – it has application in a stimulation test, usually in concert with calcium administration, to 'unmask' hypercalcitonemic states).

# 22

# HYPERCALCEMIA

## GENERAL CONSIDERATIONS

1. Because of the pivotal role of calcium in intracellular function, membrane stability and impulse conduction, hypercalcemia can be a potentially life-threatening disorder.

2. In general (and as an important endocrinologic principle), the more abrupt the development of hypercalcemia, the greater the symptomatology – indeed, the same degree of hypercalcemia in two different persons could range from an asymptomatic laboratory phenomenon to a patient with clinically life-threatening manifestations.

3. While there are multiple potential etiologies, the two commonest causes are malignancy and hyperparathyroidism. Stereotypically, hyperparathyroidism is usually detected in ambulatory patients during routine chemical screening. The hypercalcemia of malignancy is the commonest cause of in-patient hypercalcemia.

4. When hypercalcemia occurs as a result of increased bone resorption (most common mechanism) or increased intestinal absorption, the kidney is often able to compensate for this by enhanced renal excretion. Failure of renal homeostasis is the most important reason for perpetuation of the hypercalcemia. Mechanisms include:

    a. A direct effect of parathyroid hormone (PTH) or PTH-related protein (PTHrP) in enhancing tubular reabsorption of calcium (while the opposite occurs when PTH is suppressed in non-parathyroid hormone-related etiologies of hypercalcemia, these are much less frequently encountered situations).

    b. Hypercalcemia produces an antidiuretic hormone (ADH)-resistant diabetes insipidus and secondary dehydration which can enhance proximal tubular reabsorption of sodium and hence calcium.

    c. Severe dehydration can lead to a decrease in glomerular filtration rate.

    d. Hypercalcemia can dull the sensorium and decrease thirst perception and the drive for compensatory fluid intake.

    e. Immobilization, which can increase bone reabsorption, is often a concomitant.

## CLINICAL SYNDROME

1. Irrespective of the effects of hypercalcemia, manifestations related to the primary process which resulted in the hypercalcemia need to be considered.

2. Neurologic – decreased and dulled sensorium, psychiatric symptoms including depression, lethargy, muscular weakness, diminished deep tendon reflexes (DTRs).

3. Cardiovascular – shortened QT interval, bradycardia, heart block. Increased sensitivity to digitalis, and hypertension.

4. Gastrointestinal – increased gastric acid secretion (increased incidence of peptic ulcer disease in hyperparathyroidism), pancreatitis, constipation, nausea, vomiting and anorexia.

5. Renal – tubular dysfunction (renal sodium loss, nephrogenic diabetes insipidus), decreased renal blood flow and glomerular filtration rate, nephrocalcinosis.

6. Miscellaneous – pruritis, activation of coagulation cascade.

## CAUSES OF HYPERCALCEMIA

1. Hyperparathyroidism (discussed in Chapter 23).

2. The Hypercalcemia of Malignancy.

3. Granulomatous Disease.

4. Immobilization.

5. Milk–Alkali Syndrome.

6. Non-Parathyroid Endocrine Disease – Thyrotoxicosis and Addison's Disease.

7. Vitamin D Toxicity.

8. Vitamin A Toxicity.

9. Medications.

10. Familial Hypocalciuric Hypercalcemia.

11. Other – acute renal failure, idiopathic hypercalcemia in infancy.

**Hypercalcemia of Malignancy**

1. The commonest cause of hypercalcemia in hospitalized patients, the most common paraneoplastic syndrome and present in up to 20% of patients with neoplastic disease.

2. Although formerly felt to be caused by ectopic PTH production, sensitive assays now show PTH suppression except in isolated cases.

3. Certain tumors are statistically more likely to be associated with hypercalcemia than others (e.g. lung cancers, 6–16%; breast cancer, 18–42%; myeloma, 30–100%; human T-cell leukemia virus type 1, up to 100%). Other tumors include bladder cancer, renal cell carcinoma, leukemia, lymphoma and myeloma.

4. Although certain tumors may produce bony metastases (e.g. prostate), hypercalcemia is uncommon in them. Conversely, some tumors which have no bony metastases (squamous cell origin – e.g. lung, head, neck and esophagus) frequently produce hypercalcemia.

5. This ultimately led to the discovery of parathyroid hormone-related protein (PTHrP). This is comprised of three isoforms with 139, 141, and 173 amino acids each; nine of the first 13 N-terminal amino acids are identical to PTH.

6. PTHrP appears to be the primary mediator of hypercalcemia in squamous cell tumors but not in adenocarcinoma. It is physiologically present in breast tissue and milk and is increased by suckling and prolactin, while inhibited by bromocriptine. Its role in the hypercalcemia of breast cancer is presently being clarified (the hypercalcemia of breast cancer is often multifactorial). It is also present in keratinocytes and may be a local growth promoting factor.

7. PTHrP has most of the physiologic effects of PTH (including bone reabsorption, renal action on phosphate clearance, calcium reabsorption, proximal renal tubular acidosis (RTA) and increased urinary cAMP) but, it is not an inducer of 1-hydroxylase and does not result in increased levels of 1,25-dihydroxycholecalciferol $(1,25\text{-}(OH)_2D)$. Further, unlike PTH, it does not 'link' osteoclastic to osteoblastic activity. Thus, PTHrP can produce a greater degree of hypercalcemia and bone reabsorption than PTH.

8. The second major category of hypercalcemia of malignancy is local osteolytic hypercalcemia (LOH). Although tumor may be in 'direct' contact with bone, local mediators appear to be operant – e.g. transforming growth factors (TGF $\alpha$ and $\beta$), prostaglandin $E_2$, interleukin-6 and interleukin-1$\beta$ (this is the mediator of hypercalcemia in myeloma and was previously known as osteoclast-activating factor or OAF).

9. As opposed to PTHrP, LOH increases serum phosphorus, does not produce phosphaturia, and does not elevate urinary cAMP.

10. Rarely, some lymphomas can produce hypercalcemia through excessive $1,25(OH)_2$ D production.

## Granulomatous Disease

1. Best described in sarcoidosis (17% incidence) but can be associated with tuberculosis, leprosy, histoplasmosis, coccidioidomycosis, berylliosis and certain lymphomas.

2. Pathophysiology is the derangement of vitamin D metabolism. Vitamin D and 25-OH D levels are normal but $1,25 (OH)_2$ D levels are increased.

3. Macrophages activated by $\gamma$-interferon promote the hydroxylation of 25-OH D to $1,25(OH)_2$ D. This can be thwarted by glucocorticoids (chloroquine may also be effective in patients who cannot tolerate glucocorticoids).

## Immobilization

1. Patients at highest risk are those with rapid bone turnover – e.g. growing children, Paget's disease.

2. Suppressed $1,25 (OH)_2$ D and PTH levels.

3. Mobilization, if possible, is the most important physiologic adjunct to treatment.

## Milk–Alkali Syndrome

1. Associated with large milk and absorbable alkali consumption.

2. Deterioration of renal function with soft tissue calcification.

3. Rarely seen today, except that some 'over the counter' antacids have alkali and calcium. The additional use of thiazide diuretics can be potentiating.

## Non-Parathyroid Endocrine Disease

1. Thyrotoxicosis increases bone turnover with the catabolic effects predominating over the anabolic. Hypercalciuria is common but overt hypercalcemia is uncommon.

2. Adrenal insufficiency results in non-aldosterone-mediated renal enhancement of sodium reabsorption. This is paralleled by increased calcium reabsorption. There may be increased bone efflux of calcium as well.

## Vitamin D Toxicity

1. Usually a result of inadvertant oversight in treated hypoparathyroidism. Rarely is it by intent, but it may occur in 'health enthusiasts'. It has also been seen as a result of erratic fortification of milk.

2. PTH is initially suppressed but may become more elevated with progressive renal insufficiency. Indeed, renal insufficiency is a risk since the increased absorption of both calcium and phosphorus result in their solubility product being exceeded.

3. Corticosteroids are the mainstay of therapy – their use may have to be prolonged because of the long half-life of vitamin D. Hepatic enzyme induction may also be attempted (e.g. glutethimide) with acute toxic overdose.

## Vitamin A Toxicity

1. May be enhanced if some amount of vitamin D is also taken (because of their synergistic effect). Vitamin A, by itself, or in its different derivatives (e.g. even 13-cis-retinoic acid used in acne treatment) can produce hypercalcemia. Thus, use of derivatives warrants the ancillary monitoring of serum calcium levels.

2. Although medication discontinuance will eventually produce normocalcemia, corticosteroids may hasten the process.

## Medication-Mediated Hypercalcemia

1. Thiazides – the major mechanism is increased renal reabsorption of calcium, but an additional effect may be the potentiation of PTH action on bone.

   a. Conversely, chronic thiazide use may also be 'beneficial' in diminishing the risk of osteoporosis.

b. The relative decrease in renal calcium excretion also makes thiazide use a potential therapy in the treatment of idiopathic hypercalciuria and its related stone disease.

c. The ability of thiazides to produce significant hypercalcemia may be a type of 'stress test' that unmasks underlying endocrine pathology (e.g. hyperparathyroidism).

2. Lithium – the mechanism is a change in the PTH 'set point' so that a higher level of calcium is necessary for parathormone feedback suppression.

**Familial Hypocalciuric Hypercalcemia**
1. Autosomal dominant with 100% penetrance. Diagnosis is based on persistent hypercalcemia in the presence of low urinary calcium.

2. Renal function and bone density are normal. The PTH level is 'inappropriately' high for the level of hypercalcemia. Histology may show mild diffuse hyperplasia.

3. Associated hypermagnesemia.

4. Patients who inadvertantly undergo parathyroidectomy usually maintain their persistent hypercalcemia (or become hypocalcemic if extirpation is excessive – there does not seem to be any 'middle ground').

**'Other' Causes of Hypercalcemia**
1. Idiopathic Hypercalcemia in Infancy – rare syndrome perhaps caused by increased maternal vitamin D levels or sensitivity (characteristic facial features of hypoplastic mandible and low set ears; supravalvular aortic stenosis; mental retardation and abnormal dentition) – these may be mimicked by the offspring of rabbits fed large amounts of vitamin D during gestation.

2. Hypercalcemia may occur during acute renal failure – although there may be initial hypocalcemia, a transient PTH–calcium feedback 'imbalance' could result in temporary hypercalcemia.

**MANAGEMENT OF ACUTE HYPERCALCEMIA** (Table 22-1)

1. General Measures

a. Saline Diuresis – the ability to decrease serum calcium should be a 'mirror image' of the rate of its accumulation.

## TABLE 22-1. MANAGEMENT OF ACUTE HYPERCALCEMIA

---

General Measures
    Saline
    Loop Diuretics
    Treatment of Underlying Disorder
Calcitonin
Plicamycin
Gallium Nitrate
Phosphate
Bisphosphonates

---

Mechanisms of action include increase in glomerular filtration rate, reversal of proximal tubule sodium-linked calcium reabsorption and distal saline-mediated calciuresis. Initial infusion rate is up to 300–500 ml/hour (hemodynamic monitoring may be necessary).

b. Loop diuretics (they should never be administered without saline infusion or dehydration will be aggravated) – they work by inhibiting reabsorption of sodium (and calcium) in the Loop of Henle, the site of absorption of 25% of filtered calcium. They also lessen the likelihood of fluid overload and allow for maximal safe saline infusion rates. Dose: 40–80 mg of furosemide every 1–2 hours, as necessary. Concerns include hypophosphatemia, hypokalemia and hypomagnesemia. They are not a long-term solution.

c. Treatment of underlying disorder – usually not of immediate help but can be adjunctive (e.g. steroids, when appropriate).

2. Calcitonin – acts on osteoclasts and has an additional hypercalciuric effect. Dose is 2–8 IU/kg/day in two to four divided doses. A nasal preparation may be a future alternative. Acts within 2 hours with maximal effect in 6 hours. Tachyphylaxis develops but effect lasts only several days (duration may be enhanced with steroids). This tachyphylaxis, which is generally not seen when calcitonin is used to treat Paget's disease or osteoporosis, may be a function of the greater degree of bone turnover seen in acute hypercalcemic states. The drug is also expensive (up to $ 500/day).

3. Plicamycin (Mithramycin) – inhibits bone reabsorption. Dose is 25 µg/kg infused over 4–6 hours. May be repeated every 2 days. Onset: 24 hours; maximal effect: 48 hours. Toxicity – thrombocytopenia and qualitative platelet defects; renal and hepatic injury.

4. Gallium Nitrate – administered as a continuous infusion (200 mg/ m² in 1 liter of fluid daily over 5 days). Its site of action is the bone crystal. The onset in 2 days; maximal effect in 6–9 days; duration: 1 week. Side-effects are nausea, hypotension, renal insufficiency, electrolyte imbalance (hypocalcemia, hypophosphatemia) and anemia.

5. Phosphate – effective intravenously but very dangerous (calcium phosphate precipitation) and should not be considered except in dire circumstances. Oral phosphate is generally not helpful in the acute setting and, in high doses, is associated with diarrhea.

6. Bisphosphonates – this is now a very formidable class of drugs in the management of hypercalcemia. Unlike the P–O–P bond found in pyrophosphates, the P–C–P bond in bisphosphonates renders them resistant to phosphatases (hence, extremely long half-life). They are excreted unchanged, in the urine. They inhibit osteoclast function and viability. Etidronate was the first drug to be used. Pamidronate (aminohydroxypropylidene bisphosphonate, APD, Aredia) is more potent and effective. (Clodronate trials were discontinued in the USA because of possible leukemogenic effects but this was never clearly substantiated.) Generally given as a single 60–90 mg, intravenous infusion, and it is highly effective. Although initially approved for a 24-hour infusion, good outcomes have been shown when infused over much shorter periods of time. It has a 10–14-day duration of action. Side-effects include fever, hypophosphatemia, hypocalcemia and hypomagnesemia.

# 23

# PRIMARY HYPERPARATHYROIDISM

1. Etiology

   a. Generally sporadic in incidence, but prior neck irradiation appears to be a risk factor.

   b. Adenomas (which comprise 85% of cases) appear to be primarily clonal in nature and both adenomas and hyperplasia (remaining 15% of cases – carcinoma is probably no more than 1–2% of cases) are associated with abnormalities in chromosome 11. Familial cases (seen in Multiple Endocrine Neoplasia Type I, MEN-I) have a higher incidence of hyperplasia and have been associated with deletions in the q13 region of chromosome 11 – affected individuals may develop hyperparathyroidism because of an inherited defect on one chromosome and an acquired defect on another ('double hit' hypothesis).

   c. Despite hyperfunction, the disorder appears to be a 'set point' dysregulation in that parathyroid hormone (PTH) can be both stimulated and suppressed – but at a higher set point. This creates a paradox in therapy – if you place patients on a low calcium diet (to prevent hypercalcemia), you can worsen the dissolution of bone. On the other hand, trying to suppress the PTH by increasing the serum calcium (even without necessarily giving calcium – e.g. thiazide diuretics) can worsen the hypercalcemia.

2.  The prevalence is probably about 1:1000 – incidence increases with age; three times more common in women.

    a.  Although of historical interest, the 'stones, moans, and abdominal groans' are rarely seen today – rather, widespread use of 'biochemical screening' uncovers most cases.

    b.  Once diagnosed, some patients may retrospectively complain of having had subtle manifestations e.g. 'mild' constipation, history of hypertension, increased urinary frequency, pruritis, gastrointestinal symptoms (e.g. 'dyspepsia'), emotional lability, depression and other psychologic symptoms. Many patients, however, are truly asymptomatic.

    c.  Signs and symptoms can be categorized based on:

        i.   The effects of the hypercalcemia – this is summarized in Chapter 22 and includes neurologic, muscular, gastrointestinal, dermatologic and renal manifestations. Reversible left ventricular hypertrophy has also been described in a significant number of individuals.

        ii.  The effects of hyperparathyroidism on bone – deformities, tenderness, fractures, ectopic calcification (e.g. band keratopathy, chondrocalcinosis).

        iii. Propensity to nephrocalcinosis and metabolic stone disease. There also appears to be an increased incidence of myocardial and aortic and mitral valve calcification.

        iv.  Rarely is an abnormal parathyroid gland locally symptomatic or palpable on physical examination.

3.  The differential diagnosis encompasses all other etiologies of hypercalcemia including familial hypocalciuric hypercalcemia (often, the clinical context will be helpful in category elimination, but this may not be immediately apparent if asymptomatic hypercalcemia is the initial presentation).

    a.  Radiologic studies to 'rule in' hyperparathyroidism are of ancillary interest (e.g. bone cyst, demineralization – loss of bone can be generalized or produce characteristic 'salt and pepper' changes in the skull; loss of periodontal bone, resorption of distal phalangeal tufts or distal clavicles, 'widening' of the symphysis pubis and ectopic calcification).

b. The diagnosis is best secured by demonstrating an 'inappropriate' elevation of serum PTH in the presence of hypercalcemia.

   i. Multiple determinations are necessary to establish consistency.

   ii. If available, prior calcium determinations demonstrating a normal level are useful.

   iii. Ionized calcium determinations (unless there are serum protein abnormalities) are not necessary. The values would be elevated in primary hyperparathyroidism.

c. Ancillary tests may be useful for re-enforcement of diagnosis (or to rule out other etiologies), but they do not supplant the value of PTH assays. They include:

   i. Nephrogenous c'AMP – increased in primary hyperparathyroidism. A variation of this test is the demonstration of high basal levels, and failure to increase following exogenous PTH administration.

   ii. Serum phosphorus and phosphate clearance (tubular reabsorption of phosphate). Serum phosphorus levels are classically decreased and renal phosphate clearance increased (tubular reabsorption of phosphate is decreased) in primary hyperparathyroidism.

   iii. Serum alkaline phosphatase – generally increased. It is a measure of bone turnover, more specifically of the osteoblastic component.

   iv. Urine calcium excretion – tends to be increased. Since a direct tubular effect of PTH is to increase calcium reabsorption, significant hypercalcemia is needed to produce demonstrable hypercalciuria.

   v. Serum bicarbonate – can be decreased in primary hyperparathyroidism as a result of a PTH-mediated renal tubular acidosis.

   vi. Serum magnesium – generally decreased in hyperparathyroidism because of increased renal clearance and loss of bone storage, although it may be normal or even rarely increased.

vii. 'Old fashioned tests' such as 'calcium deprivation', 'phosphate deprivation', EDTA infusion, and 'calcium loading' are only of historical interest and can even be dangerous.

  d. Radiologic studies for localization include:

    i. Barium esophagram – low yield and not cost effective.

    ii. CT, MRI of neck – preoperative use of either test is an accepted standard.

    iii. Ultrasonography of neck – generally not cost effective.

    iv. Dual isotope subtraction radioscintigraphy ($^{201}$Tl is taken up by both parathyroid and thyroid tissue, $^{99m}$Tc only by thyroid) has proven more valuable in theory than in actuality.

4. Surgery is the only definitive therapy – removal of the adenoma or subtotal parathyroidectomy for hyperplasia.

  a. It should be performed by a skilled and experienced surgeon, well-cognizant of both normal and aberrant sites of pathology.

  b. Preoperative arteriography and/or venography (with sampling) is generally not indicated unless a prior procedure has been performed. (In selected cases, angiographic ablation can be used for treatment of mediastinal adenomas.)

  c. Clinically significant preoperative hypercalcemia can be managed along previously discussed medical guidelines. For the patient with less clinically significant hypercalcemia who wishes to 'temporize' prior to surgery, oral phosphate therapy may be of value (diarrhea is a potential side-effect; also, by decreasing serum calcium, PTH is augmented).

  d. Postoperatively, hypocalcemia is almost invariable, and calcium infusion will be necessary. Reasons include:

    i. 'Calcium-starved' bones.

    ii. Secondary to hypomagnesemia (correctable).

    iii. Suppression of normal parathyroid tissue (this will 'self-correct' unless too much tissue was removed for the treatment of hyperplasia or vascular supply to normal tissue was compromised).

e. Although hypocalcemia may persist following discharge and the need for oral calcium supplement may continue, 'overtreatment' with calcium and vitamin D should be avoided to allow for normal endogenous resurgence of remaining parathyroid tissue.

f. Although not relevant to the management of single adenomas, autotransplantation of parathyroid tissue to an accessible region (e.g. forearm) at the time of surgical correction of hyperplasia can both prevent postoperative hypoparathyroidism and easily correct future hyperparathyroidism

5. There is controversy as to whether patients with mild asymptomatic hyperparathyroidism require surgery.

   a. This would not be controversial if there were a safe and effective medical therapy.

   b. Prior to the advent of routine serum calcium screening, there were probably large numbers of 'undetected' patients whose health was seemingly not so compromised as to have sought medical care – is this applicable to the management of 'chemical' hyperparathyroidism today?

   c. There is controversy based on conflicting data as to the predictability of the loss of bone mass over time in hyperparathyroidism.

   d. The National Institutes of Health, NIH (Potts, J. et al., *J. Bone Min. Res. 6* – suppl. 2, 1992) developed a consensus position with the following suggested guidelines for surgery:

      i. Markedly elevated serum calcium – 1.0–1.6 mg/dl greater than normal.

      ii. History of one episode of life-threatening hypercalcemia.

      iii. Creatinine clearance reduced by at least 30%.

      iv. Presence of renal stones on abdominal radiograph.

      v. Urinary calcium excretion greater than 400 mg/24 hours.

      vi. Bone mass reduced greater than 2.0 SD below normal.

      vii. There was no consensus that hypertension and neuropsychiatric symptoms, *per se,* are surgical indications, but surgery may be preferred in some patients for the following reasons:

(a) Patient desire for 'definitive' treatment.

(b) Difficulty in consistent follow up.

(c) Coexistent illness complicating management.

(d) Patient is under age 50.

viii. On the other hand, patients who might reasonably be followed on an ongoing expectant basis include:

(a) Patients over age 50 who do not meet suggested criteria for surgical intervention.

(b) Those with precluding medical or constitutional problems, based on clinical judgement.

# 24

# HYPOCALCEMIA

Hypocalcemic States: Etiologies
Hypoparathyroidism

## HYPOCALCEMIC STATES: ETIOLOGIES

1. Hypoparathyroidism.

2. Inadequacy of vitamin D (decreased synthesis, activation, effect).

3. Malabsorption – binding of oral calcium to fatty acids producing intraluminal 'soaps'.

4. Hyperphosphatemia – e.g. renal failure, tumor lysis syndrome.

5. Pancreatitis – formation of calcium 'soaps' in areas of normal fat deposition (activated by pancreatic lipase). Inadequate parathyroid hormone (PTH) (perhaps mediated by hypomagnesemia or glucagon) is a secondary phenomenon.

6. Following parathyroid surgery – it may be transient secondary to normal parathyroid tissue suppression during the hyperparathyroid state, or permanent secondary to excessive parathyroid tissue extirpation.

7. Rapidly growing osteoblastic metastases.

8. Severe illness and toxic shock syndrome. Implicated mechanisms include hypomagnesemia, hypoalbuminemia, and renal failure.

9. Calcium chelators – e.g. citrate in anticoagulated blood, radiocontrast (usually not clinically significant but it may be 'regionally relevant').

10. Neonatal hypocalcemia – seen in prematurity, children of mothers with diabetes or primary hyperparathyroidism.

11. Hypercalcitoninemic states are not clinically relevant in producing hypocalcemia (it is the associated tumor that is clinically relevant).

## HYPOPARATHYROIDISM

1. Etiology

   a. Most commonly idiopathic – this can be sporadic or associated with multiple endocrine deficiency states (the latter tends to manifest at an earlier age, often associated with difficult-to-treat mucocutaneous candidiasis).

   b. Also seen as a complication of previous (usually extensive) neck surgery (e.g. 'total' thyroidectomy for cancer); may occur because of 'physical removal' or 'vascular compromise' of parathyroid tissue.

c. Hypoparathyroidism is associated with hypomagnesemia. Hypomagnesemia results in both a decrease in PTH response and effect.

d. Very rare causes include the production of a biologically imperfect parathyroid hormone, metastatic disease to the parathyroids and radioactive iodine therapy.

e. Parathyroid hormone resistance states:

   i. Type I – associated with an abnormal G protein. Urinary c'AMP does not increase in response to PTH. Subdivided into:

      (a) Type Ia – those with associated somatic features (short stature, obesity, mental retardation, short metacarpal or metatarsal bones – usually the fourth, and this produces a 'dimpling' on fist making).

      (b) Type Ib – those without the somatic features. The inheritance of both Type Ia and Ib may be X-linked dominant, but the genetics has not been completely resolved.

   ii. Type II – normal c'AMP response to PTH; the defect is apparently distal to c'AMP formation.

   iii. Pseudo-pseudohypoparathyroidism – those with the somatic syndrome but without the biochemical abnormalities.

   iv. 'Pseudo-hyperparathyroidism' – so designated because it is associated with osteitis fibrosa cystica.

2. The clinical features are related to the metabolic and structural effects of hypocalcemia and its severity. Effects include:

a. Bone – decreased resorption with imperfect bone remodelling and turnover (structurally most evident in bones and teeth of children who develop hypoparathyroidism when still in the active stages of physical development). A corollary is the tendency to metastatic calcification (e.g. lens, basal ganglia).

b. Kidney – decreased phosphate and increased calcium

clearance (although this may not be reflective in 'absolute' urinary concentration of calcium).

   c. Gastrointestinal – decreased absorption of calcium secondary to inhibition of active vitamin D.

3. The diagnosis is secured by confirming an inappropriately low PTH level (except for the rare causes of biologically inactive hormone or hormone resistance) in the presence of hypocalcemia (hyperphosphatemia is an invariable concomitant).

4. Treatment

   a. Ideally treated with parathyroid hormone (except if hypomagnesemia is the cause) but (despite the availability of recombinant human 1-34 PTH) there are significant logistic issues – cost, need for parenteral administration, short half-life, 'orphan drug' status.

   b. Calcium and vitamin D are the mainstays of therapy. Calcium intake should be at least 2 g/day. Although there is impairment of 'activation'of vitamin D in hypoparathyroidism, large doses may obviate this. Usual daily dose of vitamin D (the plant or pharmacologic vitamin D) is 50 000 to 200 000 International Units (IU; 40 000 Units = 1 mg). The advantages of using vitamin D rather than the activated forms (1,25-OH form is calcitriol or Rocaltrol, 1-OH form is calcifediol or Calderol) are savings in cost and a greater interim period of observation prior to the development of potential hypercalcemic toxicity. Conversely, calcitriol acts earlier and if toxicity does occur, it is shorter-lived. If calcitriol is used, dose range is 0.25–5 μg/day. Alternatively, dihydrotachysterol (which acts like 1-OH D) can be used at dose ranges of 0.2–1 mg/day (it also is expensive, and has a shorter half-life than vitamin D).

   c. A low sodium diet combined with the use of a thiazide may, by itself, obviate the need for vitamin D (calcium must continue to be taken) – an additional advantage is its potential effect on minimizing urinary calcium wastage.

   d. Note: Vitamin D (and analogs) are not a PTH replacement; they do not directly alter the hyperphosphatemia. Allowances for this must be made and something less than a normal serum calcium level (as long as there is clinical stability) may have to be accepted.

# 25

# METABOLIC BONE DISEASE

Paget's Disease of Bone
Rickets and Osteomalacia
Osteoporosis
      Relevant Clinical Issues
      Therapeutic Options

## PAGET'S DISEASE OF BONE

1.  Paget's disease is a disease of increased bone turnover (initiated by bone resorption) and remodelling but with a resultant imperfect and deformed bone, hence osteitis deformans.

2.  There is a higher incidence in males – in both sexes, the incidence increases with advanced age.

3.  The etiology is unclear.

    a.  There is clustering in families and it is more prevalent in Western Europe and the USA (it is uncommon in Africa and Asia).

    b.  Inclusion bodies are noted in osteoclasts. This raises the issue of a viral etiology: a paramyxovirus is a purported agent.

4.  As neither normal remodelling 'cues' nor boundaries are obeyed, this gives rise to two categories of manifestations:

    a. Bone

        i.   Manifestations include deformity (axial skeleton and skull are disproportionately affected), pain, pathologic fracture, increased incidence of benign (giant cell) and malignant (osteogenic sarcoma) tumors, vertebral-basilar insufficiency (secondary to platybasia) and deafness (usually associated with bony abnormalities and hence is a 'conduction' deafness as opposed to VIII Nerve compression).

        ii.  Patients may stereotypically present with increased skull size ('hats no longer fit properly') – especially in the bitemporal diameter ('old-fashioned football helmet'), 'saber shin' and 'bow legs' (genu varum).

        iii. X-rays show a characteristic appearance ('cotton wool', 'paint-brushed'), even if clinical symptoms are localized to other regions of the anatomy. Asymptomatic lesions may be noted on skeletal survey. Bone scan demonstrates increased uptake in active lesions.

        iv.  The serum calcium level is generally normal – except during immobilization. The serum alkaline phosphatase, as a marker of increased bone formation, is elevated (sometimes levels are extremely high) and is a good index of the extent of the disease. Urinary hydroxyproline excretion, as a marker of osteolysis, may be elevated as well. In response to therapy, the hydroxyproline excretion is more likely to improve earlier than the alkaline phosphatase elevation.

b. Increased circulation to the sites of the disease – as a result of increased arterio-venous anastamotic channels.

i. Local warmth and bruits are features. There is a greater propensity for Pagetic bone to bleed if surgery is performed.

ii. The resultant increase in cardiac output can produce a 'high output failure'.

5. Therapy

a. Calcitonin – synthetic salmon calcitonin is the variety most commonly used. It is given subcutaneously (self-administered) on a daily basis. Starting dose: 25–50 Medical Research Council or MRC units. The dosage can be increased to 50–100 MRC units daily – clinical and laboratory parameters are used as guidelines. Dose frequency may be decreased (e.g. to four or three times per week) and courses may be intermittent (rather than continuous). It can be given over many years. A nasal preparation may be a future alternative. Side-effects include nausea, flushing, vomiting, diarrhea and local pain – bedtime administration or decreased dosage may be ameliorative. Resistance may develop over time in a minority of patients (antibody formation) – human calcitonin or bisphosphonates may be substituted at that time.

b. Bisphosphonates – the greatest experience has been with Etidronate (5 mg/kg/day), which must be given in the absence of food to maximize absorption. When this lesser dose is used, resorption is inhibited (a greater dose of 20 mg/kg/day would inhibit both bone formation and resorption and can lead to osteoporosis). It is generally given in an intermittent pattern (duration of each cycle up to 6 months) and reinstituted when relapse occurs. Side effects include diarrhea and tendency for elevation of serum phosphate. APD (Pamidronate, amino-hydroxypropylidene bisphosphonate, Aredia) may become a preferred treatment because bone formation is not inhibited.

    c. Plicamycin (Mithramycin) – by itself, it is recommended only for episodic use for 'focused' problems (e.g. severe bone pain, nerve entrapment).

## RICKETS AND OSTEOMALACIA

1. Rickets and osteomalacia represent a syndrome complex of multiple etiologies, the common denominator being mineralization failure. If it affects the epiphyseal growth plate in children, the term, rickets, is used. Post-bone maturation, it is a 'softening' of bone or osteomalacia.

    a. The difference is not merely taxonomic, as permanent skeletal changes can occur in children with associated physical features – e.g. platybasia, 'bossing' of the skull, 'rachitic rosary' and 'Harrison's grooves', genu varum and genu valgum. These may additionally have physiologic consequences (e.g. restrictive lung disease). Prematurity gives an additional 'background of vulnerability'.

    b. Adults with osteomalacia may experience weakness, pain and pathologic fractures.

    c. Histologic features are characteristic and demonstrate a disparity between bone mineral density and osteoid. X-ray studies, especially early, may not be able to implicate impaired mineralization as the cause of decreased bone mass. The presence of 'pseudofractures', however (lines of Looser and Milkman – felt to result from bone susceptibility to schism at the site of arterial cross-over) helps to confirm the diagnosis.

2. Clinical Syndromes

    a. Vitamin D Deficiency or Inadequacy (Table 25-1)

### TABLE 25-1. ETIOLOGIES OF VITAMIN D DEFICIENCY OR INADEQUACY

| |
|---|
| Dietary |
| Malabsorption |
| Renal Disease |
| Anticonvulsant Therapy |
| Congenital Defects |

i.   May be dietary – theoretically, dietary sources are not necessary, as humans are capable of meeting their own needs. This ability decreases with age – elderly have diminished vitamin D-synthetic ability. Dark-skinned people with decreased sunlight exposure who do not have dietary adequacy (further, vitamin D supplementation of milk may be erratic and unreliable) are at highest risk. (The epidemiology of rickets at the time of the Industrial Revolution in England is a compelling example of how the convergence of risk factors can lead to overt disease.)

ii.  May be malabsorption – vitamin D is fat soluble and undergoes (with its active products) enterohepatic circulation. Thus, there may be a superimposed depletion of existing stores (in addition to a primary malabsorption of dietary Vitamin D). Calcium malabsorption can further compound the clinical picture.

iii. Renal Disease (structural or functional) – any etiology that impairs 1-hydroxylase (a crucial enzyme activator of vitamin D) activity. Renal failure further compounds the problem through phosphate retention (which is additionally inhibitory to the 1-hydroxylase enzyme). Metabolic acidosis augments demineralization of bone.

iv.  Anticonvulsant therapy (diphenylhydantoin and phenobarbital) – appears to inhibit 25-hydroxylase (another enzyme activator of vitamin D), but there may be additional effects.

v.   Congenital Defects

     (a) Type I 'Vitamin D-Dependent Rickets' – congenital 1-hydroxylase deficiency; responds to pharmacologic therapy with 1, 25-OH vitamin D (calcitriol, Rocaltrol). May be mimicked by rare tumors which elaborate a 1-hydroxylase inhibitor.

     (b) Type II – resistance to 1,25 dihydroxy vitamin D. A 'receptor defect'.

vi.  Laboratory features include a low to normal serum calcium and depressed serum phosphate levels, elevated alkaline phosphatase (all the result of secondary hyperparathyroidism – this becomes even more exaggerated with disease progression) as well as increased serum parathyroid hormone (PTH), increased urine cAMP and decreased urinary calcium. Additionally helpful are serum 25-hydroxy vitamin D and 1,25 dihydroxy vitamin D measurements (be mindful of seasonal and geographic variation and effect of bodily habitus).

vii. Therapy requires adequate calcium and vitamin D replacement but in a manner that individualizes the patients' needs. For example:

(a) Patients with renal disease may not respond to 'standard' vitamin D, but may require calcitriol.

(b) Correction of an underlying malabsorption (e.g. gluten-induced enteropathy, Crohn's disease in remission) will have a beneficial effect and may result in lowered dosages of medications. Conversely, the active phase of malabsorption-producing disease of any type may require higher dosages of calcium and vitamin D.

(c) Although the average daily recommended dietary allowance (RDA) for vitamin D is 400 International Units (IU)/day, initial therapy for simple vitamin D deficiency states should be 5000 IU/day for 2–3 months. Associated calcium intake should be at least 2–3 g/day, because the hypocalcemia can worsen early in treatment as 'starving bones' deposit calcium salts. The serum phosphorus tends to rise earlier and for that reason (as well as avoidance of worsening the hypocalcemic state), supplemental phosphorus is not indicated. Within several weeks, there should be a decrease in both PTH and alkaline phosphatase levels and with their ultimate normalization (and normalization of serum calcium and phosphorus), vitamin D supplementation can be reduced to standard daily replacement of 400 IU/day (in the elderly, 800 IU/day).

(d) If the primary cause of malabsorption cannot be corrected, the relative vitamin D deficiency must be 'overcome' with exuberant dosing (up to 200 000 IU/day, orally, but vitamin D can also be given by intramuscular or intravenous routes). By analogy, vitamin D 'resistant' states must be treated with either calcitriol or with titration of supraphysiologic doses of Vitamin D, with regular monitoring of serum calcium, phosphorus and alkaline phosphatase levels.

b.  Phosphate Deficiency

i.  Dietary inadequacy or phosphate malabsorption.

ii.  Renal phosphate wasting.

(a) Congenital X-linked disorder – may also be associated with impaired intestinal absorption of phosphate and calcium.

(b) Despite a secondary hyperparathyroidism, the phosphate wasting seen in this disorder is a primary process.

(c) Treatment requires large and frequent doses of oral phosphate (vitamin D supplementation may be helpful).

iii.  Renal Tubular Disease

(a) A wide range of congenital (e.g Fanconi's syndrome, Wilson's disease) and acquired (e.g. heavy metal toxicity, myeloma) diseases are capable of producing this.

(b) A rare phosphate-wasting syndrome has been described in certain tumors (e.g. prostate cancer, sclerosing hemangioma). As a corollary, the syndrome can be reversed if the tumor is totally extirpated. A characteristic biochemical feature is a low 1,25 dihydroxy vitamin D level.

(c) The clinical syndrome can additionally be associated with chronic acidosis, inhibitors of mineralization (e.g. bisphosphonates, fluorides, aluminum) and with hypophosphatasia. It is possible that a sustained acid load presented to the body, over time (e.g. as with a high protein diet), can lead to progressive bone demineralization, even though there is no overt metabolic acidosis.

## OSTEOPOROSIS

### Relevant Clinical Issues
1. Osteoporosis is best defined as an absolute decrease in bone mass. There are no qualitative abnormalities *per se* and the mineralized to non-mineralized ratio of bone remains unchanged.

2. In many ways, it is a 'natural' or (better said) an inexorable process of ageing. In most humans, bone mass tends to 'peak' in the thirties and there is a progressive decline thereafter. Proclivity to degree of bone loss is a function of the relationship between magnitude of maximal bone density and rate of loss (the ability to make bone decreases with time and without superimposed pathologic conditions, the degree of bone resorption remains constant).

3. Were it not for the clinical consequences of osteoporosis, this discussion would be academic. Statistics, however, related to fracture (and its associated morbidity and mortality) are staggering – e.g. 40% of women over the age of 80 have had at least one fracture; there are 1/4 million hip fractures per year in the USA, and by age 90, 32% of women and 17% of men will have had at least one hip fracture. Perhaps 10% or more of these result in perihospitalization death from ancillary complications, while a substantial number of those who survive are relegated to a nursing home existence. Societal costs are in the billions of dollars when direct and indirect costs are calculated.

4. Because most fractures are not spontaneous but rather the result of trauma (e.g. accidental fall), other factors are operant and are also more common in the elderly – e.g. problems of balance, vision, hearing and 'righting response'; muscular atrophy; ancillary diseases (e.g. cardiovascular, cerebrovascular, diabetes) and medications (e.g. medications associated with altered mental status or orthostatic hypotension). Still, the consequences of a fall could be averted with stronger bone.

5. Although idiopathic (or primary) osteoporosis has no fundamental etiology, there are risk factors that affect propensity and degree – this pattern of osteoporosis also affects trabecular bone disproportionate to cortical (hence vertebral compression fracture and hip fracture). This type of osteoporosis is sometimes referred to as Type II. Significant risk factors include (Table 25-2):

## TABLE 25-2. RISK FACTORS ASSOCIATED WITH OSTEOPOROSIS

Genetic
Race
Dietary Factors
Gastrointestinal Disease
Life-Style
Estrogen Deficiency States
Other Endocrine and Metabolic Diseases
       Thyrotoxicosis
       Hyperparathyroidism
       Glucocorticoid Excess
       Diabetes Mellitus
       Liver Disease
       Renal Failure
Juvenile Osteoporosis
Abnormalities of Collagen Synthesis
Vitamin C Deficiency
Tumor Invasion of Bone
Drugs
Cardiac Transplantation

a.  Genetics – there is a greater clustering within families.

b.  Race – Whites are more affected than Blacks.

c.  Dietary – inadequate calcium intake over time will decrease maximal bone calcium. While deficiency should be avoided, there is no indication for consumption of 'mega doses' of calcium in otherwise normal individuals as a preventive measure. Other nutritional deficiencies may be additionally relevant.

d.  Gastrointestinal Disease – malabsorption and maldigestion syndromes, cirrhosis, obstructive jaundice.

e.  Life-Style – decreased physical activity (even a 'mundane' activity such as walking can be beneficial), smoking, alcohol, caffeine intake and 'bodily thinness' increase the risk of osteoporosis.

   f.   Estrogen deficiency can be an independent cause or it can augment a pre-existing tendency – this is sometimes referred to as Type I osteopenia.

       i.   The specific cause of the estrogen deficiency is not relevant – it can be 'physiologic' (postmenopausal), primary hypogonadism (e.g. Turner's syndrome) or secondary hypogonadism (e.g. prolactinoma, hemochromatosis, exercise-mediated). Although it is an appreciated fact that a routine of active running can induce menstrual disturbances, bone mass is unaffected except when there is amenorrhea.

      ii.   Women whose irregular menstrual cycles are more normalized with cyclic medroxyprogesterone have improved bone density.

   iii.   A significant mechanism of action appears to be the 'blunting', by estrogen, of bone sensitivity to PTH.

   iv.   Because obesity produces increased (peripheral) estrogen synthesis and may augment bone 'stress' ('piezoelectrode effect'), this may help explain its beneficial effect.

      v.   Women with higher circulating endogenous estrogens tend to have high androgen levels as well – this may be an augmenting factor.

   vi.   Estrogen may play a role in enhancing 1-hydroxylation of vitamin D in osteoporosis.

   g.   Other endocrinologic and metabolic diseases associated with osteoporosis include:

       i.   Hyperthyroidism – it represents more of a problem with long-term replacement therapy 'overdose' than with Graves' disease, as bone loss in the latter is potentially reversible.

      ii.   Hyperparathyroidism – cortical bone is more significantly affected than is trabecular bone.

   iii.   Glucocorticoid Excess.

         (a) Mechanisms

             (1) Collagenolysis of bone matrix,

(2) Decreased calcium absorption with secondary hyperparathyroidism,

(3) Increased sensitivity to PTH.

(b) Osteoporosis is also a potential complication of replacement therapy in Addison's disease.

iv. Diabetes Mellitus.

v. Liver Disease.

vi. Renal Failure.

vii. Androgen Deficiency States.

h. Other associated causes include juvenile osteoporosis, abnormalities of collagen synthesis (e.g. osteogenesis imperfecta, Marfan's syndrome), immobilization states, rheumatoid arthritis, vitamin C deficiency (impaired hydroxyproline and hydroxylysine synthesis), involvement of bone by tumor (e.g. myeloma, leukemia), drugs (e.g. heparin, chemotherapy, cyclosporine) and cardiac transplantation.

6. Clinical manifestations of osteopenia are:

a. Those associated with the physical loss of bone and the manner in which the awareness of that bone loss is brought to medical attention (e.g. back pain secondary to a compression fracture, hip fracture, progressive loss of height – due to anterior 'wedging' of vertebrae resulting in a kyphotic posture).

b. Non-osseous manifestations of underlying disorders which may have either a primary or an augmenting role (e.g. other clinical features of estrogen deficiency or Cushing's syndrome).

7. Bone density can be quantified to assess the degree of osteopenia (and thus the clinical risk) as well as serve as a guideline prior to institution of a therapeutic program.

a. Examples of people who would benefit from screening include:

i. Estrogen-deficient women (for whatever reason) who would consider hormone replacement therapy based on their bone status.

    ii. Patients with 'hypercalcemia only' as a manifestation of their hyperparathyroidism, in whom a surgical procedure is being considered. The crucial issue in these and other related cases is whether a particular decision will be based upon the information obtained from bone density assessment. A bone density study in an otherwise healthy male or female, that would not result in a decision-making process, is not warranted.

  b. Technologies available for bone density:

    i. Conventional Radiography

      (a) Not clinically helpful because 30% of bone density must be lost before radiographs are 'positive'.

      (b) On the other hand, there are characteristic features seen once osteoporosis is evident.

        (1) Example no. 1 – in vertebral bodies, horizontal trabeculae are lost disproportionate to vertical trabeculae, end plates become more prominent ('picture frame effect') and concavities of opposing vertebral edges are noted because of the 'ease of protrusion' of discs into the vertebral bone ('codfish deformity').

        (2) Example no. 2 – there is a 'hierarchy' of loss of trabecular bone in the proximal femur.

    ii. Quantitative Computerized Tomography (QCT)

      (a) Measures the calcium density of trabecular bone (vertebral column). It is not affected by adjacent calcifications (e.g. bony sclerosis, 'hyperdense' collapsed vertebrae, calcific aorta). On the other hand, if the underlying disease state is associated with a greater tendency to cortical (rather than trabecular) bone loss (e.g. hyperparathyroidism, renal failure), the value of the QCT is less predictable.

      (b) It is more expensive and gives a greater radiation exposure (100 ×) than quantitative digital radiography – therefore, QCT may be helpful for initial screening but quantitative digital radiography can be used as follow up.

iii. Quantitative Digital Radiography (Also known as Dual Energy X-ray Absorptiometry or DEXA).

(a) It is best used to measure forearm bone density. It can also measure vertebral bone but, as noted above, measurements are affected by any kind of adjacent calcification.

(b) When available, it has supplanted Dual Photon Absorptiometry (DPA) – it has a shorter procedural time and is more reproducible; unlike DPA which requires radioactive $^{153}$gadolinium, DEXA uses conventional radiology.

**Therapeutic Options** (Table 25-3)

1. Avoidance of risk factors (as possible), exercise in moderation (this obviously will not be possible during the healing phase of a fracture). The role of environmental and situational factors in predisposing to falls cannot be minimized.

2. Adequacy of oral calcium intake – 2 g/day can significantly slow appendicular and axial bone loss in both normal and postmenopausal women. The monitoring of urinary calcium excretion may be helpful, as there is a subset of patients with a 'renal calcium leak':

### TABLE 25-3. THERAPEUTIC OPTIONS TO TREAT OSTEOPOROSIS

| |
|---|
| Risk Factor Avoidance |
| Adequacy of Calcium Intake |
| Vitamin D |
| Calcitonin |
| Bisphosphonates |
| Fluoride |
| Estrogens |
| Androgens |
| Parathyroid Hormone |
| Other Modalities |

    a. Patients found to be 'calcium wasters' should be placed on a low sodium diet.

    b. Secondary causes of hypercalciuria (e.g. acidosis, thyrotoxicosis) should be ruled out.

    c. These patients may benefit from thiazide therapy (hydrochlorthiazide, 50 mg, twice daily) – even patients without hypercalciuria who are placed on thiazide therapy may have an improved bone density and a decreased incidence of fracture, although this effect may be limited to the axial skeleton.

3. Vitamin D is not only of benefit when there is documented vitamin D deficiency (e.g. as with 25-hydroxy vitamin D levels less than 8 ng/ml), but in doses of 800 IU/day and with 1–2 g of supplemental calcium, it can reduce the risk of hip fracture in elderly women. Calcitriol (Rocaltrol) is best used in cases of renal insufficiency, but when used with supplemental calcium (1000 mg/day) with or without intranasal calcitonin, it can also prevent corticosteroid-mediated lumbar bone loss.

4. Calcitonin – can decrease or prevent trabecular bone loss, although probably only over the short term (1 year). It may contribute to a decrease in the risk for vertebral and hip fractures. Regular injections are required (at least 3 times/week), but calcitonin can also be absorbed through the nasal mucosa. The oral calcium intake must be adequate. An additional benefit is its analgesic effect that can facilitate earlier mobilization following fracture. It is expensive.

5. Bisphosphonates – studies have demonstrated increased vertebral (no apparent effect on cortical bone) bone density of 6% after 2 years of an intermittent treatment regime with etidronate (adequate oral calcium and vitamin D required). Etidronate is taken (400 mg/day) for 2 weeks every 3 months. The drug is poorly absorbed and must be taken on an empty stomach. Other related drugs that are potent inhibitors of bone resorption are alendronate and risendronate.

6. Fluoride – shown to increase vertebral bone density but the overall beneficial effect is controversial (e.g. trabecular bone may

benefit at the 'expense' of cortical bone and the incidence of hip fracture may be paradoxically higher). On the other hand, the use of an intermittent slow-release sodium fluoride (along with calcium citrate) increases vertebral bone density without decreasing the density of the radial shaft. Toxicities include gastrointestinal, and painful extremities (synovitis, ligamentous calcifications). It is not an approved therapy and is contraindicated in renal failure.

7. Estrogen – proven effective in prevention of bone loss from multiple sites.

   a. Recommended daily dose of at least 0.625 mg of conjugated estrogen or 25 μg of ethinyl estradiol, although transdermal estrogen appears equally effective.

   b. Can be taken with progesterone (this is necessary to prevent uterine cancer) without altering its efficacy (although some reduction in high-density lipoprotein will be a 'relative negative', with regard to lipid profile).

   c. Evidence suggests that the commitment to estrogen therapy must be long term in order to reap a sustained benefit on bone density in old age.

   d. Vertebral and hip bone density may be augmented by the combined use of estrogen and etidronate.

8. Although not discussed as widely because osteoporosis in men is less common than in women and menopause is a more gradual process, androgenic therapy can also prevent bone loss. As a corollary (androgenic side-effects notwithstanding), anabolic steroids may be beneficial in selected women.

9. Parathyroid hormone, 'paradoxically' (when combined with calcitriol), can increase trabecular bone (e.g. it can prevent estrogen deficiency-mediated bone loss in the lumbar spine of young women), but it is still an experimental protocol.

10. Potassium bicarbonate – the role of increased endogenous acid production over a lifetime (e.g. from dietary protein) and its long-term effect on bone dissolution, has resulted in studies which show increased bone formation and decreased bone dissolution with potassium bicarbonate supplement. The presumed benefit

is from its alkaline effect, but its future role in the management of osteoporosis remains to be seen.

11. Other classes of drugs under active consideration include flavonoids and non-steroidal anti-inflammatory agents.

# 26

# RENAL STONE DISEASE

General Considerations
Factors Relevant in Stone Formation
Clinical Approach to the Patient with Stone Disease
Calcium-Containing Stones
Struvite Stones
Uric Acid Stones
Cystine Stones

## GENERAL CONSIDERATIONS

1. Affects 0.2% of the population every year.

2. The necropsy prevalence of urinary tract stones is 5%, the lifetime prevalence is 10%.

3. Most stones form and pass 'silently' but larger 'staghorn' calculi remain, leading to acute and chronic complications.

4. Most renal stones are calcium containing. A corollary is their radiopacity.

5. The likelihood of recurrence with untreated pre-existing stone disease increases with time and reaches 50% at 10 years. The type of recurrent stone is usually of the same chemical nature as that of the antecedent one.

## FACTORS RELEVANT IN STONE FORMATION (Table 26-1)

1. The State of Saturation – an important therapeutic implication is the role of hydration in general therapy. It is obvious that by increasing the amount of 'dietary solvent' (i.e. water), stone solubility can increase proportionately. Supersaturation is complex and multifactorial, but increased urine volume allows for crystals, that would otherwise precipitate, to remain in solution.

### TABLE 26-1.  FACTORS ASSOCIATED WITH KIDNEY STONE DISEASE

State of Saturation
Urinary pH
Urinary Inhibitors
Urinary Promoters
Dietary Factors
Genetic Factors
Other Clinical States
       Hypercalciuric States
       Gastrointestinal Disease
       Hyperuricosuria
       Drugs and Toxins

2. Urinary pH.

   a. Calcium phosphate and ammonium phosphate/urate/ carbonate are more soluble in an acid environment.

   b. Calcium oxalate solubility is pH independent.

   c. Uric acid solubility is 80 mg/l at a pH of 4.5 and 1600 mg/l at pH of 6.5.

   d. Cystine is twice as soluble at a pH of 7.5 than at a pH of 7.0.

3. Urinary inhibitors.

   a. Citrate – capable of forming a soluble complex with calcium (more effective with calcium phosphate than calcium oxalate).

   b. Magnesium – can form a complex with oxalate.

   c. Other inhibitors include zinc, pyrophosphate, glycopeptides, glycosaminoglycans, glycoproteins and RNA.

4. Urinary Promotors.

   a. Self-promoting epitaxy is a process whereby existing stones can serve as a nidus for further crystal attachment. This is, perhaps, reminiscent of the adage, 'money goes to money'.

   b. Infection secondary to one type of stone disease can result in the secondary development of struvite stone disease. The role of bacterial urease can be significant in breaking down urea into bicarbonate and ammonia.

   c. Uric acid, a cause of stone disease itself, can also serve as a nidus for calcium stone formation.

5. Genetic Influences – these can play a 'primary' role (e.g. primary hyperoxaluria, adenine-phosphoribosyl-transferase deficiency) or, more commonly, an 'augmenting' influence (e.g. idiopathic hypercalciuria) that can allow for disease expression, given the right clinical opportunity.

   a. Distal Renal Tubular Acidosis (RTA Type I) – hypercalciuria is a feature of this syndrome.

   b. Primary Hyperoxaluria – it is of two genetic types, both disorders of glycine metabolism. The clinical syndrome results from an overproduction of oxalic acid. Although a different entity, primary hyperoxaluria resembles ethylene glycol toxicity where oxalate is generated in pathologic quantities as a result of it being the 'ultimate' breakdown product .

c. Adenine-phosphoribosyl-transferase deficiency – a 'recycling' enzyme defect analogous to deficiency of hypoxanthine-guanine-phosphoribosyl-transferase (HG-PRTase) deficiency. Adenine cannot be transformed to adenylic acid (in HG-PRTase deficiency, guanine cannot be transformed to guanylic acid). Unlike HG-PRTase deficiency, however, hypoxanthine 'recycling' is still intact so there can be inhibition of *de novo* purine synthesis. The excessive adenine is oxidized by xanthine oxidase (the same enzyme that oxidizes hypoxanthine and xanthine into uric acid) into 2,8-dihydroxyadenine.

d. Xanthinuria – it mimics the effect of allopurinol because it represents an inborn error of xanthine oxidase deficiency. Although xanthine is relatively soluble (certainly more soluble than uric acid), its absolute increase is so great in this disorder that stone formation can result.

e. Cystinuria – a defect in renal tubular reabsorption of basic amino acids: cystine, ornithine, lysine and arginine (COLA). Cystine is the least soluble of these, hence the potential for stone disease.

f. Idiopathic hypercalciuria – a physiologic consequence of disorders which produce either increased intestinal calcium absorption, or increased renal excretion. Increased effect of vitamin D appears to be the major mechanism operant in the 'hyperabsorptive' form.

6. The Role of Diet – regardless of other relevant factors, diet can play an important role in overt stone formation. Conversely, it can be a very relevant factor in therapy.

a. Fluid volume – as the physical parameter, 'solubility product' (SP), is a constant, the solubility of all stones is directly proportional to their concentration in the urine.

    i. A therapeutic corollary is that all reasonable efforts should be made to encourage patients with renal stone disease to drink substantial amounts of water.

    ii. Limitations of success may be related to relatively high concentrations of stone solute and the 'quality of life sacrifice' (e.g. polyuria, nocturia) incumbent upon the patient.

  b. A high protein intake can result in a decreased urinary pH, hypercalciuria (from bone mobilization), hypocitraturia, hyperuricosuria (from purine catabolism) and hypercystinuria (from sulfur-containing amino acids).

  c. Sodium intake (and hence excretion) parallels calcium excretion (increased sodium intake leads to hypercalciuria).

  d. Carbohydrates enhance calcium absorption.

  e. While the dietary calcium intake could theoretically affect urinary calcium excretion (e.g. in 'hyperabsorptive' hypercalciuria), it could also affect urinary oxalate through its ability to bind gut oxalate. Indeed, the overall risk of symptomatic renal stone disease in any given random population may be decreased by a high calcium diet.

  f. Plant fibers may bind calcium but also increase oxalate absorption.

  g. Oxalate intake – may be a predisposing factor to calcium oxalate stone formation, especially in inflammatory bowel disease.

7. Other Relevant Clinical States

  a. Hypercalciuric states (e.g. sarcoid, thyrotoxicosis, immobilization) – these states have the additional potential to produce hypercalcemia but the secondary suppression of parathyroid hormone (PTH) serves to prevent this. Decreased PTH, however, augments the hypercalciuria.

  b. Gastrointestinal disease (e.g. inflammatory bowel disease, small bowel resection) – crucial factors are increased oxalate absorption, dehydration and acidosis.

  c. Hyperuricosuria – increased risk of both urate- and calcium-containing stones.

  d. Drugs and toxins – ethylene glycol, triamterene, corticosteroids, vitamin D, laxative abuse (ammonium urate stones), carbonic anhydrase inhibition (resultant hypocitraturia and alkaline urine predispose to stones).

## CLINICAL APPROACH TO THE PATIENT WITH STONE DISEASE

1.  History – a thorough evaluation and pursuit of relevant detail can often be rewarding. Certainly questions related to prior stone events, ancillary medical illnesses that have linkages to stone disease, dietary patterns, medications, familial stone (and genetically associated) history and review of systems are crucial.

2.  Physical Examination – may reveal focal genitourinary manifestations (e.g. costovertebral angle and flank tenderness) as well as clinical clues as to etiologic processes (e.g. thyrotoxicosis, tophi, dehydration, clinical evidence of malabsorption state).

3.  Laboratory Evaluation
    a.  Stone analysis by spectroscopy.
    b.  Intravenous pyelography (IVP).
    c.  Complete blood count (CBC) and chemistry screening panel.
    d.  Urinalysis (personal examination and review of crystals) and urine culture and sensitivity.

4.  Supplementary chemistries are obtained as relevant:
    a.  Twenty-four-hour urine for volume, creatinine, calcium (diet must be calcium-restricted to obtain this), phosphorus, uric acid, citrate, oxalate and cystine.
    b.  Thyroid function studies.
    c.  Repeat calcium and phosphorus if initial calcium level is elevated; parathyroid hormone (PTH) level if calcium elevation persists.

5.  Clinical care includes general support, hydration, analgesia and antibiotics, as necessary.

6.  In the patient who does not spontaneously pass the stone, a urologic intervention may be necessary (e.g. extracorporeal shock wave lithotripsy, cystoscopy and retrograde ureteroscopy, nephrostomy).

## CALCIUM-CONTAINING STONES

1.  Calcium-containing stones are radiopaque and comprise a large heterogeneous group because of multiple etiologic associations:

a. Hypercalciuric states (e.g. hyperparathyroidism, idiopathic hypercalciuria, sarcoidosis, immobilization).

b. A consequence of hyperoxaluria. (Primary hyperoxaluria is always a possibility, but is very rare.) The oxalate concentration is the rate-limiting factor – attempts should therefore be made to minimize dietary oxalate (fruit juices, especially cranberry juice, are big offenders; other sources include tomatoes, spinach, rhubarb, chocolate and tea). Paradoxically, dietary calcium restriction results in less binding of oxalate within the gut. In addition, you do not substantially decrease urine calcium as calcium will be extracted from bone to maintain eucalcemia (although the PTH-mediated effect will tend to diminish urinary calcium excretion). This will leave you with the additional problem of bone demineralization. When certain bowel diseases are the culprit, therapy should be additionally directed at treatment of the primary intestinal problem (e.g. treatment of Crohn's disease, bile salt sequestrants for bile salt malabsorption).

c. Distal Renal Tubular Acidosis (Type I RTA) – systemic acidosis in the presence of inappropriate urine 'alkalosis'. In a fasting (more than 6 hours) patient with sterile urine, give 100 mg/kg of $NH_4Cl$ over 45 minutes. The patient must be given 100 ml of water/hour for 4 hours. Urine pH is measured hourly; serum $HCO_3^-$ is measured at 2 and 4 hours. If urine pH is greater than 5.4 with serum $HCO_3^-$ less than 16, the diagnosis of distal RTA is made. Potassium citrate is the therapy of choice.

2. Therapeutic Considerations

a. General – hydration, acid–base balance, dietary surveillance; treatment of ancillary problems.

b. Specific:

i. Thiazide diuretics – effective in idiopathic hypercalciuria. Augments renal calcium conservation and promotes a urine inhibitory environment (if hypokalemia is allowed to occur, the resultant decrease in urinary citrate could negate that inhibitory environment). Even when 'hyperabsorption' is the culprit in idiopathic hypercalciuria, the calcium-retentive property of the thiazides is still effective in 'thwarting' the underlying process.

ii.  Potassium citrate – effective in hypocitraturia associated with acidosis (e.g. RTA, intestinal disease) and idiopathic hypocitraturia. It is an ideal source of potassium for thiazide-mediated hypokalemia. Its effect is augmented with magnesium supplementation.

iii. Potassium orthophosphate – a second-line therapy in idiopathic hypercalciuria in patients who cannot take thiazide diuretics. It should not be used with the 'renal leak' etiology of idiopathic hypercalciuria or renal failure. Primary hyperoxaluria can be successfully treated with orthophosphate and pyridoxine.

iv.  Cellulose phosphate – a treatment for 'hyperabsorptive' hypercalciuria. Problems with this modality are that it binds inhibitors (zinc, magnesium) and increases oxalate absorption.

v.   Allopurinol – primarily used in the treatment of increased urate production, but can be a consideration in calcium stone disease if hyperuricosuria is a concomitant.

vi.  Bile Salt-Binding Resins (Cholestyramine, Colestipol) – useful for bile salt enteropathy-mediated hyperabsorptive hyperoxaluria.

## STRUVITE STONES

1.  Rather radiopaque large, and irregular stones composed of magnesium ammonium phosphate – carbonate apatite.

2.  These stones can arise as a consequence of prior structural (e.g. stone disease, anatomic defects) problems. They may serve as a nidus for future problems (e.g. recurrent infection, chronic renal disease).

3.  The stones must be removed and ancillary disease processes treated.

## URIC ACID STONES

1.  Uric acid stones are radiolucent.

2. They are seen in the context of patients with a clinical history of gout or urate deposition disease (e.g. tophi). Starvation, dehydration, concentrated acid urine and rapid tissue turnover (e.g. cancer) may be concomitants. Those patients with hyperuricemia based on impaired renal secretion are not at risk, because the kidney is 'protected'.

3. Hyperuricosuria – increased urinary uric acid could also serve as an environment for calcium stone disease.

4. Treatment is hydration, urine alkalinization (potassium citrate, 30 mEq, thrice daily, is usually adequate) to maintain pH of 6.0–6.5 (patients can monitor this with pH tape), and allopurinol. Obviously, uricosuric agents (as effective as they may be in the maintenance therapy of some forms of gout) are not only ineffective, but they can aggravate the underlying process.

## CYSTINE STONES

1. Cystine stones are rather radiopaque, with the tendency to recurrence and bilaterality.

2. Normal cystine excretion is 20 mg/day – in cystinuria, values may exceed 400 mg/day and thus obviate the need for stone analysis (crystals in urine also have a characteristic transparent, refractile and hexagonal appearance; they also give a 'positive nitroprusside test').

3. Therapy includes generous fluid intake, urine alkalinization with potassium citrate to keep the urine pH above 7.5 (night-time alkalinization and fluid intake are important, even if the resultant nocturia is disconcerting).

4. Specific medications are 'sulfhydryl binders' and include D-penicillamine, α-mercaptopropionylglycine (Thiola®) and Captopril.

# ENDOCRINOLOGY AND ONCOLOGY

# 27

# THE RELATIONSHIP BETWEEN ENDOCRINOLOGY AND NEOPLASTIC DISEASE

1.  Although hormone excess states can be mimicked by exogenous administration of the hormone (e.g. Cushing's syndrome secondary to therapeutic glucocorticoids, thyrotoxicosis factitia), these states are rarely produced endogenously without some associated neoplasia. (A corollary is that the neoplastic process, itself, can produce clinical manifestations relevant to its mass effect).

    a.  The physical superficiality of that growth will be operant in bringing the growth problem to medical attention. For example, thyroid enlargement is more likely to be noted than adrenal enlargement, notwithstanding the increasing number of adrenal 'incidentalomas' brought to medical attention because of increased use of abdominal MRI and CT.

        i.   While guidelines for clinical management of adrenal 'incidentalomas' are somewhat controversial, there is agreement that functional analysis (for steroid and catecholamine production) should be done on all lesions.

        ii.  While all functioning lesions should be removed, there is controversy as to the size of the non-functioning lesion that requires either immediate surgery or expectant follow up (it is generally accepted that follow up be every 6–12 months until no change in size is confirmed; then, every 2–3 years). All lesions greater than 6 cm should be removed initially; some recommend doing so even if the lesion is greater than 3 cm.

b. The ability of that neoplasm to affect adjacent endocrine and non-endocrine tissues (e.g. as in pituitary tumors) will also determine the clinical syndrome.

c. Some endocrine neoplasias can occur in well-defined syndromes. These are summarized as follows:

   i. Multiple Endocrine Neoplasia, Type I

     (a) Also known as the '3 Ps' because the pituitary, pancreas and parathyroid glands are primarily affected (other tumors – e.g. carcinoid, can also occur).

     (b) Autosomal dominant with 100% penetrance; linked to disorders of chromosome 11 (initial inherited defect plus an acquired defect during life: the 'double hit').

     (c) Hyperparathyroidism has a high incidence of hyperplasia (at surgery, it is often difficult to find the right 'balance' between tissue removal and the amount to leave behind – recurrence rate is high; hence, autotransplantation of parathyroid tissue, generally in the forearm, can be considered).

     (d) Pancreatic lesions are often multiple and difficult to cure (except with total pancreatectomy – but this has a significant mortality). Syndromes can now be treated pharmacologically. Lesions include gastrinomas (these may also be present in the duodenum), vasoactive intestinal peptide (VIP)-producing tumors and glucagonomas.

       (1) VIPoma Syndrome: watery diarrhea, hypokalemia, achlorhydria (Verner–Morrison Syndrome); can manufacture other hormones including serotonin, calcitonin, pancreatic polypeptide and substance P.

       (2) Glucagonoma Syndrome: characteristic rash

involving groin, thighs and perineum (necrolytic migratory erythema); weight loss; oral lesions; psychiatric manifestations; catabolic effects of glucagon (gluconeogenesis; depletion of amino acid pool) appear to be operant in the clinical syndrome.

(3) Somatostatinoma Syndrome: characterized by glucose intolerance (insulin suppression) but because glucagon is suppressed as well, severe hyperglycemia and ketonemia are rare; steatorrhea and diarrhea (malabsorption); cholelithiasis (decreased gall bladder tone and biliary stasis).

(4) Zollinger–Ellison Syndrome: severe acid hypersecretion leading to extensive peptic ulcer disease; malabsorption and diarrhea (secondary to direct intestinal mucosal injury and inactivation of pancreatic enzymes); non-suppressible hypergastrinemia (but able to be stimulated by secretin – also stimulated by calcium but this is an unnecessary and less safe test; not stimulated by a meal; these test responses help distinguish gastrinoma from other hypergastrinemic states such as achlorhydria and retained gastric antrum).

(e) Pituitary neoplasma are in the same general frequency of histologic composition and clinical presentation as when they occur sporadically.

ii. Multiple Endocrine Neoplasia (MEN) 2a and 2b both include medullary thyroid carcinoma and pheochromocytoma.

(a) Both are linked to chromosome 10.

(b) MEN 2a is associated with primary hyperparathyroidism.

(c) In MEN 2b, hyperparathyroidism is very uncommon; medullary thyroid carcinoma is more aggressive and multiple mucosal neuromas occur (lips, tongue, gastrointestinal tract); Marfanoid habitus.

2. **Non-Endocrine Neoplasia Can Have Endocrinologic Effects.**

   a. The physical replacement of endocrinologic tissue by cancer can give rise to deficiency states.

      i. This can theoretically occur in all endocrine organs but while some are more common sites of metastases (e.g. ovaries, adrenals), other organs are much less common (e.g. parathyroids).

      ii. In actuality, organ hypofunction secondary to replacement of endocrine tissue by cancer is uncommon compared to other etiologies of endocrine deficiency states (e.g. menopausal-mediated ovarian failure, idiopathic autoimmune-mediated Addison's disease).

      iii. Even if tumor were demonstrable in an organ, generally 90% of it would have to be replaced to produce a hypofunctioning state; servomechanistic feedback stimulation would act upon the remaining remnant to maintain functional normalcy (e.g. ACTH elevation in response to a decrease in adrenal function).

      iv. When prolactin inhibiting factor (PIF) transmission to the pituitary is compromised by tumor, the endocrine excess state of hyperprolactinemia can develop.

   b. The treatment of neoplastic disease could produce endocrine effects.

      i. Radiation therapy – e.g. cranial radiation producing pituitary insufficiency, gonadal radiation producing gonadal failure, neck irradiation producing hypothyroidism.

      ii. Neck irradiation can also lead to thyroid cancer (rarely, but possible, extensive follicular cancer can produce a thyrotoxic state) and even hyperparathyroidism.

      iii. Many chemotherapeutic agents (e.g. alkylating agents) can produce gonadal insufficiency.

      iv. Adrenal insufficiency can arise from use of o'p' DDD (Mitotane, Lysodren) and aminoglutethimide (Cytadren), but these may be 'desired effects' (e.g. treatment of breast cancer).

   v. Aminoglutethimide can also impair thyroid hormone synthesis.

   vi. Syndrome of inappropriate antidiuretic hormone (SIADH) can result from cyclophosphamide (Cytoxan) or vincristine (Oncovin) therapy.

   vii. Tumor localization can be facilitated using labelled hormone radioscintigraphy (e.g. somatostatin for ectopic ACTH production, VIP for intestinal tumors and metastases).

c. Endocrinologic therapies are utilized in the management of non-endocrinologic neoplasia.

   i. Prostate Cancer – use of orchidectomy, diethylstilbestrol (DES) in the past. Present standard for maximal anti-androgenic effect utilizes a peripheral androgen antagonist (Flutamide) and a gonadotropin releasing hormone (GnRH) analog (Leuprolide – sustained GnRH effect 'down regulates' the pituitary).

   ii. Breast Cancer – oophorectomy and tamoxifen used in premenopause with secondary maneuvers including androgens and medical (rarely surgical) adrenalectomy. Use of tamoxifen is common for postmenopausal use (estrogens no longer used). Other endocrinologic maneuvers have been empirically tried: the degree of response seems predicated on the estrogen receptor concentration.

   iii. Endometrial Cancer – progestational drugs used in treatment.

   iv. Corticosteroids may be used as a primary agent, invariably as part of a chemotherapeutic regime (e.g. acute leukemia, lymphoma) or in an ancillary manner (e.g. spinal cord compression, cerebral edema).

   v. Ovarian, hepatic cell, renal cell cancers and melanoma may also respond in a limited way to endocrinologic maneuvers.

d. Non-Endocrine Tumors can be associated with ectopic hormone production:

    i. Syndrome of inappropriate antidiuretic hormone (SIADH),

    ii. Hypercalcemia,

    iii. Cushing's Syndrome,

    iv. Tumor-associated hypoglycemia,

    v. Miscellaneous – human chorionic gonadotropin, calcitonin, corticotropin releasing hormone (CRH), growth hormone releasing hormone (GHRH), hypophosphatemia.

# Section H

# DISORDERS OF LIPID METABOLISM

# 28

# NORMAL LIPID METABOLISM AND RELATED DISEASE STATES

General Principles
Triglyceride Metabolism
Cholesterol Metabolism
Classifications of Lipid Disorders
The Association of Diabetes Mellitus with Hyperlipidemia
The Effect of Estrogens on Serum Lipids
The Role of Lipoprotein Deficiency States and the Predilection to
    Cardiovascular Disease
Evidence for the Association of Coronary Artery Disease and
    Lipid Abnormalities
Evidence for the Beneficial Effect of Altering Lipid Levels
Clinical Approach to Abnormal Lipid States
Therapeutic Modalities
Specific Drug Therapy

## GENERAL PRINCIPLES

1. There are four major categories of circulating lipids: triglycerides, phospholipids, free fatty acids and cholesterol. They are in a steady-state relationship with storage forms of lipids.

2. Because of their hydrophobic nature, protein carriers are necessary to maintain solubility. These carriers also exert secondary functions (e.g. low-density lipoprotein or LDL receptors recognize apolipoprotein (apo) B, apo C-II is a cofactor for lipoprotein lipase or LPL, abnormal apo E production results in elevation of intermediate density lipoproteins or IDL; apo A-I is a cofactor for lecithin cholesterol acyltransferase (LCAT), apo A-II contains cysteine which permits disulfide-bridged oligomers with apo E).

3. Lipoproteins have been empirically classified based on their electrophoretic mobility, sedimentation, density and size. As empiric as these categories are, they encompass components with unique properties and physiologic roles.

## TRIGLYCERIDE METABOLISM (Figure 28-1)

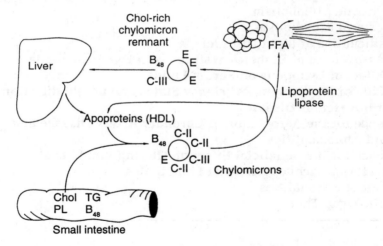

**Figure 28-1.** Transport of Exogenously Derived Lipids: $B_{48}$, apolipoprotein $B_{48}$; Chol, cholesterol; FFA, free fatty acids; HDL, high-density lipoprotein; PL, phospholipids; TG, triglycerides. Reproduced with kind permission from Ginsberg, H.N. Lipoprotein physiology and its relationship to other agenesis. *Endocrinology and Metabolism Clinics of North America*, vol. 19 no. 2, 1990, pp. 211–28

1. Triglycerides are the major form of fat storage – present throughout the body in adipose tissue storage sites as well as the liver. Energy content is 9 cal/g (as opposed to 4 cal/g, each, for carbohydrates and protein). Its efficiency as a storage form is amplified by the absence of water.

2. The source can be dietary or endogenous. Dietary sources are mechanically processed, emulsified with dietary phospholipids and endogenous bile salts and catabolized by lipase into monoacylglycerol and fatty acids. They are absorbed from the 'unstirred aqueous layer'.

3. Short-chain (less than 14 carbons) fatty acids are transported to the liver via the portal circulation. Long-chain fatty acids and monoacyl and free glycerol are reunited to form triglycerides. They are packaged with lipoproteins A-I, A-II, A-IV, and B-48 to produce chylomicrons. On average, about 100 g of triglyceride is packaged to chylomicrons daily.

4. Lipoprotein lipase allows for free fatty acid formation from chylomicrons and peripheral storage of triglycerides. This is effected by loss of phospholipid and A-I, A-II and A-IV and the taking in of cholesterol and C-I, C-II, C-III and E. Apo C-II is a necessary cofactor for lipoprotein lipase. The remaining remnant (B-48, cholesterol ester and apo E) is taken up by the liver.

5. Lipoprotein lipase activity decreases in diabetes and fasting and increases with carbohydrates.

6. Endogenous triglyceride production occurs in the liver – acetyl CoA (from CHO or other sources) is the basic building block. NADPH is the major cofactor. Endogenous triglycerides leave the liver as packaged very low density lipoproteins (VLDL); major lipoprotein carriers are B-100, C-I, C-II, C-III and E. Insulin increases fatty acid and triglyceride synthesis; corticosteroids and alcohol increase triglyceride synthesis; glucagon decreases triglyceride synthesis and increases ketogenesis (Figure 28-2).

## CHOLESTEROL METABOLISM

1. Although having a 'demonic' reputation because of the ability of its storage pool to 'spill over' into the vascular wall, cholesterol has important functions as a steroid hormone and bile salt

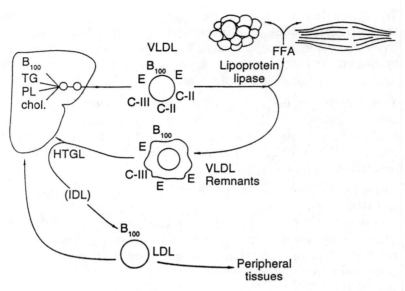

**Figure 28-2.** Transport of Endogenously Derived Lipids: FFA, free fatty acids; TG, triglycerides; VLDL, LDL, IDL, very low-, low- and intermediate-density lipoproteins; HTGL, hepatic triglyceride lipase. Reproduced with kind permission from *Endocrinology and Metabolism Clinics of North America,* vol. 19 no. 2, 1990

precursor as well as being an indispensable component of cell membranes (e.g. the abnormal acanthocytes, as seen in a-beta-lipoproteinemia, and the congenital defects associated with the rare hypocholesterolemic disorder, the Smith–Lemli–Opitz syndrome, gives credence to the importance of an 'optimal' cholesterol level).

2. Dietary cholesterol (usually esterified) is broken down into free cholesterol and a free fatty acid by a pancreatic hydrolase. Unesterified cholesterol is taken up by mixed micelles of bile acid and free fatty acid, monoglyceride or phospholipid. Only 30% of dietary cholesterol is taken up by the intestinal cells but absorption is linked to fat absorption (dietary cholesterol in 'unregulated' western diets is in the range of 0.5–1.0 g).

3. Most chylomicron cholesterol remains within the 'remnant' after lipoprotein lipase action. They are taken up by hepatocytes which they reach by passage through the space of Disse. Hepatic

receptors bind apo E sites on the remnant. Endogenous hepatocyte synthesis of cholesterol is decreased (through inhibition of 3-hydroxy-3-methyl-glutaryl coenzyme A (HMG CoA reductase)) in response to the uptake process. Most hepatic cholesterol either directly synthesized or taken up is excreted through bile as cholesterol or converted to bile acids (bile acid production is rate limited by 7 $\alpha$-hydroxylase). The sum of the bile acid and cholesterol loss (1–1.5 g/day) equals the sum of the cholesterol uptake and production.

4.  Endogenous cholesterol synthesis takes place in the liver, gastrointestinal tract and most other tissues. This cholesterol is carried in the circulation as VLDL with apo B-100, C-I, C-II, C-III and E. This cholesterol can be esterified by the action of lecithin cholesterol acyl transferase (LCAT) with high density lipoprotein (HDL) cholesterol and apo A-I functioning as substrates (intracellular esterification is effected by acyl-CoA: cholesterol acyl transferase – ACAT).

5.  After lipoprotein lipase activation, VLDL is converted to LDL with dissociation of apo C, phosphatidyl choline and unesterified cholesterol. These can interact with HDL, become esterified by LCAT and thus be 'recycled'.

6.  Peripheral cells take up LDL cholesterol via receptor-mediated pinocytosis. The greater the receptivity, the less the endogenous synthesis (HMG CoA reductase is rate-limiting). ACAT enables cholesterol to be stored in esterified form. A small amount of cholesterol is taken up via non-receptor mechanisms.

7.  HDL is pivotal in the efflux of cholesterol. LCAT and apo A-I are catalytic in esterifying the cholesterol (Figure 28-3).

    a.  Transfer proteins serve to shuttle this esterified cholesterol – the structure of this cholesterol ester transfer protein (CETP) has been recently identified.

    b.  The relevance of this transport protein has been elucidated in a patient with a deficiency of CETP who had a HDL cholesterol greater than 200 mg/100 dl yet a LDL cholesterol less than 30 mg/100 dl. It is possible that a new type of pharmacology may develop from inhibition of CETP.

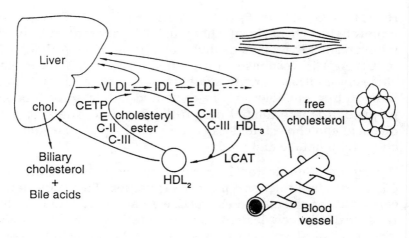

**Figure 28-3.** High-density Lipoprotein Metabolism: VLDL, LDL, IDL, HDL, very low-, low-, intermediate- and high-density lipoproteins; CETP, cholesterol ester transfer protein; LCAT, lecithin cholesterol acyltransferase. Reproduced with kind permission from *Endocrinology and Metabolism Clinics for North America*, 1990, vol. 19 no. 2, p. 224

## CLASSIFICATIONS OF LIPID DISORDERS

1. Three types of classifications are customarily used. Although each is inclusive of all lipid disorders, they use different approaches.

   a. The classification of Frederickson and Lees is based on abnormal lipoprotein electrophoretic patterns and is empirically designated (Table 28-1).

### TABLE 28-1. FREDERICKSON AND LEE'S CLASSIFICATION OF LIPID DISORDERS

| Type of Abnormality | Abnormal Lipoprotein Elevation |
|---|---|
| I | Chylomicrons |
| II a | LDL (β) |
| II b | LDL and VLDL (β and Pre-β) |
| III | 'Broad β' |
| IV | VLDL (Pre-β) |
| V | Combination of Type I and IV |

b.  Classification based on genetic abnormality – many specific genetic abnormalities are now known. For clinical correlation, however, it is best incorporated with a classification based on pathophysiology.

c.  Classification based on pathophysiology – the most meaningful in clinical medicine. It lends itself to including ancillary information codified in the other two categories.

   i.   While a substantial number of processes are of a 'primary' nature, it is important to appreciate that there are many 'secondary' problems which produce the same effect – in many cases, these 'secondary' problems are treatable (e.g. uncontrolled diabetes mellitus) and their treatment will result in correction of the underlying pathophysiology. Associated with hyperlipidemic states including glucocorticoid excess (elevated LDL, HDL and VLDL), anabolic steroids (decreased HDL), estrogen effect (increased triglycerides, decreased LDL and increased HDL), hypothyroidism (increased LDL), anorexia nervosa (increased LDL), cholestatic jaundice (increase in an abnormal LDL), immunoglobulin disorders (hypertriglyceridemia and abnormal lipoprotein production), uremia (increased VLDL), β-adrenergic blockade (increased triglycerides and decreased HDL) and thiazide diuretics (increased triglycerides and LDL).

   ii.  It is also important to understand that the concern with these hyperlipidemic states rests in their atherogenic potential. Although pancreatitis and skin lesions may be ancillary manifestations, surely disorders of lipid metabolism would not warrant such emphasis were it not for cardiovascular implications.

## THE ASSOCIATION OF DIABETES MELLITUS WITH HYPERLIPIDEMIA

1.  Insulin deficiency, relative or absolute, results in impaired lipoprotein lipase activity.

2.  Paradoxically, the hyperinsulinemia seen in Type II diabetes mellitus gives rise to increased triglyceride production. Obesity, even without overt diabetes, can do this. Because obesity is often

seen in the clinical presentation of Type II diabetes, it has an additive effect.

3. Insulin deficiency can also decrease receptor-mediated LDL degradation.

## THE EFFECT OF ESTROGENS ON SERUM LIPIDS

1. The major mechanism of increase in triglycerides secondary to estrogen is increased hepatic VLDL production. Although triglyceride removal is also enhanced, it is not of comparable magnitude.

2. Estrogens increase LDL catabolism resulting in lower serum cholesterol levels.

3. Estrogens increase hepatic HDL production (primarily the lighter $HDL_2$ subclass). This is lessened if exogenous estrogens are given by 'patch' (thus bypassing the portal circulation) and also if progestins are added to the regime.

4. Estrogens decrease plasma Lp(a) lipoprotein (a circulating factor linked to atherosclerosis) concentration and inhibit oxidation of LDL, factors which may be contributory to their beneficial cardiovascular effect.

5. The type of progestin used in concert with the estrogen is significant. Micronized 'natural' progesterone does not seem to decrease HDL. Medroxy progesterone in doses of 10 mg/day for 7-14 days/month does not decrease HDL either, even though LDL cholesterol increases slightly. 19-nor derivatives (norgestrel – present in LoOvral and Triphasil; norethindrone – present in Ortho Novum 777 and Loestrin) do reverse some estrogenic effects: i.e. they decrease HDL cholesterol and triglycerides, but they also result in a greater estrogenic effect because they increase sex hormone binding globulin levels.

## THE ROLE OF LIPOPROTEIN DEFICIENCY STATES AND THE PREDILECTION TO CARDIOVASCULAR DISEASE

1. Decreased β-lipoproteins (as in a-beta-lipoproteinemia) do not increase the risk, but they are associated with other pathologies: malabsorption, anemia with morphologic acanthocytosis, neuropathy, impaired steroid production.

2. Tangier Disease (HDL deficiency) may, but this is a very rare disease. It is associated with tonsillar lipid deposition, neuropathy and corneal opacity.

3. Relative HDL deficiency is a risk factor for premature atherosclerosis.

## EVIDENCE FOR THE ASSOCIATION OF CORONARY ARTERY DISEASE AND LIPID ABNORMALITIES

1. In patients who survive myocardial infarction, there will be disproportionate representation of a wide range of dyslipidemic states including combined familial hyperlipemia, familial hypertriglyceridemia, familial hypercholesterolemia, sporadic hypertriglyceridemia and sporadic hypercholesterolemia.

2. A study of Japanese-American men living in San Francisco (versus native Japanese men) showed five times as many San Franciscans with elevated cholesterol levels, greater than 260 mg/dl, and with a 2.8 times greater incidence of coronary heart disease (Kato *et al.*, Am. J. Epidemiol., 1973).

3. In a now classic study, Ancel Keys (Keys, A., Circulation, 1970) studied middle-aged men in seven countries and noted a correlation of coronary heart disease with fat consumption and cholesterol levels greater than 250 mg/dl.

4. The Framingham Study (Castelli, W.P., Can. J. Cardiol., 1988) showed a correlation with coronary heart disease and serum cholesterol in men over the age of 40 and serum cholesterol. In women, the total cholesterol/HDL-cholesterol was an important predictor over the age of 50.

5. Serum cholesterol levels measured early in life correlate with the risk of cardiovascular disease later in life.

6. Depressed HDL levels appear to be a risk factor for coronary vascular disease. Further, the total cholesterol:HDL ratio is felt to be a better measure of coronary heart disease risk than either parameter alone.

   a. Factors which tend to decrease HDL cholesterol levels: familial deficiency, postpuberty males and other hyperandrogenic states, some progestins, obesity, hypertriglyceridemia, Type II diabetes mellitus, sedentary state and cigarette smoking.

b. Factors which tend to increase HDL levels: familial hyper-α-lipoproteinemic states, hypotriglyceridemia, exercise, thin habitus, estrogens, alcohol, diphenylhydantoin.

7. A variant of LDL, Lp(a), contains an apoprotein: apo (a) which is homologous to plasminogen and is highly linked to atherosclerosis. Levels seem to be genetically determined and range from 0 to 100 mg/dl. Diet does not appear to influence the level and it is minimally responsive to drug therapy. Because it is structurally homologous to plasminogen, its significance lies in its potential competitive binding and prevention of plasminogen activation by tissue plasminogen activator (TPA). It may be contributory to the high atherosclerotic risk in diabetes mellitus because it is elevated in poorly controlled diabetes. On the other hand, levels are statistically higher in Blacks and this does not seem to correlate with coronary artery disease in them. Estrogen can decrease Lp(a) lipoprotein concentration.

8. As more is learned about LDL subtypes, there will be greater refinement in our understanding (e.g. the small dense type B subtype is associated with atherosclerosis, as opposed to the A). HDL subfractions will also become more relevant.

9. A note of caution – despite the fact that cholesterol reduction lessens the likelihood of coronary artery disease, lower levels in middle-aged men do not reduce their stroke morbidity or mortality. Further, neither hypercholesterolemia nor decreased HDL-cholesterol appear to affect morbidity or mortality from coronary artery disease above age 70.

10. Insofar as there may be prolonged postprandial hypertriglyceridemia in some individuals, this may result in an increased risk of coronary atherogenesis.

## EVIDENCE FOR THE BENEFICIAL EFFECT OF ALTERING LIPID LEVELS

1. In Lipid Research Clinics: Coronary Primary Prevention Trial – use of cholestyramine, even with mild lowering of serum cholesterol, resulted in a significant decrease in coronary artery disease.

2. The Leiden Intervention Trial showed the effect of a strict vegetarian diet (with concomitant improvement in lipid profile) on the prevention of coronary artery disease progression.

3. Cholesterol Lowering Atherosclerosis Study (CLAS) – Colestipol–Niacin regime is more effective than diet (albeit there were drug side-effects) in stabilizing and causing regression of coronary artery disease.

4. Helsinki Heart Study – Gemfibrozil had a significant effect on myocardial infarction and cardiac death (although, curiously, other causes of death such as stroke and accidents kept the overall mortality the same as controls).

5. Seattle study (Brown *et al.*, N. Engl. J. Med., 1990) showed a salutory effect on coronary artery disease with both lovastatin/colestipol and niacin/colestipol versus conventional therapy.

## CLINICAL APPROACH TO ABNORMAL LIPID STATES

1. Lipid screening should be universal and should be done at an early age. Particular emphasis should be placed on those with risk factors for atherosclerosis or who have had a cardiovascular event. Risk factors include male sex, family history, cigarette smoking, hypertension, diabetes mellitus or significant obesity (greater than 30% above ideal body weight).

2. Standard lipid measurements are total cholesterol, triglycerides and HDL cholesterol (HDL-cholesterol and thus the calculated LDL-cholesterol are not reliable if the triglyceride value is greater than 400 mg/dl). Measurements are made in the fasted state.

3. LDL-cholesterol (LDL-C) is calculated as follows:

$$LDL\text{-}C = Total\ Cholesterol - (HDL\text{-}C + TG/5)$$

where TG is triglycerides.

4. If an abnormality is found, secondary causes must be ruled out.

5. A hypertriglyceridemic state, with levels between 250 and 500 mg/dl is associated with a doubling of the risk of coronary artery disease, but this is probably because of its association with other risk factors. Secondary reasons including other disease states, diet and lifestyle must be analyzed. The nature of the hyper-triglyceridemia must also be addressed to see if there is a primary

lipopathy, especially one associated with coronary artery disease, that may require specific therapy.

6. With respect to cholesterol levels, guidelines have been established by the National Cholesterol Education Program (*Ann. Int. Med.*, 1988). Pharmacologic treatment is recommended under the following circumstances:

   a. With no other risk ractors, LDL-cholesterol greater than 190 mg/dl.

   b. With two risk factors, LDL-cholesterol between 160 and 190 mg/dl. An optimal LDL-cholesterol is 130 mg/dl or less.

7. To the extent possible, HDL levels should be maximized. 'Normal' range of Total cholesterol/HDL-cholesterol is 2.5–4.5.

## THERAPEUTIC MODALITIES (Table 28-2)

1. Dietary Therapy (based on Report of National Cholesterol Education Program: *Arch. Int. Med.*, 1988). Its benefit is independent of any added pharmacologic effect.

   a. Weight reduction, if necessary, is an imperative.

   b. Qualitative dietary changes include: decreased total dietary fat (less than 30% of calories), decreased saturated fatty acids (less than 10% of calories), decreased cholesterol intake (less than 300 mg/day). Additionally, polyunsaturated fatty acids

### TABLE 28-2. THEAPEUTIC MODALITIES TO TREAT HYPERLIPIDEMIAS

Dietary Therapy
Exercise
Drug Therapy
    Bile Acid-Binding Resins
    Nicotinic Acid
    Gemfibrozil
    3-Hydroxy-3-Methyl-Glutaryl-Coenzyme A
      Reductase Inhibitors
    Other Drugs
    Combination Therapy

should be less than 10% of calories with monounsaturated fatty acids comprising the remaining total fat calories. This comprises the 'Step 1' Diet. Walnut oil (polyunsaturated to saturated fat ratio of 7.1:1 – high in *n*-3 linolenic acid) may also be salutory.

c. As necessary, the 'Step 2' Diet can be introduced. This differs from the 'Step 1' in that saturated fatty acids are decreased to less than 7% of the total calories (total dietary fat is less than 20% of the total calories) and cholesterol intake is less than 200 mg/day.

d. Evidence suggests that inclusion of dietary fiber (e.g. oat bran and psyllium) can decrease LDL cholesterol an additional 10%. Although seemingly not a 'major factor', garlic (900 mg/day) can decrease total and LDL-cholesterol. Soy protein (in large quantities) can decrease total cholesterol and triglycerides.

e. So-called 'omega-3' fatty acids (e.g.eicosapentanoic) may additionally decrease atherogenic potential through their effect on prostaglandin synthesis. Potential side-effects can be worsening of Type II diabetes mellitus and an increase in bleeding time.

f. Although controversial because of concerns regarding its addictive and other negative properties, alcohol in 'moderate amounts' decreases the risk of myocardial infarction (probably by increasing $HDL_2$ and $HDL_3$).

2. Exercise is a vital adjunct because of its role in weight loss, mental well-being and improved HDL-cholesterol.

3. Dietary therapy must be given a reasonable trial period before drug therapy is additionally prescribed. (Remember: Drug therapy is an adjunct, not a substitute for dietary therapy.)

## SPECIFIC DRUG THERAPY

1. Bile Acid-Binding Resins

a. Work by diverting intestinal bile acids and cholesterol from enterohepatic recycling. The cholesterol pool is decreased in the body. The diminished bile salt pool also increases cholesterol conversion to bile salts. Hepatic LDL receptor activity increases.

b. Its major effect is to decrease LDL.

c. Usual daily dose: cholestyramine, 16–24 g; Colestipol, 15–20 g.

d. Side-effects: gastrointestinal (bloating, constipation), interference with absorption of other drugs (e.g. thyroid hormone, digoxin, phenobarbital, thiazide diuretics, tetracycline, warfarin – therefore, administer these medications at least 1 hour before or 4 hours after resin administration), elevation of triglycerides (especially if there is already basal hypertriglyceridemia).

2. Nicotinic Acid

   a. Acts by decreasing synthesis of VLDL.

   b. Can decrease VLDL and LDL but also is most effective agent in elevating HDL.

   c. Usual daily dose: up to 6–8 g/day (start with low dose as flushing may be an untoward side-effect – this may be pre-emptively mitigated with aspirin prophylaxis). A long-acting preparation is available.

   d. Additional side-effects: dyspepsia (including peptic ulcer activation), headache, itching, hyperuricemia, abnormal liver function tests (LFTs), glucose intolerance.

3. Gemfibrozil

   a. A fibric acid derivative; it is the most widely used drug in that category.

   b. It increases lipoprotein lipase activity as well as decreases hepatic triglyceride synthesis.

   c. Acts primarily on lowering VLDL cholesterol (not very effective on LDL cholesterol) and triglycerides. HDL cholesterol is increased.

   d. Usual daily dose: Gemfibrozil, 600 mg, twice daily, before meals.

   e. Side-effects: myositis leading to possible rhabdomyolysis (can be augmented if combined with an HMG CoA reductase inhibitor), cholecystitis (by increasing bile lithogenicity), potentiation of the action of vitamin K antagonists, elevated hepatic aminotransferase levels, rash and leukopenia.

4. HMG CoA Reductase Inhibitors.

   a. Lovastatin was the first available drug in this class, but now included are Fluvastatin, Simvastatin and Pravastatin. All have generally comparable efficacy.

   b. They all act by inhibiting the rate limiting step in cholesterol synthesis that is indigenous to all mammalian cells: the conversion of 3-hydroxy-3-methyl glutaryl CoA (HMG CoA) to mevalonate.

   c. A very potent secondary effect is their ability to increase LDL cholesterol receptors. Thus, they not only 'impede' cellular output of cholesterol into the circulating pool, but the increased cellular 'receptivity' to cholesterol additionally diminishes the cholesterol pool size. Total and LDL cholesterol are decreased and HDL cholesterol is increased. The hypocholesterolemic effect is amplifed with the addition of a bile acid-binding resin.

   d. In conjunction with a cholesterol-lowering diet, objective improvement in pre-existing coronary artery lesions have been demonstrated. The large Scandinavian Simvastatin Survival Study (Lancet, 1994) clearly showed improved survival in patients with coronary heart disease.

   e. Because synthesis of cholesterol *in vivo* is maximal between midnight and 03.00, all medication is best administered in the evening. Lovastatin is additionally best given with the evening meal to enhance its absorption.

   f. Usual daily dose: Lovastatin, 20–80 mg/day; Pravastatin: 10–40 mg/day; Simvastatin, 5–40 mg/day; Fluvastatin, 20–40 mg/day.

   g. Side-effects: abnormal liver function tests, myositis, gastrointestinal symptoms and possible cataracts. There may also be drug–drug interactions with immunosuppressants, erythromycin (potentiaton of rhabdomyolysis) and anti-coagulants (potentiation of warfarin).

5. Other Drugs (not regularly used)

   a. Probucol – can decrease LDL but also decreases HDL. An important property is its action as an antioxidant. It inhibits oxidative modification of LDL and lipid peroxidation. Side-effects include gastrointestinal discomfort (nausea, vomiting, diarrhea), chest pain, neuritis, headaches and dizziness. Recommended dose: 500 mg, twice daily (no titration required).

b. Neomycin – non-absorbable sterol binder that promotes sterol excretion. Decreases LDL.

c. Norethindrone and Oxandrolone – decrease chylomicrons and VLDL by enhancing activity of lipoprotein lipase, (but also decrease HDL).

6. Combination Therapy

a. This therapy is used to augment the effect on one lipid component that might not optimally respond to a single drug, or to broaden the response to include an effect on other lipid components (e.g. improve both the triglyceride and cholesterol profile).

b. Gemfibrozil can be combined with niacin to treat hypertriglyceridemia that does not normalize with either agent, alone.

c. Gemfibrozil can also be combined with an HMG CoA Reductase Inhibitor to reduce triglycerides and enhance the hypocholesterolemic effect, but myositis (potentially leading to rhabdomyolysis and renal failure) can be a complication. The onset of myositis can be sudden so that pre-emptive creatine phosphokinase monitoring may not be of value.

d. The combination of niacin and bile acid-binding resins could augment the beneficial cholesterol profile while preventing or reversing the hypertriglyceridemia that might occur with resin use alone.

e. In cases of profound elevation of LDL cholesterol, combined use of niacin, bile acid binding resins and a 3-hydroxy-3-methyl-glutaryl-CoA reductase inhibitor, is a consideration.

f. The addition of Probucol (because of its antioxidant properties) may augment the improved coronary endothelial reponse of HMG CoA reductase inhibition, in the setting of atherosclerosis.

# Section I

# DISORDERS OF EATING AND WEIGHT

**29**

# OBESITY

## OBESITY: DEFINITION AND MEASUREMENT

1. In its most simplistic definition, obesity means an excess of body fat. Excess weight, *per se*, is an inadequate definition because weight can increase as a result of increased muscle mass or fluid retention.

2. Obesity exists when body weight is 20–30% above ideal body weight as calculated by actuarial data. For practical purposes, since increased muscle mass and fluid excess are usually clinically obvious, obesity often correlates with body weight.

3. A better index of obesity is the Body Mass Index (BMI):

   $BMI = Weight\ (kg)/Height^2\ (m^2)$.

   Normal BMI = $22–25\ kg/m^2$

4. Body fat can be calculated more quantitatively by densitometry (underwater weighing), isotopic studies of body water or potassium, or using CT or MRI. These are expensive and inappropriate for general use.

5. Skinfold measurements as a function of subcutaneous fat (e.g. triceps, biceps, suprailiac and subscapular regions) give approximate measurements of body fat.

6. Obesity is not uniform throughout the body. Abdominal or 'android' obesity has a higher morbidity and mortality than 'gynoid' or lower segment obesity. The number of $\alpha 2$- to $\beta 1$-adrenergic receptors is less in the abdominal than gluteal depot – free fatty acids (FFA) are more mobilizable from the abdominal depot.

## OBESITY AS A HEALTH ISSUE

1. Obesity is unequivocally a health issue of major importance. Although any non-medical judgements or pejorative commentary about the obese person are to be condemned, there is irrefutable evidence that obesity as a medical issue is linked to serious disease. Conversely, weight loss in the obese individual results in increased longevity.

2. Hypertension is three times more common in obesity. Purported mechanisms include increased circulating catecholamines as there is both increased peripheral resistance and cardiac output. Renin, aldosterone and catecholamine levels fall with weight loss.

3. Cardiovascular disease is increased – abnormal lipid profile and hypertension are contributory. Very low density protein (VLDL) and low density lipoprotein (LDL) cholesterol and triglycerides are increased. High density lipoprotein (HDL) cholesterol is decreased. Weight variability (i.e. repeated weight loss and regain) may be an additional risk factor in selected individuals.

4. Non-insulin-dependent diabetes mellitus is increased. Insulin resistance (post-receptor) combined with inadequate pancreatic reserve can bring out overt diabetes.

5. Pulmonary function is impaired: there is ventilation–perfusion imbalance (perfusion is predominantly lower lung, ventilation is upper lung); hypoventilation and sleep apnea.

6. Additional endocrine abnormalities include increased androgen to estrogen conversion (this may be a factor in the increased risk of breast and gynecologic cancers), abnormal dexamethasone suppression, and failure of antidiuretic hormone suppression with a water load.

7. Colorectal and prostate cancers are increased in men; endometrial, cervical, breast, ovarian and biliary tract cancers are increased in women.

8. Increased risk of orthopedic problems.

9. Overweight in adolescence can predict a broad range of adverse health effects that are independent of adult weight.

## ETIOLOGIC FACTORS CONTROLLING OBESITY

1. Genetic – familial clustering; ethnic clustering (e.g. Pima Indians); Prader–Willi Syndrome (Chromosome 15 locus); Fröhlich's Syndrome; Laurence–Moon–Biedl Syndrome; the role of an 'obesity gene'; the association of obesity with abnormalities in the sensitivity of the $\beta_3$-adrenergic receptor of adipocytes.

2. Dietary Patterns – multiple studies have shown that obese people are more governed than non-obese to respond to 'environmental' cues rather than hunger; association with 'learned' behavior patterns (with reinforcing 'rewards and punishment'); conflicting societal cues (e.g. the 'desirability' of thinness versus the

pervasiveness of 'consumables') and the role of a market driven economy and ethic; difficulty of coping with appealing food presentations.

3. Body Image – inconclusive evidence of any role.

4. The prevalence of obesity increases with age and to a greater degree in women.

5. Diminished Exercise – the problem with this factor is sorting out cause versus effect.

6. Socioeconomic Factors – increased prevalence in disadvantaged socioeconomic groups, especially in women.

7. The Nature of the Adipocyte – earlier obesity is associated with an inherent increase in the number of adipocytes. These adipocytes may have increased insulin binding (when compared with the cells of a patient whose obesity appeared later in life). This, coupled with a relative increase in circulating lipoprotein lipase activity could increase fat synthesis.

8. What are the satiety signals? A number of hormones and humoral substances (e.g. glucose, cholecystokinin) have been purported. An 'anti-obesity hormone' found in mice may have future clinical implications. The medial hypothalamus is the site of the satiety center.

9. Energy Kinetics – may play a role in the context of the spectrum of weight variability in a large population, but should, in principle, be able to be overridden by patterns of consumption.

## AN INTEGRATED UNDERSTANDING OF OBESITY

1. During forced starvation, there is an increase in appetite and preoccupation with food (conscious and subconscious).

2. Likewise, there is a decrease in energy expenditure with weight loss. This appears to be related to energy expenditure as a function of lean body mass. In obesity, lean body mass is also increased, while it is decreased in the non-obese state. This decreased energy utilization with weight loss is both basal and during physical activity. Further, decreased food intake lessens the thermic effect of eating (Figure 29-1).

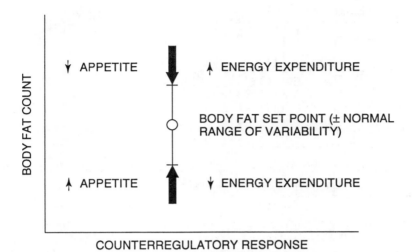

**Figure 29-1.** Counterregulatory changes that tend to keep individual weight at a certain 'set-point'. Reproduced with kind permission from The Pathophysiology of Obesity: Implications for Treatment, Weigle, D.S. (ed.) *The Endocrinologist,* 1991, vol. 1, p. 385

3. Conversely, when forcibly fed, individuals will become more easily sated (and could even experience nausea) and weight gain will level off. Increased energy expenditure associated with weight gain plays a complementary role in weight stabilization.

4. These studies and others suggested individualized 'set points' which are determined by the respective intersections of an energy consumption versus BMI curve and an energy utilization versus BMI curve. These curves need not be 'mirror images' of each other and may change under many influences, including age (Figure 29-2).

5. While the above factors do not localize specific etiologies, they support a dynamic concept of obesity and its therapeutic implications.

## THERAPEUTIC APPROACHES

1. While diet can override any innate tendency to obesity, it is rarely sustained over the lifetime of the person. The effectiveness of diet

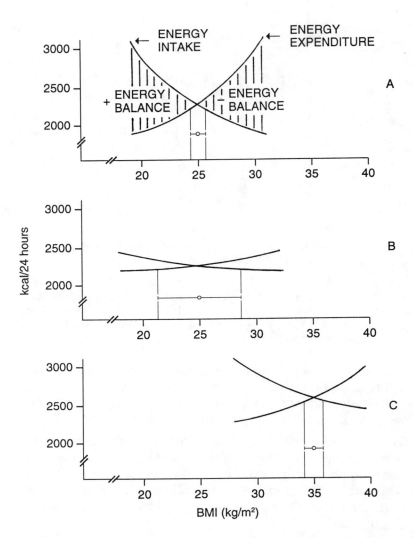

**Figure 29-2.** Relationships between energy intake, energy expenditure and body mass index (BMI) in three hypothetical individuals. (A) A non-obese individual who regulates his BMI tightly around a set-point of 25 kg/m². (B) An individual who regulates his BMI less tightly around a set-point of 25 kg/m² (this individual would be non-obese or moderately obese depending on environmental variables). (C) An obese individual who regulates his BMI tightly around a set-point of 35 kg/m². Reproduced with kind permission from The Pathophysiology of Obesity: Implications for Treatment, Weigle, D.S. (ed.) *The Endocrinologist*, 1991, vol. 1 p. 385

is further influenced by a large variability in acceptance and in the actual patterns of practice of weight reduction. Motivation, support and ancillary behavioral modification can be important adjuncts.

2. In general, the more 'realistic' the diet and the more it can be incorporated into one's 'life ethic', the more effective a tool it can be. Furthermore, combining a reduced fat diet with aerobic exercise is statistically associated with the greatest likelihood of successful weight loss, even if it does not lead to ultimate 'leaness'.

3. Starvation diets have no role in treatment. They may additionally stifle hunger because of starvation ketosis but there are significant side-effects. These include severe electrolyte imbalance, loss of lean body mass (obesity increases lean as well as adipose tissue), hyperuricemia, anemia (not associated with iron, folate, or B-12 deficiency) and orthostatic hypotension (autonomic instability). Weight loss also increases bile lithogenicity and the risk of gall bladder disease.

4. Modified fasts are of two types – both warrant medical supervision:

    a. One hundred grams of carbohydrate (400 Calories) – decreases nitrogen, sodium and potassium loss, eliminates ketosis. Nitrogen loss can be decreased still further with additional supplemental protein (e.g. 50–70 g).

    b. Protein diet (1.5 g/kg) – ketosis prone; significant fluid and sodium loss but 'nitrogen sparing' (earlier 'protein-sparing' diets were of poor quality protein which led to associated morbidity and mortality).

5. Exercise – an imperative for successful diet. It unquestionably complements the effect of weight loss by:

    a. Increased energy utilization during exercise.

    b. Weight redistribution.

    c. Mental well-being (enhanced if there is supplementary 'positive reinforcement').

    d. Appetite suppression.

    e. Increases lean body mass and thus the resting metabolic rate.

6. Surgery

   a. Jejunoileal Bypass – risks and complications outweigh benefits (early and late mortality, intractable diarrhea, oxalate kidney stones, immune complex syndromes, irritable bowel disease). No longer utilized nor recommended.

   b. Gastric exclusion procedures – seem to be effective, but have to be directed to a highly selected population.

7. Medications

   a. While some studies have suggested a beneficial (albeit adjunctive) role, their use still remains controversial.

   b. They all have sympathomimetic activity although they have been subdivided into amphetamine (e.g. dextroamphetamine, benzphetamine) and non-amphetamine (e.g. diethylpropion, phendimetrazine, fenfluramine) classes.

   c. While their potential benefit has been much discussed, weight regain after drug termination is very common.

# 30

# ANOREXIA NERVOSA AND BULIMIA NERVOSA

**Clinical Features of Anorexia Nervosa**
**Complications of Anorexia Nervosa**
**Treatment of Anorexia Nervosa**
**Clinical Features of Bulimia Nervosa**

## CLINICAL FEATURES OF ANOREXIA NERVOSA

1. Primarily a disease of young women – rarely seen in men (being male, however, does not exclude the diagnosis).

2. Disproportionately seen in higher socioeconomic environments.

3. The issue is not hunger but self-image. In fact, there is often a preoccupation with food.

4. Relevant symptoms may include abdominal pain and cold intolerance.

5. Relevant physical findings include: hypotension, bradycardia, bradypnea, hypothermia, peripheral edema, increase in body hair (lanugo), yellow hue to the skin, parotid gland enlargement and heart murmur.

6. Laboratory abnormalities include:

    a. Abnormal complete blood count (anemia, thrombocytopenia, leukopenia and lymphocytosis).

    b. Decreased plasma fibrinogen.

    c. Decreased erythrocyte sedimentation rate.

    d. Hypokalemia.

    e. Hypoalbuminemia.

    f. Elevated β-carotene.

    g. Hypercholesterolemia (low-density lipoprotein is responsible).

    h. Immunoglobulins may be decreased.

    i. Glomerular filtration rate is decreased.

7. Specific endocrine findings include:

    a. Amenorrhea (associated with decrease in gonadotropin releasing hormone and hence, with a resultant decrease in gonadotropins. Gonadotropins may not respond to exogenous gonadotropin releasing hormone stimulation unless 'primed').

    b. Growth hormone is increased (insulin-like growth factor-I is decreased).

c. Arginine vasopressin is less responsive to osmotic stimulation.

d. Prolactin response to thyrotropin releasing hormone (TRH) is diminished, while growth hormone response to TRH may be augmented.

e. Triiodothyronine is characteristically decreased (with resultant increase in reverse triiodothyronine). Thyroxine is often decreased but may be increased (thyroid stimulating hormone levels are usually normal, but there may be delayed response to TRH stimulation).

f. Evidence of adrenal cortical hyperactivity with impaired dexamethasone inhibition and diminished stimulation by corticotropin releasing factor. Yet, adrenal androgen levels are decreased.

## COMPLICATIONS OF ANOREXIA NERVOSA

1. Osteopenia – contributory factors are multiple and include inadequate sex hormone production, protein and calcium inadequacy and vitamin D deficiency.

2. Cardiac – arrhythmias including prolonged Q-T interval, myocardial dysfunction, mitral valve prolapse.

3. Psychological – related to poor and inappropriate self-image.

4. Electrolyte and related mineral imbalances (e.g. hypokalemia, hypocalcemia, hypomagnesemia, hypophosphatemia).

5. Nutritional deprivation leading to impaired physical and mental performance, emaciation and ultimately death.

## TREATMENT OF ANOREXIA NERVOSA

1. Individual psychotherapy – often difficult, prolonged and painstaking.

2. Family support – while potentially important, sometimes the existing family dynamics amplifies the underlying problem. Thus, involvement of the nuclear family in the therapeutic process is very often necessary.

3. Medications – appetite stimulants (e.g. cyproheptidine), endocrine replacement therapy and general supportive therapies (including in-patient hospialization) when acutely needed (intravenous fluids, electrolyte and nutritional therapies).

## CLINICAL FEATURES OF BULIMIA NERVOSA

1. Like anorexia nervosa, bulimia nervosa is primarily a disease of women.

2. A compulsive and irresistible drive to overeat is countered by aggressive attempts to lose excessive weight (e.g. vomiting, laxatives and diuretics).

3. Antisocial behavior (e.g. stealing, hoarding) may be committed to obtain food. Increased incidence of overt psychopathology with depression, self-mutilation and suicide as associated features.

4. The classical clinical, physical and laboratory features as seen in anorexia nervosa are often absent. Instead, features are related to specific behavioral aspects or events – e.g. physical evidence of self-mutilation, poor dental hygeine, esophageal rupture, electrolyte imbalance.

5. Treatment is best directed at the primary psychopathology.

# Section J

# REPRODUCTIVE ENDOCRINOLOGY

# 31

# NORMAL MALE REPRODUCTIVE ENDOCRINOLOGY AND RELATED DISEASE STATES

Development of the Male Reproductive Apparatus
Production of Testicular Hormones and Feedback Regulation
Male Hypogonadism
Impotence
Gynecomastia

Male reproductive function requires normal development of the reproductive apparatus and normal endocrinologic function based upon an elegant servomechanistic design.

## DEVELOPMENT OF THE MALE REPRODUCTIVE APPARATUS

1. Under the influence of the Y chromosome (as correlated with the presence of the H-Y antigen), the undifferentiated gonad develops into a primordial male gonad at approximately 6–7 weeks of gestation (the differentiation takes place several weeks later).

2. This gonad is able to produce testosterone locally (from Leydig cells which are present by 8–9 weeks gestation) and allow for growth and differentiation of Wolffian duct structures (to form male internal genitalia). Sertoli cells produce a Müllerian inhibitory factor locally which causes regression of the Müllerian ductal system (without this inhibition, the innate tendency of the internal genitalia is to femininity) – this factor is either identical with or structurally related to inhibin.

3. Testosterone also allows for differentiation of the external anlage into male structures. Although the relatively low (compared with puberty) levels *in utero* are able to produce male differentiation, the higher testosterone levels of puberty are necessary to complete the maturation of the genital apparatus for male reproductive function. Testosterone does this through its effect on genital tissue growth and development. Additional effects of testosterone are on muscular development, maturation of terminal hair (and propensity to lose hair that may be 'androgen sensitive'), stimulation of sebaceous glands, augmentation of erythropoiesis, epiphyseal and laryngeal cartilage growth, and 'androgenic behavioral patterns'.

4. Testosterone, by itself, cannot produce full bone mineralization and maturation because incomplete epiphyseal closure and diminished bone density is seen in the rare estrogen-resistance syndrome.

5. Chromosomal abnormalities can lead to impaired structural development.

   a. Klinefelter's Syndrome (Table 31-1).

      i. Affected individuals are phenotypic males and genotypically carry the Y chromosome so that there are

## TABLE 31-1.   CHARACTERISTIC FEATURES OF KLINEFELTER'S SYNDROME

Phenotypic Male With Varying Hypogonadism
Small, Firm Testes
Decreased Libido, Impotence, and Gynecomastia
Disproportionate Extremity Size
   (Height Greater Than Arm Span)
Personality and Behavioral Features
Tendency to Varicose Veins and Chronic Obstructive Pulmonary
   Disease
Borderline to Low Testosterone Levels
Elevated Gonadotropins
'Chromatin-Positive' Buccal Smear
XXY Genotypy

testes and development of internal and external genitalia along masculine lines. The presence of the 'extra X', however, (genotype is XXY) makes the testes imperfect.

ii.  This results in small, rather firm testes (small because there is inadequate spermatogenesis – the seminiferous tubules comprise the bulk of testicular volume; rather firm because this is not a 'secondary atrophy'). Leydig cells appear hyperplastic but this is a relative, not an absolute phenomenon. In actuality, Leydig cell function is poor and testosterone production is inadequate (especially since it has to be 'overdriven' by excessive levels of luteinizing hormone (LH)).

iii. The increased testicular stimulation by LH results in a disproportionate amount of testicular estrogen production. This further diminishes secondary masculinization; it also results in the tendency to decreased libido, impotence and gynecomastia. The estrogen-mediated increase in sex hormone binding globulin (SHBG) produces a higher total testosterone level making this value appear more 'normal' (but in actuality reducing the amount of free testosterone because of the high degree of binding of testosterone to SHBG).

iv. Delayed epiphyseal closure results in a disproportionate increase in extremity size (as compared with the trunk). Despite this increase in arm span, the height is still greater than the arm span because of inordinately long lower extremities. Other associated physical characteristics include the tendency to chronic obstructive pulmonary disease, varicose veins and certain types of personality and behavioral aberrancies. (Klinefelter's is a rather common chromosomal disorder with an incidence of about 1:500–700 males. It is disproportionately seen in males who have a history of mental problems, who are or who have been institutionalized, and among the homeless and alcoholic population.)

v. The diagnosis is suggested by the clinical scenario in concert with the hypogonad state (although patients may not necessarily seek medical attention because of this). A buccal smear will be 'chromatin-positive' (an eccentric nuclear mass of chromatin corroborative of a 'dormant X' chromosome) and neutrophils may carry a 'drumstick' (homologous to the Barr body). Definitive diagnosis is made by chromosomal analysis.

b. Other chromosomal abnormalities can result in abnormal testicular development.

i. The presence of increasing numbers of X chromosomes tends to not only be associated with severe primary hypogonadism but with severe mental retardation and skeletal and other bodily deformities.

ii. Conversely, mosaic configurations (e.g. XX/XXY) or 'hidden extra X' (e.g. XY males) may have more somatic normalcy.

iii. The XYY configuration has been associated with generally normal gonadal development, but with a higher incidence of behavioral abnormalities and anti-social behavior – this karyotype is often found in penal or mental institutions.

iv. A male variant of Turner's syndrome (also called Bonnevie–Ulrich or Noonan's syndrome) has an XY karyotype in a phenotypic male, but has somatic features resembling Turner's syndrome (e.g. webbed neck, increased 'carrying angle' of the forearm and short stature). Additionally, there is primary hypogonadism (high gonadotropins in the presence of a low testosterone).

v.  True hermaphroditism occurs when there is a 'chimeric' composition of two distinct sources of gonadal anlage resulting in the presence of both testicular and ovarian tissue in the same person (with resultant XY and XX chromosomal composition). This is a very rare disorder.

vi. Some genotypic (XY) males may present with a female phenotype and 'streak gonads' (gonadal dysgenesis) analogous to Turner's syndrome but without the other physical stigmata – this is indicative of the loss of XY-mediated development of a male gonad. Several potential sites of defect are possible.

## PRODUCTION OF TESTICULAR HORMONES AND FEEDBACK REGULATION

1.  Production of gonadotropins follicle stimulating hormone (FSH) and luteinizing hormone (LH) is dependent upon pulsatile stimulation of gonadotrophic cells by gonadotropin releasing hormone (GnRH).

2.  FSH is taken up by specific Sertoli cell receptors – a major activity of these Sertoli cells appears to be the production of a locally produced, specific, testosterone-binding protein. Advantage is taken of the rich local supply of testosterone produced by adjacent Leydig cells. The high testosterone concentration enables sperm maturation.

3.  To complete the feedback, inhibin is made by the Sertoli cells. It is a heterodimer with two distinct components: $\alpha$ and $\beta$, each having a MW of 32 000 – it is capable of suppression of FSH. Testosterone can also inhibit FSH. A noteworthy clinical corollary is the infertility that results when males take exogenous androgens – FSH is suppressed and Sertoli-mediated testosterone-binding protein is not made. The testicular concentration of testosterone is also reduced because Leydig cell function is suppressed by LH inhibition.

4.  LH attaches to specific Leydig cell receptors, stimulates adenylate cyclase, and ultimately activates testosterone synthesis. The feedback loop is completed by testosterone-mediated suppression

of LH. The specific mechanism by which this occurs is through the conversion of testosterone to estradiol in the hypothalamus (obviously, circulating estrogen entering the hypothalamus can also effect this as normally occurs in women). Hypothalamic conversion of testosterone to estradiol, however, does not always have to occur to suppress LH. Dihydrotestosterone, in fact, can do this and ultimately produces a decreased pulse frequency of LH (as opposed to estradiol which decreases pulse amplitude of LH).

a.   Testosterone synthesis requires a sequence of enzymatic steps starting with cholesterol. As in the synthesis of cortisol, the sequential actions of cholesterol side-chain cleavage enzyme (20,22-desmolase), 3-β hydroxysteroid dehydrogenase and 17-hydroxylase sequences must take place to produce 17-hydroxyprogesterone (Figure 31-1).

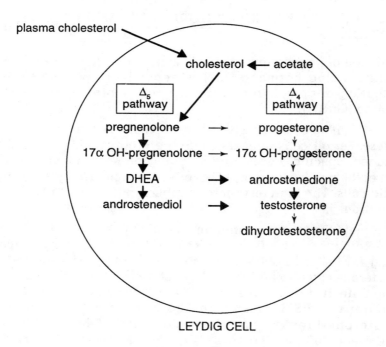

**Figure 31-1.** Diagrammatic Representation of the Androgen Synthetic Pathway in the Leydig Cells of the Testis: DHEA, dihydroepiandrosterone. Reproduced with kind permission from *Endocrinology and Metabolism*, 2nd edn., Felig, P., Baxter, J.D., Broadus, A.E. and Frohman, L.A. (eds.), McGraw-Hill Book Company

b. A crucial step in testosterone synthesis is the splitting off of a two-carbon fragment at the 17 position (17,20-desmolase) to produce androstenedione. Reduction of androstenedione by a 17-keto reductase produces testosterone. Although the term '17-ketosteroid' is often associated with androgenic activity, the most potent androgen (i.e. testosterone) is not a 17-ketosteroid. Testosterone can, itself, be converted into less potent products that are 17-ketosteroids (androsterone and etiocholanolone – although etiocholanolone does not have androgenic properties).

c. Androstenedione and testosterone are the immediate precursors (via the enzymatic action of aromatase) of the respective estrogens, estrone and estradiol (these estrogens are interconvertible).

5. Testosterone is carried in the circulation bound (about 60%) to sex hormone binding globulin (SHBG). Androgens decrease the amount of SHBG (as does growth hormone and hypothyroidism), but there is a relative increase in the free or metabolically active testosterone. Estrogens increase the SHBG (and thus the total testosterone) but decrease the free fraction. As this also occurs in thyrotoxicosis, this explains the relative hyperestrogenic state that occurs in thyrotoxic conditions.

6. The action of testosterone is to initiate nuclear transcription and thus activate the sequence of events leading to protein formation in androgen responsive cells (these are cells that have intracytoplasmic receptors for testosterone; the receptor–testosterone complex is then transported to the nucleus to begin the synthetic process).

7. Testosterone is converted to dihydrotestosterone by the enzyme, 5-α reductase. Much of the peripheral effect of testosterone can be explained by dihydrotestosterone although both testosterone and dihydrotestosterone bind to the same intracellular receptor sites and substantial levels of testosterone can seemingly take the place of dihydrotestosterone in many (but not all, e.g. prostate growth) functions. A corollary to the clinical relevance of dihydrotestosterone is the potential role of finasteride, a 5-α reductase inhibitor, in the management of prostatic hyperplasia.

8. Defects Associated with Impaired Testosterone Synthesis (all are also associated with impaired estrogen synthesis, to some degree).

a. All of these result in male pseudohermaphroditism (male sexual ambiguity or predominant female phenotype in genotypic males). Because the testes are still capable of making Müllerian inhibitory factor, there is no female internal sexual development.

b. There are three enzymatic deficiencies which also affect glucocorticoid synthesis: cholesterol side-chain cleavage defect, 3-β hydroxysteroid dehydrogenase defect and 17 hydroxylase deficiency.

   i. The first two defects additionally affect both glucocorticoid and aldosterone synthesis; the last only glucocorticoid synthesis.

   ii. The last has been traced to a genetic defect on chromosome 10. Because mineralocorticoid production is rendered excessive by the lack of cortisol-mediated suppression of ACTH, there is associated hypertension (this is classically associated with hypernatremia) and hypokalemia. Aldosterone, however, is not the active mineralocorticoid as renin is suppressed. Corticosterone and deoxycorticosterone (DOC) are excessive and are responsible for the salt retention and associated hypervolemia.

c. There are two enzymatic deficiencies associated with impaired testosterone deficiency (without defective cortisol synthesis and with normal ACTH–cortisol feedback). These are 17,20-desmolase deficiency and 17-β hydroxysteroid oxidoreductase deficiency.

   i. The former is associated with a greater array of androgen (dihydroepiandrosterone, androstenedione and testosterone) and estrogen (estrone, estradiol) deficiencies than the latter which represents a defect distal to the ability to manufacture androstenedione and estrone. Nonetheless, in the latter the androgens produced are 'weak' and are insufficient to produce complete masculinization. Affected males tend to have pseudohermaphroditism and predominantly female external genitalia, but there is also a late onset form associated with gynecomastia and hypogonadism. Affected genotypic females (XX), although they have female external genitalia, do not achieve secondary sexual maturation.

ii. Both are associated with elevated gonadotropin levels.

9. Defect Associated with Impaired Conversion of Testosterone to Dihydrotestosterone (5-α reductase deficiency)

a. Associated with sexual ambiguity at birth in genotypic, XY males (male pseudohermaphroditism). Children are initially reared as females but change to a rather unambiguous masculine phenotype at puberty – i.e. increased size of phallus (despite persistent hypospadius) and scrotal rugae development (even though the scrotum remains bifid). Affected individuals are identified (and identify themselves) at that time as males. (In the Dominican Republic where these kindreds were initially described, they are referred to as 'she–he').

b. The appearance of a masculine phenotype at the time of puberty does not occur because the defect suddenly 'self-corrects'. Rather, the defect may be an 'incomplete one' all along and the increased total gonadal androgen production that accompanies puberty may result in some production of dihydrotestosterone as well. Further, testosterone in excess can mimic some dihydrotestosterone effects (and the maternal estrogenic environment that may have thwarted this effort during fetal development is no longer present).

c. Because testosterone is capable of feedback inhibition of LH, there is no gynecomastia.

d. The prostate is notably small. (This clinical aspect has resulted in the advent of pharmacologic 5-α reductase inhibition – i.e. finasteride – to treat benign prostatic hyperplasia). Affected patients also have no hirsutism (or male pattern baldness), but pubertal voice change occurs.

10. There is a spectrum of phenotypic disorders associated with impaired peripheral androgenic effect (Receptor or Post-Receptor Defect) in genotypically (XY) normal males.

a. In the complete form (Testicular Feminization), there is

unambiguous phenotypic femininity. The vagina ends in a blind pouch, however, because Müllerian inhibition normally occurs. There are intra-abdominal testes (these should be surgically removed because of increased risk of neoplastic transformation). There are no 'masculine features' which can be seen in these normally appearing 'women' – e.g. there is scant ambisexual hair and no acne. Inheritance is X-linked recessive. (Thus, half of all genotypic male offspring of female carriers will be phenotypic females). Because testosterone is also unable to inhibit the hypothalamic–pituitary axis, LH production is increased This results in increased circulating levels of both testosterone and estradiol. The 'unopposed' estradiol will produce full feminization.

b. Partial target organ insensitivity is associated with varying degrees of sexual ambiguity. Reifenstein's syndrome is the most commonly cited syndrome (inheritance is also X-linked) but syndromes with even greater sexual ambiguity have been described by Gilbert–Dreyfus and Lubs.

## MALE HYPOGONADISM

1. Hypogonadism can occur as a result of an abnormality in any site within the sequence of events necessary for normal gonadal function.

2. The clinical syndrome may not only include hypogonadism but other additional features depending upon the nature and location of the process and the stage of life during which the process occurs.

3. Specific features are related to inability or inadequacy of sexual function. Other features are related to the lack of the extragonadal actions of androgens (habitus, bodily hair, bone maturation, voice, 'masculine personality traits'). Prepubertal hypogonadism results in absence of terminal hair growth, the tendency to a eunuchoid habitus (a disproportionate increase in extremity size, when compared with the trunk. The increased arm span is striking because of the 'additive effect' of measuring both arm lengths in calculating the arm span), lack of laryngeal maturation (and associated 'castrati voice') and lack of male pattern baldness. Because terminal hair, once grown, is resistant to regression (a

clinical issue with women as well, in different clinical settings), a beard may still be present in postpubertal hypogonadism even though the frequency of shaving is decreased – the analogy holds true with failure of regression of an already masculinized larynx or reversal of baldness.

4. Testicular size is an important aspect of the physical examination. Volume can be estimated by comparison with the standards on an orchidometer or by direct measurement using the formula: $V = 0.52 \times \text{length} \times (\text{width})^2$. Normal volume tends to be about 15–19 cm$^3$ and values are slightly higher when done with direct measurement. Primary atrophy produces smaller, firmer testes (because seminiferous tubules have not developed). Secondary atrophy, while resulting in decreased testicular volume, also decreases their firmness and resiliency.

5. Infertility can be linked to hypogonadism, *per se*, or it can occur in the absence of any other hypogonadal features.

6. Etiologies of Hypogonadism (Table 31-2):

   a. Disorders of the hypothalamus and pituitary.

      i. Etiologies have been discussed in detail in Chapter 3 and include neoplasia, infiltrative disease, infection, vascular disease, structural abnormalities, ablation, selective deficiencies, autoimmunity and idiopathic causes.

      ii. Isolated hypogonadotropic disorders can occur with Kallman's syndrome (associated with anosmia and secondary to inadequate embryologic development of

**TABLE 31-2. ETIOLOGIES OF HYPOGONADISM**

Hypothalamic Disorders
Pituitary Disorders
Gonadal Disorders
     Chromosomal Disorders
     Disorders of Testosterone Synthesis
     Myotonic Dystrophy
     Acquired Testicular Defects
Androgen-Resistance States

midline structures) and Laurence–Moon–Biedl syndrome (other features include obesity, polydactyly, mental retardation and retinitis pigmentosa).

iii. Prader–Willi is a fascinating syndrome (pronounced facial features, short stature, obesity, hypotonia, small acral appendages) in that it occurs when the source of each member of the chromosome 15 pair is from the mother.

iv. Hypogonadotropic hypogonadism can also be a feature of systemic disorders (e.g. chronic renal failure), neurologic syndromes (e.g. cerebellar ataxia), physiologic impairment of gonadotropin production (e.g. anorexia nervosa, hyperprolactinemia, possibly marijuana use), production of immunologically active but biologically incompetent LH, or it may be an 'early' pituitary hormone deficiency in a future scenario that will ultimately include other deficiency states (e.g. pituitary adenoma).

b. Gonadal Disorders – disorders in which there is inadequate gonadal function despite hypergonadotropism.

i. Chromosomal disorders – including Klinefelter's syndrome and its variants, and variant Turner's (Noonan's) syndrome.

ii. Disorders of testosterone synthesis, previously reviewed in this chapter.

iii. Myotonic dystrophy – autosomal dominant; often but not always associated with Leydig cell impairment as well as destruction of seminiferous tubules. Diffuse myopathy (face and neck are commonly involved) with characteristic myotonia (sustained contraction following stimulation). Also associated with diabetes mellitus, cataracts and mental retardation.

iv. Vanishing testes syndrome – absence of Müllerian elements, but with differentiation of Wolffian elements (albeit the phallus is generally small and there are absent testes in the scrotal sac) suggest that testicular tissue was initially present during embryogenesis.

(a) In affected males in whom the process occurs earlier in development (before 12–14 weeks) there would be ambiguous genitalia; before 8 weeks, overt feminization.

(b) Cryptorchidism, a very common entity (3% at birth, about 1% persistent through adulthood) must be ruled out. Plasma testosterone (basal or after human chorionic gonadotropin (hCG) stimulation) would be low in the vanishing testis syndrome, but not abnormal in cryptorchidism.

(Cryptorchidism should be corrected, if persistent, either by surgery or with hCG stimulation. Because of the high incidence of neoplastic degeneration in cryptorchidism, some recommend unilateral orchidectomy if only one testis is involved or careful follow up if the process is bilateral. Cryptorchidism is associated with testicular torsion, hernia and impaired sperm production; it is not clear whether cryptorchidism is the cause or effect of these problems – probably both).

(c) A 'variant' of the 'vanishing testis' syndrome is Leydig cell aplasia – testes are present but absent Leydig cells result in a hypogonadal state. Some antecedent Leydig cell function must have occurred to produce Wolffian duct maturation – alternatively, severe Leydig cell failure is associated with sexual ambiguity.

v. Acquired testicular defects – a large and multifaceted category.

(a) Viral illness – often associated with the mumps virus but may be caused by ECHO- and arborviruses, among others. The magnitude of orchitis does not necessarily predict (nor does unilaterality predict) the ultimate degree of damage; damage may be secondary to a direct trophic effect of the virus as well as the secondary effects of pressure atrophy.

(b) Radiation.

(c) Drugs – estrogens and related agents (? digitalis), testosterone synthesis inhibitors (e.g. ketoconazole, ethanol), antineoplastic agents (e.g. cyclophosphamide, methotrexate). Some antiandrogens may have an additional effect on inhibition of testosterone synthesis (e.g. cyproterone, spironolactone, cimetidine and flutamide).

(d) Infiltrative disease – e.g. granulomatous disease, hemochromatosis.

(e) Autoimmune disease.

(f) Lead toxicity.

(g) Traumatic injury or iatrogenic extirpation (e.g. for carcinoma of the prostate).

(h) Associated with systemic diseases – alcoholism and cirrhosis, chronic renal failure, sickle cell disease and cystinosis.

(i) Male climacteric – although not as abrupt a phenomenon as menopause is in women, testosterone levels decrease with age (isolated values in older men may be comparable to those of younger men, but mean values are less and older men do not demonstrate the morning peak level, usually at about 08.00, seen in younger men). The increased amount of bodily adipose tissue (a phenomenon that occurs with age) and LH elevation in response to gonadal failure results in increased estrogen levels. In addition to any direct anti-androgenic effect of the estrogen, it also stimulates SHBG production resulting in a somewhat elevated total testosterone but a decreased free level. Many of the same functional and vasomotor symptoms experienced by menopausal women can also be experienced by men.

  c.  Androgen resistance states – inborn errors and antiandrogens (e.g. spironolactone, cyproterone, cimetidine and flutamide – some of these may also inhibit androgen synthesis).

7.  Etiologies of infertility other than those discussed in the context of hypogonadism include:

  a.  Seminiferous tubule failure – an all encompassing category with multiple etiologies such as infectious disease (including viral), toxic, vascular, radiation, alcoholism, non-gonadal endocrinologic disease and systemic disease; many of these etiologies are also capable of producing Leydig cell failure.

b. Structural Disease – e.g. varicocele (the most common cause in this category), obstruction or atrophy of the epididymis or vas deferens (e.g. cystic fibrosis), disorders of the penis and prostate (e.g. Peyronie's disease).

c. Miscellaneous disorders include 'dysfunctional' or immotile sperm (e.g. as with Kartegener's syndrome), neurologic disease resulting in retrograde ejaculation and antibodies directed at sperm (although this may technically also be a component of 'female infertility').

## IMPOTENCE

1. General Issues

   a. Impotence is often a very significant manifestation of the hypogonadal state. While much of the previous discussion of hypogonadism has had an endocrinologic perspective, there are multiple etiologies of impotence with endocrinologic disease accounting for only some of them. Impotence, in addition, may be of complex or multiple etiologies (e.g. diabetes, alcoholism). Psychologic causes, while a separate category, can play an amplifying role even though the primary etiology is organic.

   b. While impotence is empirically defined as the inability to achieve vaginal penetration in 50% of the attempts, ejaculation ability is usually maintained much of the time.

   c. Initiation of the erectile process occurs via limbic system pathways, direct tactile stimulation activating neurogenic pathways, or both – parasympathetic outflow is required.

   d. The process of erection is associated with increased blood flow through the corpora cavernosum and spongiosum secondary to arteriolar dilatation. Secondary venous constriction has to take place (contraction of the ischiocavernosus muscle plays an important role) to maintain the intravascular pool of blood.

2. Causes of Impotence

   a. Systemic illness – cardiovascular disease, hepatic insufficiency, chronic renal diseae, chronic obstructive pulmonary disease.

b. Vascular disease – atherosclerosis (including Leriche syndrome), sickle cell disease, diabetic vascular disease, vasculitis.

c. Neurologic disease – central, spinal, peripheral and autonomic (multiple etiologies ranging from infarction to demyelinating disease, toxic neuropathy, diabetic neuropathy, surgical disruption of autonomic fibers).

d. Endocrinologic disease – all etiologies of hypogonadism, thyrotoxicosis and hypothyroidism, hyperprolactinemia, adrenal insufficiency, hyperestrogenic states.

e. Drug-related – major categories include estrogenic agents, agents that interfere with testosterone synthesis or action (e.g. ketoconazole, cimetidine, spironolactone), antihypertensives and drugs used in the treatment of congestive heart failure (mechanisms include autonomic dysfunction, decreased libido and hypotension), psychotropic agents (mechanisms include autonomic dysfunction, hypotension, hyperprolactinemia), anticholinergics, alcohol, tobacco use and illicit drug use (e.g. cocaine, morphine and amphetamines).

f. Psychogenic.

g. Physical Impairment of the Urogenital Apparatus – e.g. trauma, post-cancer surgery, Peyronie's disease.

3. Diagnostic Work-up

a. History – relevant information includes onset, duration, completeness, other symptoms or illnesses, presence of nocturnal or morning erections, mental status history, medications, interpersonal relationships.

b. Complete physical and focused urogenital examination.

c. Laboratory studies

i. Routine complete blood count, urinalysis, chemistry screening panel, serum electrolytes (as appropriate), urinalysis, urine culture (as appropriate).

ii. Special endocrinologic studies – testosterone (total and free), FSH, LH and prolactin levels are the 'basic' endocrinologic studies. Dihydrotestosterone, estradiol and estrone levels are additionally obtained, as appropriate. Dynamic tests that produce testicular stimulation include the use of chorionic gonadotropin, clomiphene and gonadotropin releasing hormone – they are usually not necessary.

   iii. Special studies include testing for nocturnal penile tumescence and the use of Doppler flow for penile blood pressure (this is compared with brachial blood pressure). Electromyography (by inference) may correlate regional neurologic impairment with an associated cause for the impotence. Studies which require urologic and/or vascular radiology consultation include assessment of the clinical response to intracorporeal papaverine or papaverine/phentolamine (with or without concomitant duplex scanning and penile arteriography). Cavernosometry and cavernosography can additionally monitor for venous leakage (erection is first induced with intracavernous saline – radioconstrast is added to the saline so that 'leaks' can be monitored; penile pressure is also monitored to assess the ability to sustain the erection. These interventional studies have associated morbidity and should be performed only with appropriate cause.

4. Therapeutic Options

  a. Correction of the underlying problem or disease state. When possible, it is always the most rewarding solution.

  b. Vascular reconstructive surgery – when appropriate; it may involve major vessel grafting procedures or more 'focused' procedures may be performed (e.g. empiric therapy ligating the superficial and deep dorsal veins of the penis to ameliorate venous insufficiency).

  c. Intracorporeal injection – papaverine, papaverine/phentolamine and prostaglandin $E_1$ have all been used. The effect may wane with continued usage. Ancillary oral drugs such as Yohimbine are of unclear benefit.

  d. Prosthetic devices – two general varieties: 'fixed' and 'expansile' (capable of inflation). An external portable device (combining an external vacuum effect with band-constriction) may be beneficial and acceptable (less morbidity and it obviates the need for surgery).

e.  Psychiatric evaluation and therapy, counselling and sex therapy – when appropriate.

f.  Androgenic therapy (when appropriate):

   i.  Testosterone propionate – must be given parenterally; short acting (but a useful agent when therapy is first initiated); usual dose, 50 mg three times per week.

   ii.  Oral preparations – may also be taken sublingually (methyltestosterone – Android; fluoxymesterone – Android F or Halotestin; oxymetholone – Anadrol); alkylation at 17-α position allows for oral intake but makes for potential hepatotoxicity; cannot be readily monitored with serum markers.

   iii.  Long-acting parenteral preparations (modification of 17-β hydroxyl group). Testosterone enanthate – Delatestryl; and testosterone cyclopentylpropionate or cypionate – Depo-Testosterone); general dose range: 100-200 mg every 1–4 weeks.

   iv.  A transdermal testosterone preparation is available, but it must be placed on the scrotum to maximize absorption (as a result, there is disproportionate conversion to dihydrotestosterone but this is not of clinical relevance).

   v.  Side-effects of androgenic therapy

      (a) Excessive masculinization (may be a problem in previously hypogonad males who are 'not comfortable' with the sudden change); paradoxical feminization (secondary to increased estrogen conversion).

      (b) Hepatic complications – may range from asymptomatic abnormalities of liver function tests to peliosis hepatica (blood-filled hepatic cysts) and hepatoma.

      (c) Increased tendency to polycythemia (corollary is the pharmacologic use of androgens to treat some types of refractory anemia) and exacerbation of sleep apnea.

    (d) May precipitate benign prostatic hyperplasia or act as a growth factor for pre-existing (and perhaps undiagnosed) prostate cancer.

    (e) Additional side-effects include premature epiphyseal fusion, gynecomastia, water retention and hypertension.

## GYNECOMASTIA

1. Literally, feminization of the male breast. Although lactation (galactorrhea) may occur at the same time, the pathophysiology of galactorrhea is usually distinctly different.

2. Etiologies of gynecomastia include:

    a. Physiologic – associated with an estrogen/testosterone imbalance. Seen neonatally, during puberty, and in the elderly (where it may be a concomitant of the 'ageing process').

    b. Endocrine dysfunction – hypogonadism, HCG-producing tumor states (e.g. testicular tumors, bronchogenic carcinoma), hyperestrogenic states (neoplastic, pharmacologic, pathologic), thyrotoxicosis.

    c. Systemic disease processes – e.g. alcohol abuse, liver disease, renal failure, starvation-mediated.

    d. Pharmacologic – androgen inhibitory agents (at any site in androgen synthesis or action), estrogen agonists, agents which enhance Leydig cell stimulation (e.g. HCG, clomiphene), anti-ulcer medication (e.g. cimetidine, ranitidine, omeprazole), antibiotics (e.g. ketoconazole, INH, metronidazole), and miscellaneous agents (e.g. antidepressants, calcium-channel blocking agents, opiates, marijuana, penicillamine, meprobamate, busulfan).

3. The characteristic physical finding is a firm mass or 'nubbin' of glandular tissue which can be of variable size and can be bilateral or unilateral. Other breast lesions (e.g. tumors, cysts) may present as breast enlargement. 'Pseudogynecomastia', secondary to adipose tissue deposition, should not be confused with true gynecomastia.

4. The diagnostic evaluation can be 'directed' to specific categories, based upon history and ancillary physical findings.

5. Treatment is generally directed toward specific etiologies (e.g. extirpation of a causal tumor, correction of an endocrinopathy, removal of an offending drug).

6. Even if a correctable problem is treated (and certainly if no specific cause is found), a surgical reduction procedure is often required. This may be necessary because of physical discomfort or because of the psychologic stigmata associated with breast enlargement in the male.

# 32

# NORMAL FEMALE REPRODUCTIVE ENDOCRINOLOGY AND RELATED DISEASE STATES

Fundamental Embryologic Principles
The Normal Menstrual Cycle
Amenorrhea
Hirsutism
The Menopause

## FUNDAMENTAL EMBRYOLOGIC PRINCIPLES

1.  In the absence of the Y chromosome influence, no testis will form, Müllerian duct development will proceed, and Wolffian development will not take place. Phenotype will be along female lines.

2.  An 'active' X chromosome is required for ovarian development (one X remains 'dormant' in the process). Otherwise, 'streaks' are the only remnant of the primordial gonad. With the XX configuration, germ cells are able to seed the undifferentiated gonad (compared with testicular differentiation, ovarian differentiation occurs substantially later at 77–84 days).

3.  By the sixth month of gestation, there are 6–7 million oocytes within the ovary. Meiosis actually begins *in utero* with increase in the DNA content of the nucleus to 4n (the first meiotic division occurs at ovulation, the second after fertilization). At birth, the number of oocytes declines to 1–3 million.

4.  Although gonadotropin-releasing hormone (GnRH) remains suppressed from late gestation until puberty, fetal GnRH is activated up to the first 150 days of gestation. This allows for fetal gonadal stimulation which will eventually lead to feedback suppression of GnRH.

## THE NORMAL MENSTRUAL CYCLE

1.  Under the pulsatile and cyclic stimulation of GnRH, pituitary gonadotropins are made.

    a.  Gonadotropin-releasing hormone (GnRH) is the only known hypothalamic stimulator of both follicle stimulating hormone (FSH) and luteinizing hormone (LH). Its release is stimulated by epinephrine and norepinephrine and inhibited by serotonin, dopamine and endogenous opioids – its ability to stimulate selectively FSH and LH is a function of the particular receptivity of the gonadotroph at that time. The frequency and duration of this stimulation determine whether FSH production is augmented or diminished. The prevailing endocrine environment (e.g. estrogen concentration) also plays an important role.

b.  FSH levels are generally low except for a midcycle (ovulatory) 'spurt' (coincident with the LH 'spurt') and a gradual (but low level) increase beginning premenstrually and continuing through the early portion of the follicular stage of the cycle.

  i.  Because FSH (which acts on granulosa cells) stimulates estradiol production, the gradual but progressive increase in this estradiol acts as a feedbck inhibitor to FSH – hence, there is a decline in FSH in the preovulatory portion of the follicular phase.

  ii.  Ironically, when a 'critical' level of estradiol is achieved, it becomes a stimulus to FSH – this corresponds to the midcycle 'peak'.

  iii. With the progressive decline in estradiol as the cycle nears an end (premenstrual), this again begins the stimulus to FSH production.

c.  LH levels gradually rise (albeit slightly) in the follicular phase of the cycle until a midcycle 'peak' is achieved. Levels then abruptly decline and continue to decrease further until a gradual increase begins premenstrually.

  i.  The LH 'peak' is the stimulatory impetus to ovulation and the subsequent development of the corpus luteum.

  ii.  The production of progesterone by the corpus luteum results in hypothalamic 'down regulation' and thus decreased frequency of GnRH – this is responsible for the decline in LH and lasts until the latter part of the luteal phase of the cycle when the corpus luteum is no longer able to produce progesterone (at this point, LH levels start their gradual increase).

2.  Estradiol achieves two 'peaks' during the cycle: a midcycle 'peak' (but this increase actually starts before midcycle as it is responsible for FSH and LH stimulation) and a lesser midluteal phase 'peak'. Unlike LH 'peaks', these are of longer duration (lasting several days with gradual up and down slopes). The midluteal 'peak' is of lower magnitude, but of longer duration than the preovulatory 'peak'.

3.  Progesterone levels are very low until progesterone is made by the corpus luteum (following ovulation). Peak progesterone values

occur midway through the luteal phase and then decline rapidly, commensurate with the degeneration of the corpus luteum (forming a corpus albicans).

4. The structural concomitants of the menstrual cycle are:

   a. The primary, secondary and tertiary follicles of the preovulatory phase – maturation changes are the appearance of a well-defined zona pellucida surrounding the oocyte, the proliferation of granulosa cells that surround the zona pellucida (and the late development of a follicular antrum filled with liquor folliculi – at this stage, the follicle can be considered a preovulatory or Graafian follicle) and a well-defined theca (internal and external) that surrounds the basement membrane underlying the granulosa cells.

   b. The oocyte is 'liberated' during ovulation surrounded by a 'halo' of granulosa cells (the 'corona radiata'). There is some intrafollicular bleeding (this may 'leak' into the peritoneum producing local irritation and associated 'Mittelschmerz'). Luteal cells can now 'invade' the remaining granulosa tissue – granulosa cells concomitantly change (becoming 'luteinized') and the entire complex is called a corpus luteum.

   c. Estrogen production appears to be the result of androgenic synthesis by theca cells and then aromatization to estrogen by granulosa cells (Figure 32-1).

      i. While estradiol is made primarily in this fashion, estrone can also be made this way but is additionally synthesized by peripheral conversion of androgenic precursors (primarily androstenedione).

      ii. A major effect of LH appears to be on the theca cells to synthesize androstenedione from cholesterol. FSH, on the other hand, appears to play a predominant role in the aromatization of the androstenedione that 'traverses' the basement membrane, to manufacture estrone and ultimately estradiol.

   d. Progesterone is made by the granulosa–lutein cell complex.

5. Circulating hormones are transported in the plasma, primarily in the bound state.

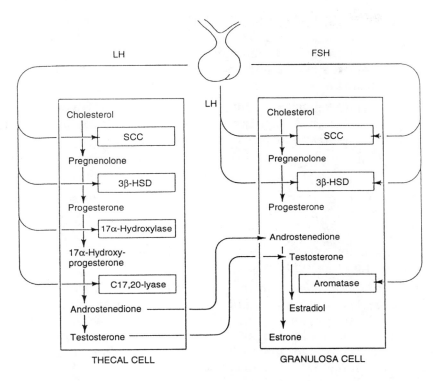

**Figure 32-1.** Biosynthesis of Ovarian Steroids: LH, luteinizing hormone; FSH, follicle stimulating hormone; SCC, cholesterol side-chain cleavage enzyme; HSD, 3β-hydroxysteroid dehydrogenase. Reproduced with kind permission from *Textbook of Endocrine Physiology*, Griffin, J.E. and Ojeda, S. (eds.), p. 135, Oxford: Oxford University Press, 1988

a. Estradiol is carried by albumin (60%) and sex hormone binding globulin, SHBG (38%) with only 2% circulating in free form.

   i. Estrogens stimulate hepatic synthesis of SHBG.

   ii. As opposed to albumin which is a 'high capacity, low affinity' binder, SHBG is a 'high affinity, low capacity' binder of sex steroids.

   iii. The chemical structure of SHBG is a glycoprotein with MW of 95 000.

   iv. SHBG binds dihydrotestosterone, testosterone and estradiol in descending order of affinity.

v. A corollary is that this hierarchy of binding affinity 'amplifies' the effect of increasing estrogen levels by not only the 'direct' effect of estrogen but by decreasing the relative availability of free testosterone and dihydro-testosterone.

   (a) The thyrotoxic state, by augmenting SHBG synthesis, can produce a hyperestrogenic state (even producing clinical effects such as gynecomastia).

   (b) Hypothyroidism, obesity, growth hormone (HGH), and androgens decrease SHBG synthesis.

   b. Progesterone is carried by both albumin and cortisol-binding globulin (CBG).

6. Estrogen affects responsive tissues through its ability to bind to specific cytoplasmic receptor sites and initiate the transcriptional phase of protein synthesis.

   a. Estrogenic effects on the female reproductive tract include overall growth and maturation, endometrial proliferation, thickening of the vaginal mucosa and production of large quantities of a relatively watery mucus. This glycogen-rich mucus allows for the generation of lactic acid (and an acidic vaginal pH) by the action of lactobacilli (Döderlein's bacillus).

      i. The unopposed estrogenic effect on vaginal epithelium results in stimulation of large numbers of 'superficial cells' (flat, mature, pyknotic and small nucleus).

      ii. Estrogen deficiency results in a more prominent 'basal–parabasal cell' vaginal cytology (smaller, rounder cells with larger more vesicular nuclei).

   b. The estrogenic effect on the breast is primarily on ductal development and areolar pigmentation. Estrogens also stimulate labial pigmentation and pigment production in non-genital areas – e.g. 'mask of pregnancy' (which can also be seen with use of oral contraceptives) and 'linea negra'.

   c. Estrogenic effects elsewhere in the body include enhancement of bone growth, density and maturation (leading to epiphyseal closure) in both men and women, fat redistribution along 'female lines', hepatic stimulation of proteins (e.g. high-density and very low-density lipoproteins (HDL, VLDL);

pro-coagulants II, VII, IX, and X, transport proteins such as ceruloplasmin, thyroxine-binding globulin, and SHBG), decreased bone sensitivity to parathyroid hormone (this appears to be an important mechanism in its 'anti-osteoporotic' effect), decreased gut motility, secondary renal sodium retention (because of a 'functional hypovolemia') and a 'feminine psyche' and 'female behavioral patterns'.

7. Progesterone has reproductive and non-reproductive effects as well.

   a. It fosters a secretory endometrium (thus preparing it for ovum implantation) and alters the composition of cervical mucus (decreased volume but increased viscosity). While unopposed estrogen maximizes 'ferning' (a characteristic pattern of dried mucus), the presence of progesterone diminishes this. *Spinnbarkeit* is also maximal at the time of ovulation (prior to progesterone effect). The classic vaginal cytology seen with an adequate progesterone effect is an 'intermediate cell' (larger cell, but with a well-formed nucleus and mature cytoplasm).

   b. The primary effect on breast tissue is alveolar growth and development.

   c. The major peripheral effects of progesterone are aldosterone antagonism (this may be compensated by increased aldosterone production), increased sensitivity to $p_{CO_2}$ (this has some application in the treatment of hypoventilation or sleep apnea syndromes), diminished peripheral sensitivity to insulin and increased basal body temperature.

8. The co-ordinated contributions of estrogen and progesterone lead to the various structural and functional properties of the endometrial lining (and the timing of their occurrence) during the normal menstrual cycle.

   a. These include gland mitoses, stromal mitoses, nuclear pseudostratification, stromal edema, leukocytic infiltration and basal vacuolation.

   b. The dependency of the endometrium for its sustenance on continued sex steroid hormone stimulation results in the cyclical desquamation of the functional (as opposed to the basal) layer when stimulation ceases (the basal layer remains intact).

   i. This occurs physiologically when the elevated postovulation estrogen and progesterone levels wane – this is true menstruation. Desquamation can also be brought on 'synthetically' by utilizing and then withdrawing exogenous estrogen and progesterone (e.g. oral contraceptives).

   ii. Estrogen withdrawal by itself (without any progesterone effect) can produce bleeding (but it is usually of a lesser magnitude because of the absence of a secretory endometrium). The character, timing and amount of blood loss, however, can be quite variable.

9. Feedback inhibition of both FSH and LH can be accomplished by estrogen – conversely, estrogen deficiency causes elevation of both FSH and LH, although FSH is the more sensitive of the two (hence a useful marker for early ovarian failure).

   a. While inhibin (a peptide heterodimer with an $\alpha$ (A) and $\beta$ (B) subunit that is made by granulosa cells) can also inhibit FSH, the magnitude of its significance is not clear.

   b. Ironically, a very similar protein, Activin (composed of 2 $\beta$ subunits) can be a stimulus to FSH.

   c. These peptide regulators may even have extragonadal effects (e.g. hematopoiesis).

**AMENORRHEA** (Table 32-1)

1. General Considerations:

   a. Because menstruation, itself, is the obvious clinical consequence of the normal harmony of the menstrual cycle, its presence is indicative of anatomic and physiologic normalcy.

   b. Nonetheless, since it is the final common end-point of a carefully orchestrated sequence of events, amenorrhea (the absence of menstruation) can occur as a result of any number of potential derangements in that long sequence.

### TABLE 32-1.   ETIOLOGIES OF AMENORRHEA

---

Hypothalamic Disorders
    Idiopathic Deficiency of Gonadotropin-Releasing Hormone
    Anorexia Nervosa
    Destructive Lesions
    'Hypothalamic Amenorrhea'

Pituitary Disorders
    Pituitary Tumors
    Empty Sella Syndrome
    Other Hypopituitary States:
        Other Tumors, Infiltrative Disease, Infection,
          Vascular Disease,
        Structural Abnormalities, Ablative, Autoimmune,
          Idiopathic,
        Selective Deficiency

Ovarian Disease
    Turner's Syndrome
    Variant Turner's Syndrome
    Testicular Feminization Syndrome
    Enzymatic Defects in Estrogen Synthesis
    Ovarian Failure
    Estrogen-Producing Tumors
    Androgen Excess States
    Polycystic Ovarian Syndrome

Disorders of the Reproductive Tract

---

  c.  Furthermore, it should be looked upon as a symptom of a more primal pathologic process – i.e. it is not the disease, *per se,* but a clinical manifestation.

  d.  Amenorrhea is empirically defined as the failure to achieve menses before age 16 (primary amenorrhea) or absence of menses for the prior 6 months in a woman who has already achieved regular menses (secondary amenorrhea). This distinction is not merely academic because etiologies can be different for each category and secondary sexual maturation is often (but certainly not always) absent in primary amenorrhea.

e. The clinical syndrome is a compendium of those features associated with the site of pathologic dysfunction as well as the consequences of that pathologic process. It is best approached by dividing amenorrhea into the categories of hypothalamic, pituitary, ovarian and reproductive tract disorders.

2. Hypothalamic Disorders

   a. Idiopathic Deficiency of GnRH

      i. Primary amenorrhea.

      ii. May be associated with 'midline' facial defects including anosmia (Kallman's Syndrome), hearing loss and color blindness.

      iii. Multiple inheritance patterns noted – a basic defect is impaired migration of GnRH neurons from an 'olfactory site' to the hypothalamus.

   b. Anorexia Nervosa

      i. Amenorrhea is one feature of a complex syndrome associated with behavioral abnormalities, inappropriate perception of body image (with eating patterns that prevent weight gain beyond a perceived threshold) and yet a paradoxical preoccupation with food. Accompanying systemic features include body temperature dysregulation, hypotension, hypercarotenemia, increased bodily lanugo hair, hypercholesterolemia, impaired renal concentration ability, elevated plasma cortisol (decreased clearance), decreased triiodothyronine, increased HGH (but low insulin-like growth factor-I) and HGH stimulation by TRH (but diminished prolactin stimulation by TRH).

      ii. Amenorrhea can also be seen in bulimia nervosa, but it is much less common.

      iii. Loss of GnRH can result in absent gonadotropin production or in a prepubertal pattern in which LH pulses occur only during sleep. Exogenous GnRH can stimulate gonadotropin production and thus 'bypass' the defect, but prior priming may be necessary.

    iv. When seen in men (albeit less frequently than in women), gonadotropins are also low and low testosterone levels contribute to the clinical syndrome.

    v. There appears to be a 'critical' weight loss in each person above which menses will resume. Improvement in the patient's 'mental profile' can also initiate normal menses – these two factors are not mutually exclusive because weight gain will usually accompany an 'improved mental profile'.

c. Hypothalamic Destruction

    i. Space-occupying lesion – includes primary neoplasia (e.g. craniopharyngioma, meningioma), ectopic tumors (e.g. pinealoma), metastatic tumors, teratoma; reticuloendothelioses (e.g. eosinophilic granuloma, Hand–Schuller–Christian disease); infectious (e.g. tuberculosis) and non-infectious (e.g. sarcoidosis) granulomatous disease; vascular abnormalities.

    ii. Head trauma – primary or secondary to hemorrhagic or ischemic processes.

    iii. Radiation – because of the greater sensitivity to radiation of hypothalamic than pituitary tissue, postirradiation hypopituitarism is invariably a hypothalamic problem.

d. 'Hypothalamic Amenorrhea'

    i. A large category that is composed of multiple etiologies. It is a common cause of primary amenorrhea and the most common cause of secondary amenorrhea.

    ii. Gonadotropin and GnRH stimulation patterns are variable.

    iii. Concomitant clinical scenarios include reduction diet and weight loss, vigorous athletic conditioning – usually aerobic (e.g. jogging) and stress.

    iv. Purported mechanisms include:

        (a) Endorphin and dopamine stimulation – both of these are inhibitory to GnRH.

        (b) The role of melatonin is less well-defined, but levels are elevated in hypothalamic amenorrhea. In pinealoma, clinical findings and gonadotropic hormone deficiencies can correlate with the secretion of melatonin.

3. Pituitary Disorders

   a. Pituitary Tumors

      i. Prolactin-producing tumors are the most common pituitary tumor and the most common cause of pituitary tumor-mediated amenorrhea. They may account for 30% of cases of all women who present with amenorrhea.

      ii. While direct pituitary destruction is a possible mechanism (with macro-, but not microadenomas), the cause is related to prolactin-mediated GnRH suppression.

   b. Additional etiologies include other space-occupying lesions (e.g tumor, infectious, structural, infiltrative), iatrogenic, immunologic, vascular and idiopathic disease processes.

      i. Gonadotropin loss tends to occur 'early' in the hierarchy of pituitary hormone loss that leads to complete hypopituitarism.

      ii. If infarction occurs postpartum (which is a time of increased vulnerability), the clinical presentation may range from 'subtle' (e.g. failure of normal menses to resume) to catastrophic (e.g. hypotension and shock).

   c. The 'empty sella' syndrome may rarely produce gonadotropin deficiency. In actuality, the skull X-ray, CT, or MRI usually demonstrate an anatomic abnormality excessively disproportionate to the clinical scenario.

4. Ovarian Disease

   a. Turner's Syndrome (Gonadal Dysgenesis)

      i. A chromosomal disorder (XO) with consequential ovarian agenesis because an additional X chromosome is necessary for ovarian development (according to the Lyon hypothesis, one X chromosome must always be 'dormant').

      ii. Primary amenorrhea

iii. Internal and external genitalia are always female:

(a) There is no testicular tissue to either inhibit Müllerian or stimulate Wolffian ductal development.

(b) Ovarian hormone deficiency prevents sexual maturation.

iv. Extragonadal facets of 'classic' Turner's syndrome include somatic features (short stature, low set ears, 'webbed neck', 'shield chest', congenital lymphedema, short fourth metacarpal bones, low set ears, high arched palate, micrognathia, epicanthal folds, low hairline, cubitus valgus and genu valgum), renal developmental abnormalities, cardiac manifestations (e.g. coarctation of the aorta, bicuspid aortic valve), predisposition to otitis media, tendency to keloid formation and metabolic abnormalities (Hashimoto's thyroiditis, diabetes mellitus and obesity).

v. The uterus is capable of response to exogenous estrogen/ progesterone therapy and regular withdrawal shedding. Estrogen can be growth promoting as well (with ultimate epiphyseal closure), but HGH has also been used with success.

b. Variant Turner's Syndrome – important to identify because the chromatin and actual chromosome pattern may be variable (depending on the degree of mosaicism). The karyotype can even be XX or XY (Swyer Syndrome). The clinical features include variable degrees of sexual ambiguity and variable non-genital somatic accompaniments.

c. Testicular Feminization Syndrome

i. Although a 'male' disorder of sexual differentiation, it most often presents as primary amenorrhea in a phenotypic female. Inheritance is X-linked.

ii. As the fundamental defect is target tissue insensitivity to androgens, the clinical appearance is a result of unopposed feminization void of any masculine features in a phenotypic female. Puberty proceeds with appropriate sexual maturation, but with sparse ambisexual bodily hair.

iii. Androgen insensitivity also takes place at the hypothalamic–pituitary level, with resultant elevation in LH and a secondary augmentation of testosterone and estradiol levels. This results in further amplification of the estrogen effect.

iv. The testes remain intra-abdominal. Because they still make Müllerian inhibitory factor (which, unlike testosterone, is effective), internal female genitalia do not develop and the vagina ends in a 'blind pouch'. Because internal (in addition to external) male genitalia develop in response to androgen stimulation, Wolffian differentiation does not occur.

v. To the extent that individuals with other related 'androgen-resistant' syndromes are also raised as women, they, too, would present with primary amenorrhea.

d. Enzymatic Defects in Estrogen Synthesis

i. The 17α-hydroxylase and 17,20-lyase (desmolase) deficiencies have already been discussed because they produce androgen deficiency states in genetic males.

ii. As estrogens require androgenic precursors, phenotypic women will have primary amenorrhea secondary to an estrogen deficiency state.

iii. The ability to make progesterone will not be impaired, but:

(a) The lack of ovulation (and inability to form a corpus luteum) will result in chronically low progesterone levels.

(b) Even if present, progesterone, by itself, will not render an endometrium capable of menstrual flow, nor will it produce the feminization associated with full sexual maturation.

e. Ovarian Failure

i. Obviously 'physiologic' if it occurs at the time of anticipated menopause.

ii. Can be premature (defined as occurring prior to age 40).

(a) Alone or in association with autoimmune and other

endocrine deficiency states (e.g. hypothyroidism, Addison's disease, Type I diabetes mellitus).

(b) The result of radiation (the threshold for ovarian failure is generally accepted at 800 rads) or chemotherapy; ovarian infection; galactosemia (effect of galactose-1-phosphate deposition in the ovary).

iii. Ovarian Resistance Syndrome (Savage Syndrome) – elevated gonadotropins in the presence of histologically normal ovarian tissue; very difficult to reverse.

f. Estrogen-Producing Tumors

i. The sustained estrogenic effect of these tumors will prevent ovulation and a normal secretory endometrium. There may be erratic and episodic shedding, however, of proliferative endometrium – bleeding may even be substantial.

ii. The abnormality can be mimicked by the use of exogenous estrogens.

iii. Neither lack of feminization nor of sexual maturation (in the prepubescent patient) is a clinical issue. On the contrary, sexual precocity may be a presenting feature.

iv. Mechanisms of hyperestrogenism include:

(a) Excessive human chorionic gonadotropin (HCG) production– seen in germ cell tumors such as germinomas, gonadoblastomas and teratomas.

(b) Primary production of estrogen – seen in tumors of mesenchymal (sex cord) components of the ovary (e.g. granulosa-theca cell tumors and Sertoli–Leydig cell tumors), and even in cystadenomas, Krukenberg and Brenner tumors. Androgens may also be made in varying amounts – these may additionally be peripherally converted to estrogens.

g. Androgen Excess States – include androgen-producing neoplasms of adrenal glands and ovaries, congenital adrenal hyperplasia, Cushing's syndrome and exogenous androgens.

h. Polycystic Ovarian Syndrome (Table 32-2)

## TABLE 32-2.   FEATURES OF THE POLYCYSTIC OVARIAN SYNDROME

Anovulation or Infrequent Ovulation
Elevated Circulating Androgens and
   Variable Clinical Androgenization
Elevated Circulating Estrogens
Elevated Luteinizing Hormone
Suppressed Follicle-Stimulating Hormone
Insulin Resistance
Association With Elevated Prolactin
Structural Ovarian Changes

i.  Because of the many facets of this syndrome, it could easily have been listed as one of the entities of either the estrogen or androgen excess states under the heading of ovarian disease. It could also have been listed under the heading of hypothalamic or pituitary disease. It is often referred to as the Stein–Leventhal Syndrome. This underscores the multiple facets of the syndrome as well as its importance and clinical relevance. There are still issues of the polycystic ovarian syndrome that require clearer understanding and ultimate resolution.

ii.  The hallmarks of the syndrome are anovulation or infrequent ovulation associated with a hyperandrogenic state.

iii.  All major androgens are elevated. Testosterone and androstenedione are primarily of testicular origin and dehydroepiandrosterone and dehydroepiandrosterone sulfate (DHEA and DHEAS) of adrenal origin. Androgenization is rarely so severe as to produce overt masculinization (virilization).

iv.  Mean total circulating estrogens are elevated.

(a)  You do not see the two distinct phases of estradiol as occurs in normal cycles and 'average' estradiol levels are reduced.

(b)  Estrone levels, however, are substantially elevated secondary to increased peripheral conversion from precursor ovarian androgens.

v. The ability of theca cells to produce androgens but the inability of granulosa cells to aromatize them to estrogens may explain the altered androgen/estrogen relationships of this syndrome.

vi. Mean LH levels are elevated and FSH levels are suppressed.

    (a) The chronic hyperestrogen state results in 'positive' feedback stimulation of GnRH resulting in more frequent bursts of LH – note, this is not the LH 'spike' of ovulation (which does not occur in this anovulatory condition) but rather episodic pulses of LH whose high amplitude and frequency result in a higher mean sustained level.

    (b) The effect of heightened GnRH activity is inhibitory to FSH (resulting in lower mean values).

vii. Insulin resistance may play a role in the pathophysiology.

    (a) Theca cells may not be as resistant to insulin as are other tissues, and insulin may disproportionately act on these cells through their elaboration of insulin-like growth factor-I.

    (b) This may explain the frequent association of polycystic ovarian syndrome with obesity (an insulin-resistant state). Acanthosis nigricans (seen with this syndrome) may also be the result of an insulin-augmented process.

    (c) Hyperprolactinemia is often seen, but its exact role is unclear. It does augment adrenal production of DHEA and DHEAS, but the reason behind its primary elevation is not known.

viii. The fact that the disease process returns after treatment with GnRH agonist therapy (instituted to 'shut down' the pituitary) suggests a primary ovarian cause. Likewise, a 'trigger' of pubertal adrenal androgens induced by 'stress' has been postulated as an initiating event.

    (a) Dysregulation of 11-$\beta$-hydroxysteroid dehydrogenase, which causes increased oxidation of hydrocortisone to cortisone, results in increased adrenal secretion of both hydrocortisone and androgens.

(b) There is a disproportionate incidence of polycystic ovary disease in women who take valproate for epilepsy (notwithstanding the increased incidence of reproductive endocrine dysfunction in both men and women who have a history of epilepsy).

ix. Structural ovarian concomitants include: a glistening and smooth, thickened ovarian capsule; multiple follicular cysts; hyperthecosis and stromal hyperplasia; and a diminished numbers of corpora albicans.

5. Disorders of the Reproductive Tract

a. Primary Disorders – developmental dysfunction of the Müllerian ductal system ranging from severe agenesis (e.g. Mayer–Rokitansky–Kuster–Hauser Syndrome) at one extreme of the spectrum to more easily correctible focal abnormalities such as imperforate hymen.

b. Acquired Disorders – endometrial scarring (Asherman's Syndrome); causes include repeat curettage procedures and infection.

6. Clinical Work-up of Amenorrhea

a. History – very helpful and important! Among information to be gleaned include primary versus secondary amenorrhea, age of onset, other associated conditions, symptoms or signs, medications, androgenic manifestations, antecedent gynecologic history, growth and development, emotional and psychodynamic history, and family history.

b. Physical Examination – equally helpful! General examination and special focus on bodily build, habitus, sexual maturity, unusual somatic features, evidence of androgenization, breast examination, neurologic examination (including visual fields), pelvic and genital examination.

c. Relevant Screening Laboratory Tests include a general 'screening battery' (complete blood count, Chemistry Panel, Urinalysis and Thyroid Function Studies) for assessment of overall health (if not recently done).

i. More specific initial studies include β-HCG (never forget its simplicity and utility), FSH, LH and Prolactin.

ii. A very helpful 'clinical trial' is a 'progesterone challenge' (medroxyprogesterone, 10 mg by mouth daily, for 7 days or a single 200 mg intramuscular injection of progesterone). Withdrawal bleeding will generally rule out both the estrogen deficiency and reproductive tract defect categories.

iii. If no bleeding occurs, a combined estrogen/progesterone test is helpful (conjugated estrogens, 2.5 mg by mouth, daily or ethinyl estradiol, 50 µg, by mouth, daily for 21 days with medroxyprogesterone, 10 mg, by mouth, daily on days 15–21). Withdrawal bleeding following this test strongly suggests an estrogen deficiency state, but will also rule out a structural reproductive tract defect.

d. The additional work-up then becomes 'focused' with the multiple facets of data already obtained directing the physician to the proper additional testing. These may include such studies as central nervous system imaging (MRI, CT), evaluation of other hormone excess or deficiency states, androgen (testosterone, androstenedione, DHEAS) and estrogen (estradiol, estrone) levels, buccal smear (and karyotype) and pelvic ultrasound.

e. Treatment is also 'focused' and will depend on multiple factors including available therapeutic options (e.g. there is no 'primary' treatment for Turner's syndrome), treatment goals (e.g. fertility), ancillary disorders (e.g. hypopituitarism secondary to a pituitary tumor), hormonal excess states (e.g. hypercortisolemia, androgen excess states), associated estrogen deficiency (e.g. premature ovarian failure), concern regarding neoplasia (e.g. ovarian tumor, intra-abdominal testes) and self-image and life-style (e.g. obesity and hirsutism in polycystic ovarian syndrome, anorexia nervosa, 'athletic conditioning', and a 'high stress' personal/workplace environment).

f. Additional concerns include the need to prevent unopposed estrogenic stimulation of the uterus (e.g. regular progestin or estrogen/progestin use in polycystic ovarian syndrome) and the issue of contraception in those woman who may have some interspersed normal ovulatory cycles with their amenorrhea or whose cycles may become more regular with treatment of the disorder.

## HIRSUTISM

1. Bodily hair is a normal epidermal appendage in both sexes. Hirsutism as an entity deals with bodily hair of such excess and distribution that it becomes a clinical concern.

2. Hair is classified into two categories based upon type:

   a. Vellous hair is soft, fine, unpigmented and found (with few exceptions – e.g. lips, palms and soles) throughout the body.

   b. Terminal hair is found only in selected locations.

      i. Terminal hair present at birth (scalp and eyebrows) is not under androgenic influence. (Ironically, scalp hair is also influenced by androgens in a 'negative way' as 'male pattern baldness' is an androgen-associated process).

      ii. Beginning with the pubertal production of androgens, vellous hair can be converted into terminal hair.

         (a) The most important androgens in this process are testosterone and dihydrotestosterone. While testosterone in men is primarily of testicular origin, only 5–25% is of ovarian origin in women (5–25% is of adrenal origin and the remainder is converted in peripheral tissues from precursor androstenedione). The androstenedione, itself, is primarily of ovarian origin, but about one-third is derived from the adrenals. The hair follicle is capable of converting androstenedione to testosterone and of reducing the testosterone to dihydrotestosterone. It is the dihydrotestosterone that is considered the primary stimulus to terminal hair formation.

         (b) At normal physiologic levels of androgens in women, terminal hair will develop in 'ambisexual' areas (extremities, axillary and pubic regions).

         (c) There is a 'hierarchy' of terminal hair growth based on 'regional sensitivity' (e.g. it is not uncommon for women to have some hair on the upper lip and periareolar chest). Hair on the sternal chest and upper abdomen and back, however, is abnormal and is indicative of extensive hirsutism that is probably present in other bodily regions, as well.

(d) The propensity for terminal hair growth is a function of the amount and type of circulating androgens, the ability of hair follicles to generate dihydrotestosterone and target organ 'sensitivity' to this androgen (because aromatase is also present in hair follicles, androgen to estrogen conversion may play a mollifying role).

(e) The 'integrated nature' of the pilo-sebaceous unit results in the tendency for acne to often parallel the development of hirsutism (although acne as an independent entity can occur without hirsutism).

3. Hirsutism is but one feature, albeit an 'early one' in a spectrum of manifestations of the hyperandrogenic state that can ultimately lead to overt virilization. As the degree of androgenicity ensues, there can be ovulatory dysfunction, clitoromegaly, altered bodily habitus, voice change and temporal balding.

4. The cosmetic features of hirsutism, notwithstanding, associated concerns are other hyperandrogenic manifestations and the gravity of the underlying process (e.g. ovarian tumor, congenital adrenal hyperplasia). Therapeutic options require understanding of these factors. Treatment goals must consider primary disease processes as well as the overt manifestations of excessive hair.

5. Etiologies (Table 32-3)

### TABLE 32-3.   ETIOLOGIES OF HIRSUTISM

Adrenal
>Congenital Adrenal Hyperplasia
>Cushing's Syndrome
>Hyperprolactinemia
>Adrenal Tumors

Ovarian
>Polycystic Ovarian Syndrome
>Hyperthecosis
>Ovarian Tumors

Idiopathic

Exogenous Androgens

'Non-Endocrine'Etiologies

a. Adrenal

   i. Congenital adrenal hyperplasia – the result of enzymatic defects associated with inadequate cortisol production and secondary augmentation of ACTH because of failure of feedback inhibition. If the defect is 'distal' to androgen synthesis (i.e. either a 21- or 11-hydroxylase deficiency), androgen production is increased.

   ii. Cushing's syndrome – multiple clinical and laboratory features secondary to excessive glucocorticoid effect, but hirsutism can also be one of the features.

   iii. Hyperprolactinemia – previously cited in the discussion of polycystic ovarian syndrome as a stimulus for adrenal synthesis of DHEA and DHEAS. Yet, many women who present with hyperprolactinemia (e.g. secondary to medications, microadenoma) are not hirsute.

   iv. Adrenal tumors – marked elevations of DHEA and DHEAS are characteristic (but some tumors may lack the sulfatase necessary for DHEAS production and other tumors can elaborate 17-hydroxy desoxycorticosterone and testosterone).

b. Ovarian

   i. Polycystic ovarian syndrome – previously discussed.

   ii. Hyperthecosis is considered a variant of polycystic ovarian syndrome that may have a greater degree of associated androgenization and 'normal sized' ovaries.

   iii. Ovarian tumors – androstenedione and testosterone levels may be markedly elevated; often associated with estrogen elevation as well (e.g. granulosa–theca cell tumor, Sertoli–Leydig cell tumor). Virilization may be pronounced.

c. Idiopathic

   i. Circulating androgens (DHEAS, testosterone, androstenedione) may be elevated in this syndrome. They are generally of ovarian origin (there can also be a 'mixed' adrenal pattern), and the elevations are of a mild to moderate degree.

ii. Hirsutism, however, could also be secondary to increased target organ sensitivity. In that case, androstanediol sulfate, a metabolite of dihydrotestosterone, may be elevated and indicative of increased testosterone to dihydrotestosterone conversion.

d. Exogenous androgens can produce hirsutism – danazol and other 'anabolic steroids' are common offenders in this category.

e. 'Non-endocrine' causes of hirsutism include drugs (e.g. dilantin, diazoxide), persistent trauma or skin 'irritation' (etiology is usually obvious, but can also be a manifestation of such entities as porphyria cutanea tarda) and rare familial syndromes (e.g. Gonzales syndrome).

6. Work-up of hirsutism

a. Recommended baseline studies (after a comprehensive as well as focused history and physical examination, and baseline general laboratory screening studies) are plasma testosterone, androstenedione, DHEAS, and 17-hydroxy progesterone. Optional tests are either a urine free cortisol or overnight dexamethasone suppression test (if there is a suspicion of Cushing's Syndrome based on clinical presentation) and a prolactin level. Urinary 17-keto steroids are generally not of additional value.

b. Moderate to marked elevation of DHEAS could be secondary to Cushing's syndrome, congenital adrenal hyperplasia, or an adrenal tumor. Adrenal suppression testing should be done to rule out Cushing's syndrome. Long-term (7 day), high-dose (8 mg/day) dexamethasone suppression with repeat DHEAS (imaging studies, as necessary) would rule out an adrenal tumor.

c. Either basal (if elevated) or an ACTH-stimulated 17-hydroxy progesterone level would screen for 21-hydroxylase deficiency. This can be part of the initial work-up and should be done irrespective of the magnitude of the DHEAS elevation.

d. If the DHEAS is normal or only 'moderately' elevated:

i. High testosterone levels should warrant ovarian (first) and then adrenal imaging studies (selective venous sampling, to follow, may be necessary).

    ii. A moderate testosterone elevation can warrant a trial of estrogen/progesterone suppression to rule out polycystic ovarian syndrome – failure to suppress could suggest an adrenal (or 'idiopathic') cause. Evidence of suppression of these androgens, by dexamethasone, would indicate an adrenal origin and would also suggest the potential therapeutic benefit of continued dexamethasone use. Any ambiguity in responses would warrant ovarian and adrenal imaging.

  e. Hirsutism that is clinically disproportionate to laboratory studies (e.g. normal free testosterone) is suggestive of an enhanced peripheral effect of androgens as an etiology of hirsutism. Elevation of serum androstanediol sulfate (a metabolite of dihydrotestosterone) would distinguish increased dihydrotestosterone production from 'true' peripheral sensitivity ('idiopathic').

7. Therapeutic options – the following are considerations for those situations where there is not a definable cause that is directly remediable (e.g. ovarian tumor, congenital adrenal hyperplasia).

  a. General – it is important to be supportive, sympathetic and understanding of the patients' concerns, irrespective of how extensive the hirsutism may appear. At the same time, patients with 'limited' hirsutism should be encouraged to use 'safer and simpler' approaches. All patients should be apprised of the need for 'reasonable' periods of time before drawing any conclusions about therapeutic efficacy and of the overall difficulty in completely 'normalizing' a previously hirsute state.

  b. Cosmetic approach – although it does not treat the basic problem, it is the safest modality (and should always be considered adjunctively, even if specific drugs are employed). Options include depilatories, waxing, shaving and electrolysis.

  c. Oral contraceptives

    i. This will work best in those individuals demonstrating androgenic suppression with its use.

    ii. 'Bonus' effects are an increased SHBG (thus decreasing

'free' testosterone), decreased dihydrotestosterone–receptor binding and, perhaps, decreased adrenal androgen production.

d. Glucocorticoids

   i. Surely, the drug of choice in congenital adrenal hyperplasia.

   ii. This should be used only in those patients who demonstrate androgen suppression with it.

   (a) Patients should be given a trial of oral contraceptives (if acceptable to them) prior to glucocorticoid use, even if they do not demonstrate chemical androgenic suppression. Their clinical course should be followed. If the response is not acceptable, then glucocorticoids can be tried.

   (b) The usual prescribing pattern is to take the lowest effective dose (e.g. dexamethasone, 0.25–0.50 mg by mouth at bedtime). Morning plasma androgen levels should be the chemical determinants of response (in concert with the clinical response).

   (c) Iatrogenic Cushing's syndrome (even when the dexamethasone is administered in this manner) is a potential complication.

   (d) At times of physiologic stress (e.g. intercurrent illness, surgical procedures), any patient on this regime has to be considered a 'treated Addisonian' with 'stress dose' steroid supplement to be administered, as necessary.

e. Antiandrogens

   i. Spironolactone

   (a) Peripheral androgen antagonist, but it also inhibits 17α-hydroxylase.

   (b) Side-effects include hypotension, diarrhea, irregular uterine bleeding and hyperkalemia (be very cautious if the patient is also taking potassium supplement).

   (c) Dose range: 50–200 mg/day.

    ii. Ketoconazole

       (a) Antifungal agent that also inhibits cholesterol synthesis, 17,20-desmolase and 11-hydroxylase.

       (b) It can also produce some degree of adrenal insufficiency.

       (c) Side-effects include gastrointestinal discomfort, abnormal liver function studies and pruritis.

       (d) Dose range: 400–1000 mg/day.

    iii. Cyproterone

       (a) Peripheral testosterone antagonist.

       (b) Side-effects include weight gain, headaches and breast tenderness.

       (c) Dose range: 10–100 mg/day (not available for use in the USA).

    iv. GnRH analogs – limited use at present; expensive; to prevent an estrogen deficiency state, they would have to be combined with an estrogen/progesterone regime.

## THE MENOPAUSE

1. The clinical state following the last cycle of ovulation-associated menstrual bleeding.

   a. The variability of age of onset is large but is usually within the 'early forties – later fifties' time span. Premature menopause (usually pathologic) occurs before age forty.

   b. Even prior to the finality of menstrual cessation, a variety of physiologic changes are occurring.

      i. There is a decrease in the ovarian oocyte pool. Fewer than 10 000 oocytes remain out of the maximal number of up to 7 000 000 that were present during the second trimester of gestation (the decline is inexorable following that 'peak value' with fewer than half a million at menarche). Mathematically, only 500–600 oocytes could have ever achieved ovulation.

ii. Gonadotropin levels increase with FSH being the earlier and more sensitive of the two. This is associated with:

(a) Decreased follicular responsiveness to FSH.

(b) A tendency to decreased cycle length, primarily because of a decreased length of the follicular phase.

(c) Cycle length, however, may be variable because menses uncommonly cease abruptly. Rather, they are often interspersed with anovulatory cycles. These anovulatory cycles may have only scant flow (because progesterone will not have been made and estrogen stimulates a proliferative but not a secretory endometrium). Conversely, the flow can also be substantial and sustained (because of protracted and unopposed estrogen stimulation).

c. Clinical manifestations are mediated in large part by estrogen deficiency (Table 32-4).

i. The ovary ceases to make significant quantities of estradiol, the most potent estrogen (estrone production is also severely curtailed). Estrone, however, can be made peripherally because ovarian androstenedione continues to be made (the adrenal is also a significant source) and this is peripherally converted (adipose tissue plays an important role) to estrone.

ii. The estrone produced is not of substantial potency to mitigate menopausal symptoms.

iii. Genitourinary symptoms are common and are related to epithelial atrophy and diminished vaginal secretion.

### TABLE 32-4.   CLINICAL MANIFESTATIONS OF THE MENOPAUSE

---

'Hot Flushes'
Symptoms Related to Mood and Emotion
Dermatologic Changes
Increased Incidence of Cardiovascular Disease
Increased Risk of Osteoporosis
Genitourinary Symptoms

---

Included are burning, dryness and irritation (with symptomatic pain, discomfort, dyspareunia and a secondary vaginal discharge). Because the distal urethral epithelium is also trophic for estrogen, dysuria (culture-negative) and urinary frequency can occur. The role of estrogen in maintaining sphincter control and support has been cited as an operant factor in menopausal incontinence (urgency and stress).

iv. 'Hot flushes' are an estrogen-deficiency-mediated phenomenon.

   (a) 'Abruptness of change' is relevant in the clinical syndrome as women with gonadal dysgenesis do not experience 'flushes'. Conversely, women who have had a surgical menopause have a higher incidence of 'flushes' than do women who have had a 'natural' menopause. In virtually all women who experience 'flushes', estrogen replacement therapy is ameliorative.

   (b) GnRH and gonadotropins have been implicated in the pathophysiology, but 'flushes' have occurred in their absence.

   (c) Norepinephrine appears to play an 'initiating' role in the clinical syndrome.

   (d) Clinically, there is an acute subjective sensation of warmth (the 'hot flash') which is followed by a 'flush', a measurable increase in body temperature, skin redness and 'convection waves' of heat emanating from the skin. The 'flush' lasts 10–20 minutes and is usually terminated by sweating (indicating 'normalization' of the thermostat). Ironically, this may lead to a brief episode of chills.

v. Symptoms related to emotion include depression, anxiety, altered mood and irritability. The causes may be multifactorial, but in those women most affected, estrogen replacement therapy appears beneficial. A particular reason may be the ability of estrogen to improve sleep (decreasing sleep latency and increasing rapid eye movement sleep) by preventing nocturnal 'hot flushes'.

vi. Dermatologic changes include fine wrinkles (not major

skin creases) – noted particularly around the eyes and lips ('rhagades'). There is a tendency for terminal hair growth ('unopposed' androgen effect ?) on the chin and upper lip, but there is also decreased pubic and axillary hair.

vii. The incidence of cardiovascular disease increases following menopause (the earlier the menopause, the more the 'lead time' in its promulgation). While the loss of a 'favorable' lipid profile is felt to be a major factor, the loss of other estrogen-mediated effects (e.g. local endothelial effect, effect on decreasing plasma Lp(a), and the effect on inhibition of oxidation of low-density lipoproteins) may also be relevant.

viii. Menopause is a distinct risk factor for osteoporosis. Trabecular bone is disproportionately affected. Conversely, estrogen therapy can arrest bone loss, but doses less than 0.625 mg/day of conjugated estrogen (or its equivalent) are generally considered ineffective. The effect of estrogen on bone integrity is enhanced when combined with calcium supplement.

2. Estrogen Replacement Therapy

   a. Benefits

      i. There is no controversy regarding the benefit of estrogen in relief of 'hot flushes' or in normalizing genitourinary epithelium. Estrogen will additionally improve the general condition of the skin (it does increase collagen content and thickness of skin and its effect is most evident in those women with the greatest deficiency).

      ii. There is also no controversy regarding its effect on arresting bone loss. There are other risk factors, however, that are operant in bone loss (e.g. thin bodily habitus, sedentary life style, white race, smoking and alcohol use). As there is individual variability in bone density, a quantitative bone density study should be done before estrogen therapy is initiated based on 'bone status' alone.

      iii. Estrogen therapy can also improve emotional symptoms and cognitive function in symptomatic women. As noted above, this may be a direct or indirect effect.

iv. Estrogen can decrease the cardiovascular risk profile, decrease the risk of stroke and increase peripheral blood flow.

b. Risks

    i. When used alone, it is associated with an increased risk of endometrial carcinoma. When used with a progestin, this risk is nullified. Further, uterine 'shedding' may not be necessary to nullify the risk, as one accepted regime uses combined estrogen/progesterone on a daily basis. In women who have had a hysterectomy, it is not necessary to add a progestational agent.

    ii. In menopausal woman, there is no increased risk of the cardiovascular complications seen in women on oral contraceptive pills (especially women past age 35 who smoke, although smoking under any circumstances is to be discouraged). Indeed, the majority of studies have suggested a beneficial effect of estrogen in cardiovascular disease prevention when used in the postmenopausal state.

    (a) The beneficial effect of unopposed estrogen on lipoproteins (increased HDL, decreased LDL) is lessened when progestational agents are used, but this varies with the type of progestin.

    (b) Even with the use of an added progestin, however, the total cholesterol/HDL ratio remains 'more favorable' than if nothing is done because the opposing effect of the progestin is outweighed by the beneficial effect of the estrogen.

    (c) When all factors in the cardiovascular risk profile are considered (e.g. subfractionation of HDL, fasting serum glucose, insulin levels, Lp(a), fibrinogen, antithrombin III and all other purported actions of estrogens), estrogen combined with a progestin actually gives a more favorable profile than estrogen alone.

    (d) Transdermal estrogens (because they 'avoid' the 'first-pass' portal circulation) have no effect on serum lipids.

    (e) There is no apparent increased tendency to hypertension or venous thromboembolic disease secondary to menopausal estrogens. A history of prior thromboembolic disease, however, is a contraindication to its use.

iii. High-dose estrogens may be associated with insulin resistance and glucose intolerance.

iv. There may be a slightly increased risk of breast cancer in women currently taking an estrogen preparation. Past use, irrespective of duration, does not appear to increase the risk.

(a) Certainly women at risk (family history of breast cancer, fibrocystic disease) should be highly cautious regarding its use.

(b) An intangible benefit may be in 'sensitizing' women to be more cognizant of 'preventive measures' (e.g. self-examination and regular medical examination; mammography).

(c) In actuality, it has not been clearly established that postmenopausal estrogen replacement therapy in women with a prior history of breast cancer is truly contraindicated.

(d) The frequency of postmenopausal hot flushes in women (and men) can be substantially decreased by the use of the non-estrogen, megestrol acetate.

v. Additional untoward effects may be nausea, headaches (migraines may be exacerbated), mastodynia and hyperpigmentation (these symptoms may abate if either dose or preparation is changed). There is a higher incidence of gall-bladder disease (decreased gall-bladder motility?, lithogenic bile?). Estrogens can produce abnormal liver function studies (active liver disease is a contraindication to use).

c. Estrogen preparations available (and average daily dosage).

i. Conjugated estrogens (Premarin) – 0.625–1.25 mg.

ii. Ethinyl estradiol – 10–20 μg (oral contraceptives generally have somewhat larger amounts).

   iii. Micronized estradiol (Estrace) – 1 mg.

   iv. Transdermal estradiol patch – 0.05 mg (10 cm).

   v. Estropipate (formerly piperazine estrone sulfate; Ogen) – 0.625–2.5 mg.

   vi. The most commonly used regimes are:

     (a) Daily (or patch) estrogen for the first 25 days of each calendar month with a progestin (e.g. medroxyprogesterone, 10 mg) added for days 16–25.

     (b) 'Variations' of this regime are: 4-week cycles (so that the starting day of the week always remains the same) or continuous daily estrogen (both regimes with cycled progesterone as above).

     (c) Withdrawal bleeding can be an annoyance but is generally tolerated. Breakthrough bleeding requires gynecologic evaluation.

     (d) Continuous estrogen/progesterone (e.g. 0.625 mg/day of conjugated estrogen with 2.5 mg of medroxyprogesterone) may obviate the problem of cyclic withdrawal bleeding, but there may be a higher incidence of breakthrough bleeding and (because of the relative newness of this approach) the long-term risk/benefit effects await further evaluation.

   vii. While estrogen cream had been used in the past (and it actually exerted its action through absorption across the vaginal epithelium), intravaginal administration of estriol prevents urinary tract infection in postmenopausal women and appears to exert its effect through modification of the vaginal flora.

# Section K

# ILLUSTRATIVE CLINICAL CASES AND COMMENTARY

# 33

# ILLUSTRATIVE CLINICAL CASES

## CLINICAL CASE #1

A 61-year-old man has noticed progressive swelling of his hands and feet. He can no longer take off his ring at night, and old shoes that once felt comfortable to him now feel tight. On careful questioning, he has been experiencing a 'dull aching' in his head. Libido and sexual function have declined, a finding he attributes to his 'age'.

1.  What additional history might you expect from him with 'focused questions'?

2.  What might you note on physical examination?

3.  He was told he was 'borderline diabetic' 5 years ago. What might be the present state of his diabetes and why? What might be his serum phosphorus and urinary calcium excretion?

4.  What endocrinologic studies are most useful in establishing the diagnosis? What are other important endocrinologic and radiologic studies?

5.  What might explain his loss of libido and sexual function?

6.  What are his treatment options?

## CLINICAL CASE #2

A 35-year-old woman has noted persistent galactorrhea for 3 months following the weaning of her now 9-month-old daughter. She has one other child, a 4-year-old son, whom she also breastfed for 6 months. In the case of her son, milk production ceased completely within 2 weeks of weaning and menses had returned to normal, even while she was breast feeding. At present, menses have not been regular and flow is scanty. There is no other endocrinologic history of relevance. She jogs three times a week for 2 miles each run. She also has a history of 'gastritis' which was treated with a course of Cimetidine 2 years ago. She had been on the oral contraceptive pill in the remote past and had a brief delay of return of menses following its cessation, but with subsequent normal and regular resumption since (until her recent state). Other than easily expressible milk from both breasts, there are no striking physical findings.

1. What constitutes an appropriate work-up at this time?

2. What is included in the differential diagnosis of this clinical presentation?

3. How comprehensive should a supplemental work-up be?

4. Assuming the most likely diagnosis, what is the clinical management?

5. What would you advise regarding future pregnancies?

## CLINICAL CASE #3

An 83-year-old woman develops an acute respiratory infection and chooses to be treated at home with antibiotics rather then being admitted to the hospital. Because of her general frailty and low-grade dementia, she lives with her daughter who has recently taken additional time off from work to provide a greater intensity of care. The patient had been anorectic for the past 3 days and her daughter, concerned about her mother's fluid intake, has been 'forcing liquids'. Additional history regarding the patient includes hypertension well controlled on hydrochlorthiazide, breast cancer treated with surgery and adjuvant chemotherapy 8 years prior, and a 60-pack/year smoking history. Over the ensuing 3 days of her illness, the patient becomes progressively more confused and lethargic, ultimately necessitating her hospitalization.

In the Emergency Room, she is very somnolent and disoriented; temperature, 99.8 °F (37.7 °C); blood pressure, 138/74; pulse, 68/minute; respirations, 16/minute. She appears thin and frail, but neither edematous nor dehydrated. Pertinent physical findings include only evidence of her previous right mastectomy but no adenopathy or tumor recurrence, and decreased percussive resonance with course rhonchi in the right lower lung field. There are no lateralizing neurologic deficits. Among other routine admission studies, her serum laboratory values reveal the following: Na, 116 mEq/l; K, 3.9 mEq/l; $HCO_3^-$, 20 mEq/l; chloride, 82 mEq/l; glucose, 126 mg/dl; blood urea nitrogen, 18 mg/dl; and creatinine, 1.0 mg/dl. Urine specific gravity was 1.022.

1. How can her clinical picture best be explained? Why was she so symptomatic?

2. What are appropriate management strategies?

3. If the syndrome of inappropriate antidiuretic hormone were to persist and fluid restriction is of limited effect, are there other treatment strategies?

## CLINICAL CASE #4

A 71-year-old woman is admitted to the hospital with the acute onset of atrial fibrillation. She was generally comfortable and able to maintain a satisfactory blood pressure despite a heart rate of 156. On full digitalization, her heart rate was reduced to 126. Recent history is unremarkable except for mild lethargy. She has not lost weight and her appetite is described as 'very good'. She had an unremarkable prior medical history and was on no medications at the time of admission. The 4th year medical student assigned to her case astutely thought of thyrotoxicosis. He did not note any obvious goiter, but the thyroid gland felt 'irregular', and non-tender. Physical examination, except for her rapid heart rate, was otherwise 'normal'. Total thyroxine level was 10.9 µg/dl (normal: 4-12 µg/dl).

1. Are other endocrine studies warranted?

2. She has no exophthalmos, her skin is not very smooth or moist, and there is no history of heat intolerance or hyper-defecation. Does this make the diagnosis of thyrotoxicosis less likely?

3. If she is thyrotoxic, what is the therapy of choice?

4. Is pretreatment warranted prior to definitive treatment?

5. If antithyroid drug therapy is used during her treatment course, is propylthiouracil (PTU) preferable to methimazole (Tapazole)?

## CLINICAL CASE #5

A 26-year-old woman has noted excessive mood swings, anxiety and heat intolerance for the past 6 weeks beginning about 1 month postpartum. She has experienced 'fluttering' of her heart and continued weight loss despite good appetite.

1. What endocrinologic problem might she have, and what laboratory studies would be helpful in establishing the diagnosis?

2. What would you expect the value of the 24-hour Radioactive Iodine Uptake to be?

3. Would you expect neck tenderness on physical examination?

4. Is her medical syndrome associated with any particular HLA haplotype?

5. What can be the expected natural course of events and what type of therapy is indicated?

6. How might you counsel her regarding future pregnancies?

## CLINICAL CASE #6

A 21-year-old college student has been concerned about recent weight gain over the past 6 months, particularly in her abdominal girth. She has also experienced some generalized weakness, irregular menses and has noticed an increased tendency to bruise.

1.  In addition to your usual comprehensive history and physical examination, what other study or studies might be in order at this time?

2.  Assuming your test results were positive, what other clinical and laboratory features might you expect?

3.  What other studies would you perform to elucidate a specific etiology?

4.  If testing proves compatible with ACTH-mediated hypercortisolism, but cranial MRI (even with gadolinium enhancement) is equivocal, what diagnostic procedure might be in order?

5.  If bilateral adrenalectomy is performed for Cushing's disease (ACTH-producing pituitary adenoma), how might a subsequent syndrome that includes headache, visual field defect and hyperpigmentation be explained?

## CLINICAL CASE #7

A 41-year-old woman has been experiencing weight loss, fatigue, abdominal cramps and light-headedness for the past 6–8 months. She initially attributed it to domestic stress, but symptoms continue to worsen. A friend recently commented to her regarding her 'suntanned appearance'.

1. What studies would be included in her medical work-up at this time?

2. Once the diagnosis is made, what is the strategy of hormone replacement therapy?

3. She feels improved following therapy, but notices that menses have become sporadic and she is experiencing 'hot flushes'. How might this be explained? What diagnostic test(s) would be in order?

4. Following a subsequent automobile accident in which the patient sustained a fractured humerus and pelvis, she is admitted to the hospital. What are her special medical needs?

## CLINICAL CASE #8

A 45-year-old woman has had progressive fatigue, lethargy and muscular weakness for the past 2 months. She has been taking a thiazide diuretic, but only intermittently, for premenstrual fluid retention. No potassium supplement was prescribed, but she was told to 'eat a banana' on the day she uses the diuretic. Six months ago, her blood pressure was 144/92 on routine examination and she was told to 'cut down on salt intake', but this has been difficult to achieve.

On physical examination, she is non-obese, and rather passive and lethargic with obvious muscular weakness. There is no overt edema. Blood pressure, 168/98; pulse, 88/minute (no change with posture); respirations, 10/minute; weight, 118 lb (53.5 kg); height, 62" (1.57 m).

Pertinent physical findings include absence of peripheral edema, arteriolar narrowing on funduscopic examination, a prominent apical heart impulse with a prominent S1, A2 and S4 gallop. Lung fields are clear. Deep tendon reflexes (DTRs) are diminished. Included in laboratory tests are: Na, 142 mEq/l; K, 2.2 mEq/l; Cl, 95 mEq/l; $HCO_3^-$, 35 mEq/l; and fasting blood sugar, 154 mg/dl.

1.  How might her clinical presentation and laboratory values be best explained?
2.  How should the work-up proceed?
3.  What should be done for diagnostic confirmation?
4.  Once there is diagnostic confirmation, where do we go from here?

## CLINICAL CASE #9

A 28-year-old man has complained of 'pounding' in his chest, episodic sweating and headache. He has generally tended to be a nervous person, but he feels his anxiety level has definitely increased over the past year. He has also lost 15 lb (6.8 kg) despite adequate food intake. Family history is relevant for a maternal uncle who had a 'calcium problem' and a sister who had surgery for thyroid cancer. On physical examination, he appears rather tremulous and diaphoretic; blood pressure, 154/98; pulse, 102.

1. What diagnostic studies are in order?

2. If there is a familial association regarding his sister's thyroid cancer, what studies should be performed on him to rule it out?

3. Would you have expected him to have mucosal neuromas or a 'Marfanoid' habitus? Why (or why not)?

4. What other diseases are associated with the most likely cause of his hypertension?

5. What is the 'Rule of Tens'?

## CLINICAL CASE #10

A 46-year-old woman with diabetes mellitus for the past 28 years and on twice daily split dose neutral protamine Hagedorn (NPH)/regular insulin has noticed increasing pre-breakfast blood glucose values.

1. What are possible causes?

2. She has been noted to have 'mild' proteinuria as far back as 13 years ago. She has been noticing recent increased fatigue and a decreased work capacity. Some recent dreams have been 'strange' and when she's awoken, she has found herself in a 'pool of sweat'. How might her diabetic control now be explained and what can be done for substantiation?

3. She has had four pregnancies, but only two of her children are living. What types of obstetrical problems might she have had?

4. She has an identical twin. What is the likelihood of that twin also being a diabetic?

5. What major histocompatibility complex (MHC) markers might that twin have?

6. Concomitant with this woman's tiredness, she has noticed an increased tendency to cold intolerance and a 'deepening' of her voice. What might she be developing and what studies would be in order?

## CLINICAL CASE #11

A 58-year-old man who has been generally healthy sees you for routine medical check-up. On blood test screening, you obtain a serum calcium of 12.1 mg/dl.

1. In retrospect, what symptoms might the patient have had if questions were asked of him in a very focused manner?

2. His last serum calcium was measured 2 years prior? What might that value have been?

3. What is the appropriate work-up at this time?

4. After chemical work-up, the diagnosis of primary hyperparathyroidism is strongly suspected. What imaging procedures might be additionally helpful?

5. The patient is very fearful of having surgery. What studies might be convincing in underscoring its need? What is he at risk for if surgery is not performed?

6. In the course of a subsequent bout of acute gastroenteritis, he becomes very lethargic, dehydrated and then obtunded. How might his underlying endocrinoloic problem be operant? How would you know? What is appropriate therapy and what is not?

## CLINICAL CASE #12

A 46-year-old man with a history of chronic alcohol abuse is brought to the Emergency Room. He is profoundly weak and has experienced spontaneous carpal–pedal spasm. His nutritional status had deteriorated over the past 2 months and there has been progressive weight loss. Striking physical findings, in addition to his poor state of nutrition, include 4 cm hepatomegaly, mild icterus, spider angiomata, diminished motor tone, exaggerated deep tendon reflexes (DTRs) and spontaneous facial twitches and carpal–pedal spasm. Chvostek's sign is present. Included among his laboratory studies are a serum calcium of 6.3 mg/dl, phosphorus of 2.2 mg/dl and alkaline phosphatase of 264 (normal: 35–110 IU).

1. What are reasonable explanations for these laboratory values?

2. Are other studies indicated for confirmation?

3. What are the most reasonable and cost-effective diagnostic and therapeutic options?

## CLINICAL CASE #13

A 53-year-old white woman has recently learned that her non-identical twin sister has sustained a vertebral compression fracture following a fall on ice. This patient is 3 years postmenopause and was never enthusiastic about taking estrogens because she has been minimally symptomatic of the menopause and her maternal aunt died of breast cancer. She is thin, had been sedentary throughout her adult life, smoked one pack of cigarettes per day until 5 years ago, continues to drink alcohol 'socially' and has a lifelong history of lactose intolerance.

1. What do you advise her to do? What are her therapeutic options?

2. After reviewing the database and her treatment options, she accepts an estrogen/progesterone regime and tolerates it well. Is radiologic follow-up necessary?

3. Her cousin, who is a laboratory technician, runs a 'screening profile' on a blood sample of this patient and then tells her she has an 'overactive thyroid gland'. How might you explain this?

## CLINICAL CASE #14

A 51-year-old woman calls you for the first time and is in distress because she had a 'cholesterol test' given by a 'health food' store as part of 'Health Awareness Day' at a local mall. The value told to her was 306. She has a history of long-standing obesity, is taking a combination of a β-blocking agent and a thiazide diuretic for hypertension, and was recently started on an estrogen patch and oral progesterone for postmenopausal symptoms. Her family history is relevant for a 55-year-old brother who had a recent coronary artery bypass graft (CABG) procedure and a father who died of a 'heart attack' at age 57.

1. What do you do at this point?

2. When she sees you in your office, you obtain the following laboratory studies: fasting blood sugar, 134 mg/dl, thyroxine, 5.8 µg/dl; thyroid-stimulating hormone (TSH), 13.2 µU/ml; total cholesterol, 312 mg/dl; low-density lipoprotein (LDL) cholesterol, 216 mg/dl; high-density lipoprotein (HDL) cholesterol, 37 mg/dl; total cholesterol/HDL cholesterol, 8.4; triglycerides, 295 mg/dl. Other than moderate obesity and a blood pressure of 148/94 (supine and after rest), mild arteriolar narrowing on funduscopic examination and a borderline heart size, her physical examination is normal. What is your next course of action?

3. She takes your clinical advice and the treatment regime you have prescribed. Four months later, her blood pressure is now 128/82. Laboratory studies include: thyroid-stimulating hormone (TSH), 2.4 µU/ml; fasting blood sugar, 102 mg/dl; triglycerides are now normal and her LDL cholesterol is 172 mg/dl with a total cholesterol/HDL of 4.8. Is a lipid-lowering agent indicated at this time? If so, what kind?

## CLINICAL CASE #15

A 23-year-old woman consults you because of amenorrhea. She has never had menses despite normal adolescent growth and development. She also has had mature secondary sexual maturation in a clear and unambiguous female pattern. She does not experience either *Mittelschmerz* or molimina and her bodily (but not scalp) hair is sparse and scanty. On pelvic examination, her vagina is noted to end in a 'blind pouch' without palpable cervix or uterine fundus, although bilateral 'ovaries' seem to be palpable in the adnexal region.

1. What is the differential diagnosis as well as the most likely diagnosis?

2. What constitutes an appropriate work-up?

3. What are the long-term management objectives? What is the likelihood of fertility?

## CLINICAL CASE #16

A 34-year-old woman sees you for oligo-amenorrhea and infertility. She has been trying, unsuccessfully, to conceive for the past 3 years. Menses throughout her teenage years had been generally irregular, but she had been on the oral contraceptive pill for 10 years prior to 3 years ago. She has a long-standing history of overweight with recent exaggeration of bodily hirsutism, but no masculinization.

1. In addition to a complete medical and gynecologic examination, what endocrinologic studies would be in order?

2. If a pelvic ultrasound were done and it demonstrated multiple small cysts, bilateral ovarian enlargement and a thickened capsule, what would be the expected results (when compared with normal) of the following hormone levels: follicle stimulating hormone (FSH), luteinizing hormone (LH), testosterone, androstenedione, dehydroepiandrosterone sulfate (DHEAS), prolactin, estradiol, estrone?

3. Why did this patient only recently have exaggeration of her hirsutism?

4. Why was she not virilized?

5. If a glucose tolerance test were done on this patient, what might her insulin levels be when compared with her corresponding glucose values?

# 34

# COMMENTARY

## CLINICAL CASE #1

1.  This case is very suggestive of acromegaly. The clinical syndrome is caused by the consequences of sustained and unabated growth hormone (HGH) excess as well as the mass effects of a pituitary tumor.

    As a result of the HGH excess, this patient may have symptoms related to malocclusion, exaggerated facial features (that he or someone he is close to is aware of), arthropathy, carpal and tarsal tunnel syndromes, hyperhidrosis, weight gain and sleep apnea. To the degree that the adenoma is space occupying in 'very limited confines', clinical manifestations can include pituitary hormone deficiency states and visual and other neurologic deficits. Specific pituitary function loss can result in lethargy, weakness, fatigue, fasting hypoglycemia, mental sluggishness, cold intolerance, deepening of his voice, loss of libido and impotence, and hypopigmentation.

2.  Physical findings would reflect the somatic and constitutional effects of acromegaly. There might be a broadening of the nose and thickening of the lips, frontal bossing and malocclusion and exaggeration of the facial furrows ('leonine facies'). Hands, soles and digits could be thick and prominent, there might be increased bodily perspiration (nullified perhaps by associated hypothyroidism) and skin oiliness; there might also be an increase in skin tags and other cutaneous growths. Hypertension could be present and there might be obvious visceromegaly (e.g. liver, thyroid). Kyphosis could be noted. There could be testicular atrophy and delay in deep tendon reflexes as well as clinical evidence of carpal tunnel or tarsal tunnel syndromes. Visual field loss could be present.

    In rare cases not associated with pituitary adenomas, other features might be present (e.g. bony protuberances as might occur with fibrous dysplasia).

3.  As HGH is antagonistic to insulin, you might expect a worsening of his glucose tolerance. Serum phosphorus and urine calcium excretion are often both elevated.

4.  Because HGH production is subject to natural cycles, is affected by many stimuli, and has a short half-life, dynamic testing is crucial for laboratory diagnosis. Failure to suppress HGH to less

than 5 ng/ml, 60 minutes after an oral glucose load of 100 g is considered diagnostic. As an ancillary test, an elevated basal insulin-like growth factor I (somatomedin C) level is also considered diagnostic. Supplementary studies which show altered HGH dynamics in acromegaly (i.e. loss of nocturnal HGH 'pulse', thyrotropin-releasing hormone and gonadotropin-releasing hormone stimulation of HGH, and L-DOPA and bromocriptine inhibition of HGH) are not additionally helpful and add needless cost to the evaluation. It is important to evaluate for pituitary insufficiency. Basal follicle-stimulating hormone, luteinizing hormone and testosterone would test the intactness of the pituitary–gonadal axis. Thyroid-stimulating hormone and thyroxine would measure thyroid function. A definitive test of the pituitary–adrenal axis is the measurement of the cortisol response to insulin-mediated hypoglycemia. Demonstration of adequate urinary concentrating ability should rule out posterior pituitary insufficiency.

Comprehensive testing can be delayed if surgery is performed (as long as the patient is 'covered' with glucocorticoids and there is no significant hypothyroidism) as deficiencies might be present postoperatively that were not present before. A prolactin level is helpful because prolactin might be concomitantly produced by an HGH-producing adenoma, or prolactin could be elevated secondary to loss of tonic hypothalamic inhibition. In extensive pituitary insufficiency, prolactin values would be low or undetectable.

The most important radiologic study is pituitary imaging and MRI is the modality of choice. Other radiologic studies (e.g. skull, soft tissue or extremities) might demonstrate features of the clinical syndrome (a plain skull X-ray could also demonstrate enlargement of the sella), but are redundant (notwithstanding the findings that might be seen with uncommon etiologies of acromegaly – e.g. fibrous dysplasia).

5. The loss of libido and sexual dysfunction could be secondary to the physical loss of gonadotropin-producing cells or by their inhibition secondary to hyperprolactinemia. Hypothyroidism and hypoadrenalcorticism could play supplementary roles (hypothyroidism could also elevate prolactin).

6. Surgery is the recommended primary treatment. Initial success

can as high as 80% using the transsphenoidal approach. Postoperative follow-up requires evaluation for pituitary hormonal deficiencies and documentation of the normalization of the insulin-like growth factor I and suppression of post-glucose HGH to less than 2 ng/ml.

Radiation therapy is a consideration for recurrent disease or surgical failure. The success rate can also be as high as 80%, but the effect is often delayed and hypopituitarism occurs in up to 50% of the cases.

Octreotide has proven to be an effective medical treatment, but it represents an ongoing and expensive commitment. In certain cases, it can be distinctly beneficial. Bromocriptine may reduce HGH levels, but true 'normalization' is uncommon.

Endocrine replacement therapy is required for all deficiency states. Glucocorticoids and L-thyroxine will suffice as treatment for their trophic hormone deficiency states. Unless fertility is desired, parenteral testosterone (injection or transdermal patch) should suffice for androgen replacement therapy.

## CLINICAL CASE #2

1.  This case is highly suggestive of hyperprolactinemia, most likely the result of a pituitary adenoma. This is supported by her persistent galactorrhea, even after weaning, and her amenorrhea 9 months postpartum. While intense athletic activity can produce amenorrhea, it is unlikely that 6 miles of running per week would be operant. Likewise, although cimetidine, an H-2 blocker, can increase prolactin levels, she has long since discontinued that medication and its hyperprolactinemic effect is not presently relevant. There is no apparent use of other medications (e.g. phenothiazides) or clinical states (e.g. chronic renal failure, hypothyroidism) which could result in hyperprolactinemia. Her presumed adenoma would most likely be a microadenoma (less than 1 cm) becaue of her relatively recent syndrome (she did not have persistent galactorrhea after her first child was born and had no difficulty in conceiving her second child). Further, she has no evidence of visual field compromise, other cranial nerve impairment or pituitary insufficiency.

    The most helpful screening test is the basal prolactin level. Although stimulating and suppressive tests have been devised, they have no added advantage. Values greater than 200 ng/ml are almost always associated with prolactinomas, but tumors can occur with values substantially less. Thus, any inexplicable elevation in prolactin would warrant a follow-up MRI of the sella. A complete history and physical examination would also help exclude non-pituitary etiologies and would additionally provide visual field and funduscopic evaluation. While a complete pituitary work-up would be initially unnecessary, thyroxine and thyroid-stimulating hormone levels would be useful and should be obtained prior to an MRI.

2.  The differential diagnosis of hyperprolactinemia includes pituitary adenoma, organic disease (e.g. renal failure, hypothyroidism), hyperestrogenism, medications (e.g. opioids, H-2 blockers and dopamine antagonists or depletors including phenothiazides, butyrophenones, metoclopramide, reserpine, and α-methyl DOPA), and physiologic influences (e.g. chest-wall stimulation).

3.  If studies substantiate the etiology of hyperprolactinemia as secondary to a microadenoma, panhypopituitarism is highly

unlikely and formal testing of pituitary function is generally not necessary (thyroxine and thyroid-stimulating hormone measurements are obtained to rule out hypothyroidism as a cause of the elevated prolactin rather than to presuppose hypopituitary hypothyroidism). Macroadenomas, however, should produce sella enlargement and can produce varying degrees of hypopituitarism. This would warrant more formal pituitary testing which can be done postoperatively as long as essential hormone deficiencies are covered in the perioperative period.

4. Bromocriptine is a highly effective dopaminergic medication that can normalize serum prolactin levels in the majority of patients with both microadenomas and macroadenomas. Side-effects are generally minimal after acclimation. Bromocriptine (or pergolide, a related agent) is the medical treatment of choice. Other than side-effects, which may persist to some degree, the major drawback is the need for indefinite use (and its associated cost) and the realization that a 'definitive resolution' is lacking.

    Surgery can produce a permanent cure and is the primary treatment option for large and medically non-responsive lesions. Recurrence (over time) and hypopituitarism, however, are significant drawbacks.

    Radiation therapy is generally considered adjunctive. Response can be delayed and hypopituitarism can eventually ensue.

5. Bromocriptine is not a contraindication for future pregnancy. Once conception takes place, bromocriptine can be discontinued (the elevated prolactin level does not adversely affect the fetus) and the mother then followed clinically for any evidence of tumor growth (e.g. headache, change in visual fields, evidence of hypopituitarism). In reported instances when bromocriptine was administered during pregnancy, there was no evidence of significant harm to the fetus.

# CLINICAL CASE #3

1. The patient's 'basal frailty and low-grade dementia' notwithstanding, the 3 days prior to hospitalization represented a significant change in her mental status, manifest primarily by lethargy and mental deterioration. In the absence of any other obvious cause, the hyponatremia (and associated serum hypo-osmolality) appears the cause. The 'abruptness of change' which brought her from a (presumably) normal serum sodium to a value of 118 would contribute to the magnitude of her symptoms. Her 'inappropriate' urine specific gravity of 1.022 at a time when the urine should have been dilute is supportive of the syndrome of inappropriate antidiuretic hormone (SIADH). It is not relevant that her urine is not maximally concentrated – it is only relevant that the urine specific gravity is inappropriately high.

   There are several potential reasons for the development of hyponatremia. Her clinical picture supports a new pneumonic process. She could also have an underlying malignancy (small cell carcinoma is associated with SIADH) with or without a superimposed pneumonia. Central nervous system disease resulting in an organic etiology for her dementia as well as metastatic disease to the brain could be additionally operant. Her anorexia would make her less likely to clear free water (decreased solute intake) and her thiazide diuretic, by inhibiting the 'cortical diluting segment', would also inhibit free water clearance. By 'forcing liquids', she was consuming more free water than she was able to clear. Characteristically, those who have SIADH are not edematous (unless there are other underlying reasons for the edema).

2. Certainly, the thiazide diuretic should be discontinued. Unless she is in 'grave danger', it is reasonable to merely restrict water intake while seeing that her oral electrolyte intake is commensurate with progressive improvement in her electrolyte status (and, of course, her clinical condition). As increased ADH (or its effect) can only produce a positive water balance if that water is first 'brought into the body', she can 'self correct' with voluntary restraint. Further, this would not be creating a hardship of excessive thirst, because she should not be thirsty as long as she were neither hyperosmotic nor hypovolemic.

If there were more serious clinical issues (e.g. more profound mental changes, seizures), she could be treated with judicious use of hypertonic (e.g. 3%) saline and loop diuretics. Isotonic saline, alone, will not correct her electrolyte problem as the urine osmolality reflects a greater level of electrolyte concentration than that present in the correcting solution. Loop diuretics are helpful because they prevent chloride and sodium reabsorption in the thick ascending limb. This prevents medullary hypertonicity. Even with enhanced ADH or its effect, water cannot be 'forced' into the medulla if the 'osmotic environment' is not conducive to its absorption. Thiazide diuretics, on the other hand, are not only of no therapeutic benefit, but are downright dangerous. In this patient, it is possible that significant improvement would follow discontinuance of her hydrochlorthiazide and its substitution with another effective antihypertensive (if necessary). If even after her acute treatment, the underlying process causing the SIADH persists, then fluid restriction should maintain serum iso-osmolality.

3. Both demethylchlortetracycline (Declomycin) and lithium could decrease renal sensitivity to ADH. Lithium is too toxic to be a consideration, but Declomycin can be a helpful agent.

# CLINICAL CASE #4

1. Although the differential diagnosis of atrial fibrillation is large, thyrotoxicosis is clearly a potential cause. A total thyroxine $(T_4)$ value in the 'normal range' does not rule out thyrotoxicosis. The wide range of normal total $T_4$ values is based on population variability. Crucial for any given $T_4$ value is whether the 'pituitary set point' is satisfied. This is ascertained by measurement of the thyroid-stimulating hormone (TSH), a highly sensitive determinant of the thyrometabolic state.

   In addition, this patient could have isolated triiodothyronine $(T_3)$ thyrotoxicosis in which case the $T_3$ is elevated in the presence of a normal $T_4$. If this patient has a suppressed TSH, a serum $T_3$ level is indicated. A less likely possibility of normal $T_4$ in this patient would be excessive thyroid hormone production in the context of decreased or inhibited thyroid hormone binding by its binding proteins. This issue can be clarified by obtaining a free $T_4$ level (or by its calculated equivalent, the free thyroxine index (FTI) or thyroid hormone binding index (THBI) – the product of the total $T_4$ and the 'resin uptake' test).

2. While many overt manifestations of thyrotoxicosis are usually common in younger individuals, they may be subtle or even absent in the older population. Also, in older patients, cardiovascular manifestations tend to predominate. Atrial fibrillation, poorly responsive to digoxin, is a helpful clue. The etiology of thyrotoxicosis tends to be different in the older population and is generally caused by autonomous thyroid disease (as opposed to Graves' disease, which is more often seen at a younger age). Hence, the absence of ophthalmopathy, dermopathy and a clearly defined goiter in this patient does not rule out thyrotoxicosis.

   The thyroid gland 'irregularity' suggests a multinodular gland, even if enlargement is not overt. The radioactive iodine uptake test could provide useful information. The uptake could be done in concert with a scan to delineate foci of autonomous function. In autonomous disease, the uptake would be elevated (although often not as high as is seen in Graves' disease). The uptake and scan are also helpful in determining dosimetry if radioactive iodine therapy is to be used. While seemingly unlikely in this patient, inflammatory thyroid disease (or thyrotoxicosis factitia) would result in suppressed uptake values.

3. If the diagnosis is autonomous thyrotoxicosis, radioactive iodine is the therapy of choice. While surgery can also be definitive, it is not necessary. Antithyroid drug therapy can control the thyrotoxic state while the drug is taken, but the effect is lost once the medication is discontinued. Hence, it is not a definitive option for long-term cure. The only major side-effect of radioactive iodine is inevitable hypothyroidism. This can be effectively anticipated and pre-empted when thyroid gland failure ensues. Persistent TSH elevation would be diagnostic of thyroid gland failure.

4. It may be advisable to initially pre-treat this patient with antithyroid drug therapy. In dealing with this patient's unstable cardiovascular status (and the potential need for both antiarrhythmic and antithrombotic medication), a distinct advantage of antithyroid drug therapy is the predictability of restoration of the euthyroid state. Further, when radioactive iodine is finally given, there would be less likelihood of precipitating a thyrotoxic crisis resulting from liberation of pre-formed thyroid hormone. If necesssary, antithyroid drugs can also be reinstituted following radioactive iodine to maintain the euthyroid state until the full effect of the radioactive iodine is achieved.

5. Both propylthiouracil (PTU) and methimazole (Tapazole) are effective antithyroid agents that work by blocking synthesis of thyroid hormone. Methimazole has a longer pharmacologic and metabolic half-life and has a lower (and dose-related) incidence of agranulocytosis. On the other hand, PTU has the additional effect of decreasing $T_4$ to $T_3$ conversion, and this could theoretically diminish the magnitude of the thyrometabolic state.

## CLINICAL CASE #5

1. The diagnosis is strongly suggestive of chronic thyroiditis (also known as painless thyroiditis, subacute lymphocytic thyroiditis and postpartum thyroiditis). It is commonly seen in young women, but is certainly not uncommmon in men. The process is a generally painless inflammatory state that results in excessive liberation of thyroid hormone. Total thyroxine ($T_4$) and free thyroxine ($fT_4$) levels are increased. Although not necessary for screening, triiodothyronine ($T_3$) levels would also be elevated. Specific clinical abnormalities associated with thyrotoxicosis would appear as a function of the extent and degree of hormonal excess. Because the thyrotropic 'set-point' would have been exceeded, thyroid stimulating hormone (TSH) levels would be depressed.

2. The hyperthyroxinemia is the result of a 'liberation process' of thyroid hormone from an inflamed gland. It is not because the 'hormone-producing process' is accelerated. Thus, the 24-hour Radioactive Iodine Uptake (RAIU) would be suppressed.

3. Although a goiter might be present, it is usually small and characteristically non-tender (and thus, not generally perceived by the patient). It may persist following acute disease resolution. Subacute or granulomatous thyroiditis (de Quervain's thyroiditis), on the other hand, is associated with significant thyroid pain and tenderness, and more generalized constitutional symptoms.

4. Chronic thyroiditis is associated with HLA-DR3 and -DR5 haplotypes.

5. Chronic thyroiditis is generally a self-limiting disease and treatment is largely supportive and symptomatic (e.g. β-adrenergic blockade). Indeed, if the pathophysiology is release of pre-formed hormone, neither classic antithyroid drugs nor radioactive iodine would be expected to work. Affected persons may go through a secondary hypothyroid phase. It may be compelling to treat the hypothyroid phase with thyroid hormone, but restraint is best advised, as only a small percentage of those affected will have permanent hypothyroidism. Alternatively, if it is necesssary to treat the hypothyroidism, future testing is indicated, because permanent hypothyroidism requires a lifetime commitment of thyroid hormone therapy.

6.  This type of condition has the tendency to recur following future pregnancies (even following therapeutic abortions). Thus, both the patient and her physician must be sensitized to this possibility.

## CLINICAL CASE #6

1. There is a need to rule out Cushing's syndrome in this patient. While obesity is a common medical problem, the presence of additional features warrants further work-up. The obesity of Cushing's syndrome is centripetal or truncal and it involves the face, abdomen and 'scruff' of the neck. Irregular menses occur because of a relative hyperandrogenism (hirsutism and acne can be associated features). The weakness should be objectified and is largely a proximal myopathy. Easy bruisability is caused by increased vulnerability of capillaries and other small vessels. There may be associated wide red striae and 'easy peeling' of the skin.

   The overnight dexamethasone suppression test is a simple and cost-effective screening tool. While an abnormal test does not rule in Cushing's syndrome, a normal test rules it out.

   Alternatively, the 24-hour urine free cortisol is also an excellent screening test and can be a valuable follow up to a dexamethasone suppression test that may be falsely positive.

2. In addition to features of Cushing's syndrome already discussed is osteoporosis, which might not have yet resulted in clinical consequences in this woman, but which might be ascertained using bone density studies. Other features include hypertension, glucose intolerance (with or without overt diabetes), increased intraocular pressure, depressed immune function and psychiatric manifestations.

   Relevant laboratory features would include leukocytosis with neutrophilia, lymphopenia and eosinopenia; polycythemia; hypokalemia and increased very low-, high- and low-density lipoprotein concentrations. Coagulation factors V and VIII might be elevated, and hypercalciuria might be an additional finding.

3. Cushing's syndrome can be categorized based upon ACTH dependence or independence. An ACTH level can distinguish between these two categories as the level is low or undetectable in all ACTH-independent etiologies, but elevated in both Cushing's disease (pituitary-mediated Cushing's syndrome) and the ectopic ACTH syndrome. ACTH levels are characteristically higher in ectopic Cushing's than in pituitary-mediated Cushing's syndrome. When an immunoradiometric assay (IRMA) is used,

which is highly specific for pituitary ACTH, values in the ectopic syndrome are either low or undetectable.

The classic sequence to distinguish between Cushing's disease and other causes of Cushing's syndrome involves structured low- and high-dose dexamethasone testing. The low-dose test utilizes 2 mg of dexamethasone and the high-dose test utilizes 8 mg of dexamethasone, each given daily in divided doses over a 2-day period. Plasma cortisol levels or urine metabolites are used to monitor suppression. The test rationale is that no one with Cushing's syndrome should suppress on low-dose dexamethasone, while those with pituitary-mediated Cushing's syndrome (Cushing's disease) will demonstrate high-dose suppression.

Supplemental testing (primarily of historical interest) takes cognizance of the fact that adrenal adenomas will generally produce disproportionately higher amounts of urinary 17-hydroxy corticosteroids than 17-keto steroids, while the converse would occur with adrenal carcinoma. When corticotropin releasing hormone (CRH) is used as a diagnostic tool, it is able to increase ACTH levels in Cushing's disease (but not in pituitary-independent etiologies and very rarely with ectopic ACTH syndromes). Metyrapone stimulation is capable of increasing serum deoxycortisol in ACTH-dependent Cushing's syndrome (but not in other etiologies).

Imaging studies for structural delineation include adrenal CT and cranial MRI (the preferred modality to assess pituitary structure).

4.  Inferior petrosal sinus sampling can be a powerful tool to resolve ambiguity regarding a primary pituitary etiology for ACTH-dependent Cushing's syndrome. The rationale is that there should be a disparity between pituitary and peripheral ACTH levels if the origin is pituitary. An additional benefit of this test is its ability to lateralize the lesion.

5.  Bilateral adrenalectomy can result in symptomatic enlargement of the pituitary adenoma responsible for Cushing's disease (Nelson's syndrome). The syndrome can include symptoms secondary to the mass effect of the tumor (e.g. visual field deficits), increased ACTH elaboration (hyperpigmentation) and pituitary insufficiency.

## CLINICAL CASE #7

1. Although symptoms such as weight loss, fatigue, abdominal cramps and light-headedness can apply to a large number of clinical entities, including Addison's disease, the presence of this patient's 'suntanned appearance' makes the screening for Addison's disease an imperative.

A complete history and physical examination can provide additional clues. Her hyperpigmentation, while making her appear 'suntanned', would also be present in non-solar-exposed areas. These include her skin creases and gingiva and buccal mucosa. She would tend to be hypotensive (relative to her basal level) and orthostasis would be common. Her heart would be 'small and quiet'. There could be symptoms of fasting hypoglycemia, decreased bodily hair and irregular menses. Psychiatric manifestations, although again 'non-specific', would complete the picture. Rarely might there be costrovertebral angle tenderness (Rogoff's sign) and calcification of her ears (Thorn's sign).

Associated laboratory findings include hyponatremia and hyperkalemia, a non-anion gap metabolic acidosis and inappropriate urine sodium wasting in the presence of hyponatremia and hypovolemia. The complete blood count could reveal a low-grade normocytic (perhaps macrocytic) anemia with a mild neutropenia, eosinophilia and relative lymphocytosis. There might also be hypoglycemia, azotemia, and mild hypercalcemia. Chest X-ray would demonstrate a relative decrease in heart size; ECG often reveals only 'non-specific' changes.

The crucial endocrinologic test is measurement of her plasma cortisol before and after ACTH stimulation. Plasma cortisol levels are obtained before and after a 250 µg intravenous bolus of a synthetic corticotropin, cosyntropin. Plasma levels less than 20 µg/dl effectively rule out Addison's disease. In reality, patients with Addison's disease have substantially lower values.

Hyperpigmentation is an important clinical clue that suggests she would have primary Addison's disease. Melanocyte-stimulating hormones are part of the 'ACTH package' and are increased in primary Addison's disease, even though diurnal variation is still maintained.

2.  Ideally, the replacement regime would mimic the normal adrenal circadian cycle of cortisol levels which are highest in the early morning and lowest in the late afternoon. Replacement has traditionally consisted of giving two-thirds of the daily dose of glucocorticoid upon awakening in the morning (e.g. 20 mg of hydrocortisone) and one-third in the late afternoon (e.g. 10 mg of hydrocortisone). Some patients even take the entire glucocorticoid replacement in the morning because normal afternoon cortisol production is so low. A drawback to this approach is that the normal morning surge of cortisol is 'not truly mimicked' because that ACTH-mediated surge takes place prior to awakening. Thus, there is both an unopposed stimulus to hyperpigmentation and lingering morning constitutional symptoms until the morning dose of glucocorticoid 'kicks in'.

    An alternative replacement regime is with a longer acting glucocorticoid (e.g. dexamethasone or prednisone) given at bedtime. Unfortunately, this could produce an inappropriately high steroid level during the night and result in insomnia. Further, the steroid effect may 'wear off' prematurely during the day.

    Mineralocorticoid replacement can be accomplished with fludrocortisone (Florinef), 0.05–0.2 mg/day. While serum electrolytes can be useful for monitoring, blood pressure (basal and postural), weight and presence or absence of edema are very practical (and readily accessible) parameters to follow.

3.  While irregular menses can be part of the Addisonian syndrome, her 'hot flushes' suggest significant estrogen withdrawal. The most common etiology of Addison's disease today is autoimmune (idiopathic) and there is linkage with this and the occurrence of other autoimmune diseases. Included are gonadal failure, immunologic thyroid disease, Type I diabetes mellitus, vitiligo, hypoparathyroidism and pernicious anemia. Although we are not given clinical information, there is nothing in this case that suggests other etiologies of Addison's disease (e.g. tuberculosis or fungal disease, HIV-associated disease, metastatic disease or any of the other less common causes).

    The follicle-stimulating hormone (FSH) level is the most sensitive predictor of early menopause and its elevation would support a diagnosis of primary ovarian failure. Vaginal cytology additionally confirm estrogen deficiency. While 41 years is not an exceptionally young age to experience menopause, it might be inappropriately young in her case, and the result of immunologically-mediated premature ovarian failure.

4. Acute physiologic stress warrants the same substantial level of glucocorticoid that she would endogenously produce were her own adrenal glands functional. Typically, steroid doses of four to six times basal replacement are given over the first 24 hours followed by tapering doses as the inciting event abates. Considering the severity of her injury, a reasonable regime would be hydrocortisone, 100 mg, intravenously, every 8 hours for the first 24 hours (this could also cover her throughout any anticipated surgical procedure). Assuming an otherwise uneventful recovery, the tapering process could be completed within 5 days. Adequate hydration with isotonic saline is essential. Because of this fluid replacement and the mineralocorticoid effect of the glucocorticoid in the dose administered, independent mineralocorticoid administration is generally not necessary.

## CLINICAL CASE #8

1. This case is compelling for the potential diagnosis of primary hyperaldosteronism. The patient has severe symptomatic hypokalemia as manifest by overt muscular weakness, lethargy, loss of baroreceptor-mediated postural changes in pulse, and blunting of her deep tendon reflexes. It is very unlikely that the thiazide diuretic she was intermittently taking could explain her state (although the thiazide would have to be discontinued and restoration of normokalemia sought to see if it played any role). Furthermore, 'eating a banana' on the day one is taking the diuretic would have little effect in ensuring potassium balance. The arteriolar narrowing and clinical findings on cardiac examination confirm both the magnitude and relative duration of the hypertension. The hypertension of primary hyperaldosteronism is 'volume-mediated'. Yet, as in her case, peripheral edema is unusual. Glucose intolerance, as might be inferred by her blood sugar of 154, is also a feature of hyperaldosteronism and correlates with the hypokalemia.

2. Although it is both futile and inappropriate to screen all hypertensive patients for primary hyperaldosteronism, it is highly appropriate that this patient be screened. The ability to maintain normokalemia after thiazide discontinuance (and after pharmacologic potassium replenishment), while a reasonable and cost-effective screening test, is unlikely to occur in this patient. It is also important that this patient's hypertension be treated, even as testing proceeds. Prazosin and related drugs (terazosin, doxazosin) are very effective agents that are not likely to affect test results.

   One specific screening measure requires demonstration of inappropriate kaliuresis with a suppressed plasma renin and an increased serum aldosterone:renin ratio while on a liberal sodium diet (at least 100 mEq/day). Her condition may be too unsettled to carry this out, but merely demonstrating an inappropriately suppressed upright plasma renin in the presence of an increased aldosterone:renin ratio will still be quite useful. An ancillary test requires the administration of 25–50 mg of Captopril and demonstration of persistence of the elevated plasma aldosterone : renin ratio 60–120 minutes after drug administration. Potassium replenishment can continue during testing and certainly is a desired treatment goal.

3. The rationale for diagnostic confirmation is that functional autonomy cannot be suppressed by normal physiologic suppressors. If this patient demonstrates inappropriate elevation of aldosterone after either intravenous or oral sodium challenge, then aldosterone production is autonomous. Of the available test protocols, administration of normal saline, 2 liters intravenously, over 4 hours, is the most expeditious (the patient should be recumbent and should have fasted overnight). Blood pressures are to be monitored during the procedure. A resultant plasma aldosterone greater than 10 ng/dl is highly likely to be diagnostic of primary hyperaldosteronism.

4. Subset identification is important at this point because surgical removal of an aldosterone-producing adenoma (or an intact carcinoma or unilateral hyperplasia) will correct the electrolyte imbalance and generally the hypertension, as well. An additional benefit is that the contralateral adrenal gland remains to assume all other adrenal functions. Conversely, bilateral adrenalectomy for hyperplasia will not cure the hypertension and will additionally render the patient Addisonian.

   Features often seen with adenoma, as opposed to hyperplasia, are a younger age, a greater severity of hypertension and hypokalemia and a higher aldosterone level (which does not increase when changing from a recumbent to an upright posture). While helpful and interesting, this information cannot substitute for quantitative data.

   CT imaging can usually identify the nature of the lesion by defining its anatomic structure. Supplemental imaging with MRI or radioscintigraphy with iodo-cholesterol may be additionally helpful. If there is ambiguity, selective adrenal vein sampling can be done. The aldosterone : cortisol ratios of each side are compared during an intravenous Cosyntropin infusion.

   If the lesion is unilateral, surgical extirpation should suffice, but additional antihypertensive therapy may be necessary. If the lesion is bilateral hyperplasia, spironolactone can correct the electrolyte imbalance (the potassium-sparing diuretics such as amiloride and triamterine may be adjunctively helpful) but additional antihypertensive therapy will invariably be required. A very rare cause of hyperplasia that is glucocorticoid suppressible (associated with elevations of 18-oxocortisol and 18-hydroxycortisol) can be treated with glucocorticoids.

## CLINICAL CASE #9

1. A case is made in this patient for the possibility of pheochromocytoma. While diagnostic studies for pheochromocytoma are not indicated in the routine evaluation of hypertension, there are compelling features in this patient which justify the search. He complains of headache, and increased nervousness. Hypermetabolism is suggested by his weight loss despite adequate food intake. He has noticed increased perspiration, which is confirmed on physical examination. Physical examination also establishes his hypertension, tremulousness and tachycardia. Additional relevant information comes from his family history of a 'calcium problem' and of thyroid cancer.

   Considering the constellation of problems that can produce overlapping cardiac, endocrine and neuropsychiatric manifestations, the differential diagnosis is large. A 24-hour urine determination for metanephrines and free catecholamines, however, is a very sensitive and specific assay, especially if the hypertension is sustained. Plasma metanephrines are also a sensitive assay. Modern assay procedures avoid most of the diagnostic pitfalls of the past and pheochromocytomas are generally associated with substantially elevated values. If his hypertension is sporadic, however, a 24-hour urine determination may be normal. In that case, obtaining a 'spot urine' and comparing the metanephrine and catecholamine to creatinine ratios in that sample can be discriminatory.

2. There is an association between medullary carcinoma of the thyroid and pheochromocytoma. Both can be found in the autosomal dominant Multiple Endocrine Neoplasia (MEN) Types IIa and IIb. Both entities can additionally be independently familial. If his sister had medullary carcinoma of the thyroid, even if he proves not to have a pheochromocytoma, he should be screened for medullary carcinoma with a basal and pentagastrin/calcium-provoked calcitonin level. His uncle's 'calcium problem' ought to be better identified. If it were hyperparathyroidism, it would be compatible with inheritance of a MEN Type IIa pattern. Two basal serum calcium levels would comprise effective screening. If he proves to have hypercalcemia, this should be followed with a parathyroid hormone level as part of his screening process.

3. MEN Type IIa is not associated with a Marfanoid habitus (while IIb is). If the propensity to pheochromocytoma were genetically based (and his uncle had hyperparathyroidism), he would not be expected to have a Marfanoid habitus because his MEN pattern would be Type IIa.

4. In addition to the MEN Type II syndromes, other entities associated with pheochromocytoma include: von Hippel–Lindau disease, von Recklinghausen's disease, Sturge–Weber syndrome, ataxia telangiectasia, tuberous sclerosis, Carney's triad, renal artery stenosis and cholelithiasis.

5. The 'Rule of Tens' alludes to the approximate 10% likelihood of pheochromocytoma occurring in the following patterns: familial, chidhood, multiple, bilateral, malignant, extra-adrenal and recurrence following surgery.

## CLINICAL CASE #10

1.  This woman's morning hypoglycemia could be secondary to insulin inadequacy, or it could represent reactive hyperglycemia in response to nocturnal hypoglycemia (Somogyi phenomenon). Possible causes of inadequate glycemic control include weight gain, increased caloric consumption at dinner, cessation of a prior evening exercise pattern (and/or a more general decline in physical activity), development of insulin resistance, subclinical infection (or other etiologies of increased physiologic stress), or insufficient insulin dosing. Conversely, nocturnal hypoglycemia could be secondary to increased insulin sensitivity (e.g. as a result of weight loss, renal failure, or other endocrine deficiency states), insufficient food intake at dinner (or avoidance of a previously consumed bedtime snack), or excessive insulin dosing.

2.  The history suggests that this patient might be experiencing nocturnal hypoglycemia and that her morning hyperglycemia represents the effect of augmented counterregulation. Although relatively uncommon, the situation could be greatly clarified with nocturnal blood glucose values. The patient should deliberately be awoken during the night and her finger stick blood glucose determinations recorded. If there is sufficient concern about the severity, and therefore potential danger, of nocturnal hypoglycemia, prudence would suggest empiric lowering of her afternoon insulin dose, even before this data collection is undertaken.

    There is suggestive evidence in her history that deterioration of renal status could be a factor. Her long-standing diabetes, antecedent proteinuria and more recent fatigue and decreased work capacity are compatible with this. Certainly, her renal status should be investigated.

3.  Diabetes mellitus is associated with an increased risk of fetal congenital abnormalities. These particularly involve the cardiovascular, neurologic, renal and gastrointestinal systems. Neonatal offspring of diabetic mothers are also more prone to hypoglycemia, hypocalcemia and hyperbilirubinemia. The pregnancy can additionally be marked by polyhydramnios, hypertension and toxemia, and fetal macrosomia is a frequent concomitant.

4. This patient most likely has Type I diabetes mellitus. The concordance rate for this type of diabetes is 50%.

5. Major histocompatibility complex (MHC) markers associated with Type I diabetes mellitus are DR3 and DR4 Class II antigens and B8, B15, and B18 Class I antigens.

6. Among other entities that can produce tiredness, cold intolerance and a 'deepening' of her voice, hypothyroidism should be a serious consideration. There is a clear association between Type I diabetes mellitus and other autoimmune diseases including hypothyroidism. While a serum thyroxine ($T_4$) level would be a helpful index for general screening, the thyroid-stimulating hormone (TSH) measurement is much more discriminatory and is clearly indicated.

## CLINICAL CASE #11

1. By present day standards, most cases of primary hyperparathyroidism are recognized through screening serum calcium determinations on otherwise asymptomatic individuals. The 'classic' or 'textbook' presentations of 'stones, moans and abdominal groans' are seemingly relegated to medical folklore, except for the occasional patient who might fall outside the screen. Nonetheless, there might be subtle clinical features of hyperparathyroidism that could be present even in 'asymptomatic' individuals. Sometimes, they are so subtle that they are only best appreciated retrospectively, after cure of the disease. In this patient, perhaps a fleeting episode of flank colic could have been caused by the passage of a kidney stone. He might have been diagnosed as being 'borderline hypertensive' or he could have experienced increased urinary frequency or pruritis, gastrointestinal symptoms, or psychologic symptoms such as emotional lability or depression. An elderly person might be more vulnerable to pathologic fractures.

2. Although we will never know what were the values of prior calcium determinations, it is very possible that he exhibited hypercalcemia in the past, even if his levels were only 'borderline' abnormal. The natural course for many cases of hyperparathyroidism is a drawn-out, but unrelenting course. If his calcium level 2 years ago were truly normal, it would still be compatible with the present diagnosis of primary hyperparathyroidism. In all presentations of hypercalcemia, however, all reasonable causes should be considered part of the differential diagnosis.

3. The most important test at this time is a serum parathyroid hormone (PTH) determination, done in concert with a serum calcium, on at least two separate occasions. The importance of clinical history, physical examination and basic laboratory studies, which would form part of a comprehensive general examination, cannot be minimized. There might be subtle corroborates of hyperparathyroidism (e.g. hypophosphatemia, elevated alkaline phosphatase, increased serum chloride and decreased bicarbonate), or such studies might uncover (however asymptomatic the patient) other etiologies of hypercalcemia (e.g. history of lithium use, hyperglobulinemia).

A sensitive parathyroid hormone (PTH) assay will distinguish between primary hyperparathyroidism and all the other major etiologies of hypercalcemia. Unless there is a serum protein abnormality, there is no need to obtain ionized calcium levels. Other laboratory testing for hyperparathyroidism is unnecessary, with the exception of a 24-hour urine for calcium determination to rule out the rare syndrome of familial hypocalciuric hypercalcemia (the serum magnesium is elevated in this syndrome as well). A phosphorus measurement in that same sample could be useful for the measurement of renal phosphate clearance (which is increased in primary hyperparathyroidism).

4. Either CT or MRI of the neck is an accepted standard for preoperative investigation, and surgery is the only definitive therapy. Studies such as barium esophagram, neck ultrasonography and dual isotope subtraction scintigraphy are only sporadically (and unpredictably) of value and are not cost effective.

5. Demonstration that he might already have 'silent' renal calculi or objective quantification of decreased bone mass (e.g. using dual energy X-Ray absorptiometry (DEXA)) would be very helpful in his decision-making process. Any other developing or concomitant manifestation (e.g. band keratopathy, early peptic ulcer disease, hypertension, left ventricular hypertrophy, psychologic symptoms – the last perhaps noted by family members even if he were not aware of them) would also be useful. Furthermore, he would be at risk for future development of these manifestations.

6. These clinical findings are compatible with acute, superimposed hypercalcemia. The demonstration of a substantially higher serum calcium than was recently noted would be confirmatory. This problem was precipitated by gastrointestinal fluid and electrolyte losses. Hypercalcemia can also induce anorexia, nausea and vomiting and antidiuretic hormone resistance, all capable of augmenting the process.

The most important therapy is intravenous fluid and electrolyte replacement. Intravenous saline would not only correct the dehydration, but would also promote calciuresis. Loop diuretics would additionally promote calcium excretion, but their use would necessitate careful monitoring of his volume status.

Thiazide diuretics should never be used – they would only aggravate the hypercalcemia. Additional therapies are available (e.g. Pamidronate, calcitonin), but may not be necessary if fluid and electrolyte replenishment could 'take him back' to how he was before his gastrointestinal illness 'tipped him over'. Other agents listed in the management of hypercalcemia are not indicated. Plicamycin is an antineoplastic agent and is potentially toxic. Gallium nitrate is also toxic and it also has a delayed onset and peak effect. Intravenous phosphate can be very dangerous and could result in renal failure and disseminated calcification.

Once stable, it would be both opportune and important to impress upon this man the need for a definitive surgical procedure.

## CLINICAL CASE #12

1. There are many potential medical problems seen in the patient with chronic alcohol abuse and hypocalcemia is clearly one of them. Possible mechanisms include poor nutrition, decreased exposure to sunlight and decreased intestinal absorption of both calcium and vitamin D. Intestinal mucosal disease and pancreatic insufficiency contribute to the decreased intestinal absorption. The elevated alkaline phosphatase and hypophosphatemia are supportive of vitamin D deficiency and are the result of a secondary hyperparathyroidism. Liver disease could also elevate the serum alkaline phosphatase, and hypophosphatemia can additionally be secondary to dietary inadequacy.

   Alcoholic patients can also be magnesium-depleted secondary to dietary inadequacy, malabsorption and increased renal wastage. This results in a secondary hypoparathyroidism (decreased parathyroid hormone synthesis and response). The total calcium could also be artifactually depressed by associated hypoalbuminemia.

2. A serum magnesium level and 25-hydroxy vitamin D would be very important. Additional studies include other tests of liver function. Serum glutamic-oxaloacetic transaminase, serum glutamic-pyruvic transaminase, lactate dehydrogenase and the albumin : globulin ratio would measure hepatocellular integrity and synthetic function. Ambiguity as to the cause of the alkaline phosphatase elevation could be clarified with a serum gamma-glutamyl transpeptidase (GGT) level (although this could be elevated by alcohol excess), or a 5' nucleotidase. A serum amylase or lipase would be a measure of active inflammatory disease of the pancreas, although demonstration of pancreatic calcifications on abdominal X-ray would be suggestive of chronic pancreatitis. A quantitative stool fat determination would be a measure of maldigestion/malabsorption. The need for additional tests for malabsorption would be predicated on the evolving clinical scenario, with appropriate therapies instituted, as necessary.

3. All reasonable efforts should be made to insure dietary adequacy. Unfortunately, these are often easier to theorize than to accomplish, once the patient leaves the hospital setting. Proven hypocalcemia and hypomagnesemia should be treated with

intravenous calcium and magnesium. This patient should also be observed for evidence of alcohol withdrawal and treated accordingly (any seizure diathesis would be worsened by the hypocalcemic state). To the extent that pancreatic disease and malabsorption, as culprits, are mediated by his alcohol abuse, abstinence should help mucosal healing and pancreatic restitution. Permanent pancreatic insufficiency will require exocrine enzyme replacement.

Proven vitamin D deficiency (as confirmed by a low 25-hydroxy vitamin D level) should be treated with daily oral doses of 5000 International Units (IU) of vitamin D and 2–3 g of calcium. In the absence of renal disease or fat malabsorption, there is no reason to give a more active form of the vitamin. As serum calcium, phosphorus and alkaline phosphatase values normalize, the dose of vitamin D can be decreased to daily maintenance of 400 IU. To the extent that malabsorption persists, higher doses of vitamin D will be necessary. If future dietary intake of calcium and magnesium are uncertain, 1500 mg of calcium and 400–500 mg of magnesium must be added as daily supplements.

## CLINICAL CASE #13

1.  This patient clearly has multiple risk factors for osteoporosis. Family history can be inferred because of the fracture that her sister sustained, although it is not clear to what extent this was trauma-induced. Her race, thin stature, sedentary life-style, cigarette smoking (even though she discontinued 5 years earlier) and her alcohol intake have added to her risk. As milk products are the most important dietary source of calcium, her lactose intolerance presumably resulted in a sustained period of decreased calcium intake. Finally, her postmenopausal state leaves her without the beneficial effect of estrogen on bone preservation.

    Following a complete medical evaluation including general screening laboratory studies, and assuming no significant abnormalities, realistic recommendations would include adequate (1500 mg/day) supplementary calcium and vitamin D, 400 Units/day. She should also be advised to limit or curtail her alcohol intake and to exercise actively. Because the issue of estrogen replacement therapy is complex and multifactorial, she should be apprised of its advantages and disadvantages. If risk for pathologic fracture is an important determinant in her consideration of estrogen replacement, then a bone density study is indicated (the dual energy X-ray absorptiometry (DEXA) is the most appropriate, but a quantitative computerized tomography (QCT) would also be acceptable, and would additionally not be affected by non-bony calcifications adjacent to her bone). If estrogen replacement is not a consideration, she should be made aware that there are other approaches to osteoporosis including bisphosphonate, fluoride and calcitonin, but they should be presented in the context of the prevailing consensus and controversy regarding their value and their availability. If she would consider any of those other approaches, then again, a bone density study is justified to provide important baseline information.

2.  The DEXA can provide helpful follow-up, but it should not be done until after a year of active therapy. The patient should not be disheartened if bone density does not 'improve' because a major effect of therapy is to thwart the acceleration of bone loss. Not having had an antecedent radiographic study prior to her initial baseline limits the information base and full appreciation

of the effect of her therapy. On the other hand, follow-up studies could show improvement in her bone mineralization by comparison with age-matched controls.

3. It is possible that her 'screening profile' included a total serum thyroxine ($T_4$), but no free $T_4$, thyroid hormone binding index (THBI) or thyroid-stimulating hormone (TSH). By increasing the concentration of thyroxine-binding globulin (TBG), estrogen can increase the total $T_4$, but would not affect the other three parameters or the thyrometabolic status of the patient. The degree of elevation of the total $T_4$, however, would be affected by the dose of the estrogen. The resin uptake test, which is one of the two tests on which the THBI is based, is depressed if the TBG is elevated, but the product of the total $T_4$ and the resin uptake, i.e. the THBI, would be normal (the THBI is also known as the free thyroxine index, or FTI).

## CLINICAL CASE #14

1.  This patient has an elevated total serum cholesterol and a medical response to it is clearly in order. She also has a significant family history of coronary artery disease and this puts her at statistical risk, although it is unclear whether the basis for this risk is hypercholesterolemia. The total cholesterol screen that this patient had is inadequate and a full lipid profile (cholesterol fractionation and triglycerides) is indicated. If she has an elevated low-density lipoprotein (LDL) cholesterol, whether or not the high-density lipoprotein (HDL) cholesterol is depressed, there are measures to take to try to change it. An elevated HDL cholesterol could also be contributory to the total cholesterol, but it is unlikely, in light of the magnitude of the total cholesterol, to be a significant constituent.

    Fundamental recommendations to consider, even while your work-up is in progress, relate to her weight, her antihypertensive medication and her estrogen replacement therapy. Weight reduction is a difficult, but important problem to discuss. It must be handled with support and sensitivity and in a non-judgemental context. Further, her long-standing obesity renders her at statistical risk for recidivism, even if there is initial success. Thiazide diuretics and β-blocking agents both contribute to an unfavorable lipid profile, and there are clearly other available and very effective antihypertensive agents (e.g. ACE inhibitors, calcium channel blockers) that will not have an adverse effect on her lipid status. Her estrogen patch may be well accepted, but substitution with an oral agent, by its transport through her portal circulation, will improve her lipid profile (decreasing the LDL cholesterol and increasing the HDL-cholesterol, particularly the HDL$_2$ subclass). Although estrogen can also elevate her serum triglycerides, any adverse effect of this is outweighed by a dominant effect of estrogen on reducing the LDL cholesterol. While concomitant use of a progestin could theoretically negate the beneficial effects of the oral estrogen, the magnitude of this 'negative effect' is also outweighed by the benefits of the estrogen. The progestin is necessary to reduce the risk of endometrial hyperplasia and cancer.

    For completeness of assessment, consideration should be given to secondary causes of hypercholesterolemia (e.g. liver disease, paraproteinemia, diabetes mellitus, hypothyroidism).

2. This patient clearly has an unfavorable lipid profile and significant hypertension. While her total thyroxine is within the normal range, her thyroid-stimulating hormone is clearly elevated. Treatment with L-thyroxine is in order, even if the hypothyroidism does not totally explain her hypercholesterolemic profile. Dietary counselling is now a clear imperative and she should consider changing to an oral estrogen preparation. Her antihypertensive medication must effectively control her blood pressure without untoward side-effects. Her blood sugar is 'high normal', but follow-up determinations are all that is indicated for now (the thiazide diuretic and β-blocking agent could both have played 'facilitatory roles' in the tendency to hyperglycemia).

3. Now euthyroid and on medication that would not adversely affect her lipid profile, she still has an abnormal (but improved) lipid profile. If there is a greater role for diet and weight loss, this is to be strongly encouraged. The Step I diet requires a decrease of daily fat intake to less than 30% of total calories, decreased saturated fat intake to less than 10% of total calories, and decreased cholesterol intake to less than 300 mg. Additionally, polyunsaturated fats should be less than 10% of calories with monosaturated fats comprising the remaining total fat calories.

If she has already made strides at weight reduction and is committed to her present diet, then a Step 2 Diet can be recommended. It requires a significant commitment on the part of the patient and it differs from the Step 1 Diet by decreasing the saturated fats to less than 7% of total calories and cholesterol intake to less than 200 mg/day. If this can reduce her LDL-cholesterol to less than 160 mg/dl and place her total cholesterol/LDL cholesterol in the 'normal range' (2.5–4.5), then continued medical follow up without medication, can suffice. This is important because family history and hypertension represent two distinct risk factors for coronary artery disease. If this diet is unacceptable or ineffective, the prevailing consensus would be to place her on a lipid-lowering regime. Bile salt sequestrants, whose major effect is to decrease LDL, are an option. They can produce unpleasant gastrointestinal side-effects and also interfere with the absorption of L-thyroxine (the thyroxine should be taken either several hours before or after a resin dose). Nicotinic acid, also an option, acts by decreasing LDL synthesis (it also increases HDL synthesis). Untoward side-effects include dyspepsia, flushing, hyperuricemia, abnormal liver function tests and (particularly relevant in her case), abnormal glucose tolerance. 3-Hydroxy-3-methyl glutaryl coenzyme A (HMG CoA) reductase inhibitors, a third option, also decrease LDL and increase HDL cholesterol. Potential side-effects include abnormal liver function tests, myositis, gastrointestinal symptoms and cataracts.

## CLINICAL CASE #15

1. The differential diagnosis in this patient is that of primary amenorrhea. Major categories to consider are hypothalamic disorders, pituitary disorders, disorders of the reproductive tract, and ovarian disease. Realistic entities within the category of hypothalamic disorders include idiopathic deficiency of gonadotropin-releasing hormone (GnRH), anorexia nervosa, hypothalamic destructive lesions and 'hypothalamic amenorrhea'. GnRH deficiency is unlikely because secondary sexual maturation would not have taken place. Likewise, there should be a characteristic 'pathologic thinness' were she to have anorexia nervosa and there might be other clinical (e.g. increased bodily lanugo hair, carotene deposition in her skin, hypotension and temperature dysregulation) and laboratory (e.g. low triiodothyronine ($T_3$), impaired renal concentrating ability, hypercholesterolemia) concomitants. A hypothalamic destructive process should be evident by history and by evidence of more extensive loss of hypothalamic function (e.g. as evidenced by other pituitary deficiencies). 'Hypothalamic amenorrhea' is generally associated with certain scenarios (e.g. vigorous aerobic conditioning, 'stress') and it is unusual for it to be of such sustained duration.

   Pituitary disorders should produce syndromes related to the mass effect of lesions and associated endocrine excess (e.g. as produced by 'functioning lesions') and endocrine deficiency states.

   Disorders of the reproductive tract are possible in this patient. Indeed, even if there were an intact uterus, the vagina ending in a 'blind pouch' would impede any menstrual flow.

   Of the potential ovarian causes of amenorrhea, testicular feminization is the most likely diagnosis. Indeed, it is the most likely entity in the entire differential diagnosis. Turner's syndrome, as a cause of primary amenorrhea, is associated with well-defined somatic features (the small stature and facial features are generally very striking) and thus can be ruled out. If the diagnosis were 'ovarian failure', this would almost invariably occur after menarche (and would thus be a 'secondary amenorrhea'). Enzymatic defects in estrogen synthesis would produce a 'hypoestrogenic state' and an estrogen-producing tumor would produce sexual precocity if it developed prior to puberty, and secondary amenorrhea after puberty. Further, the associated mass lesion should be noted on pelvic examination, and the clinical course should not have been this prolonged. Polycystic ovarian syndrome generally results in either secondary amenorrhea or in irregular menses. Furthermore, this syndrome (or other hyperandrogenic states) would be expected to produce some degree of androgenization (at least some degree of hirsutism). Indeed, one notes the opposite in this patient.

Factors which rule in testicular feminization include her primary amenorrhea, secondary sexual maturation in an unambiguous female pattern (the estrogen made by this 'genotypic male' would be 'unopposed' because her androgen is ineffective), sparse bodily hair (ambisexual bodily hair is under strong androgenic influence in both sexes), and absence of a palpable uterus (she is able to make Müllerian inhibitory factor). Her female phenotypy results from the 'natural tendency to femininity' that cannot be overridden by her ineffectual androgens. She has abdominal testes (these are her 'bilateral ovaries'), but there is target tissue insensitivity to their androgenic products.

2. Clearly, a comprehensive history and physical examination can be invaluable. Additional laboratory tests would include luteinizing hormone (LH), testosterone and estradiol levels (all of which would be elevated because of failure of hypothalamic-pituitary inhibition). The buccal smear (for Barr body presence) or karyotype delineation, although not necessary, would confirm the anticipated genotype. A pelvic ultrasound would demonstrate the intra-abdominal testes. A progesterone alone or estrogen/progesterone 'clinical trial' for withdrawal bleeding would be of no value.

3. The overriding management objective is to maintain normal femininity in this phenotypic woman. She should always be considered a woman in the course of her personal, social, or sexual conduct.

For diagnostic confirmation, and to eliminate any possibility of gonadal cancer, the testes should be removed. As this would result in the loss of estrogen (the androgen loss would not be relevant), she should be maintained on full estrogen replacement therapy (it can be given on a continuous basis). She will never ovulate or have menses, and thus is incapable of fertility.

## CLINICAL CASE #16

1.  This patient has clinical evidence of a hyperandrogenic state. It appears to be long standing and of relatively 'mild to moderate' severity in that she continues to menstruate (albeit irregularly) and there is no overt masculinization. If exogenous androgenic causes are ruled out, potential etiologies are adrenal, ovarian and idiopathic.

    Adrenal causes include congenital adrenal hyperplasia, Cushing's syndrome, hyperprolactinemia and adrenal tumors. The two enzymatic deficiencies of cortisol synthesis that produce excessive androgens are the 21- and 11-hydroxylase deficiencies. The 21-hydroxylase is the more common deficiency and can be associated with salt-wasting whereas the 11-hydroxylase deficiency (because desoxycorticosterone is produced in excess) results in salt retention (hypertension and hypokalemia can be concomitants). In Cushing's syndrome, there should be reasonably obvious clinical features of glucocorticoid excess with androgenic excess a 'superimposed' facet. Hyperprolactinemia can be a stimulus for increased adrenal androgen dehydroepiandrosterone (DHEA) and dehydroepiandrosterone sulfate (DHEA-S) production, but many women with hyperprolactinemia are not hirsute, and hyperprolactinemia can be an additional feature of the polycystic ovarian syndrome (PCOS). An androgen-producing adrenal tumor is a possible cause, but would be unlikely because her long-standing androgen excess dates back to the time of menarche.

    Ovarian causes are PCOS (hyperthecosis can be considered a variant) and ovarian tumors. An idiopathic cause always remains a possibility.

    The value of a complete history, general physical examination and gynecologic examination cannot be overstated. Appropriate baseline endocrinologic studies include plasma 17-hydroxy progesterone, DHEA-S, testosterone, and androstenedione. The 17-hydroxy progesterone is the basic screening test for congenital adrenal hyperplasia. While a basal level should be appropriate, an early morning determination takes advantage of the endogenous ACTH stimulation. Conversely, the determination can be made following exogenous ACTH stimulation. Adrenal tumors would be commonly associated with marked elevation of

DHEA-S while ovarian tumors would tend to have high levels of androstenedione and testosterone (along with pronounced virilization). If Cushing's syndrome is suspected, both the dexamethasone suppression test and the 24-hour free cortisol are excellent screening studies. Moderate to marked elevation of DHEA-S can occur in Cushing's syndrome, but this test should not be the determinant for diagnosis. Idiopathic hirsutism can be associated with mild elevations of all androgens.

If the work-up is normal and measured androgens are not elevated, there might be increased peripheral sensitivity to testosterone. This results from increased conversion of testosterone to dihydrotestosterone (DHT). Androstanediol sulfate, a metabolite of dihydrotestosterone, would be elevated and could serve as a useful marker.

2. Polycystic ovarian disease is a rather common cause of androgenization and is the likely diagnosis in this patient. The protracted history and associated weight excess are common features. Multiple ovarian cysts are generally found on routine pelvic examination, but the pelvic ultrasound would be more quantitative and specific. The ultrasound can also be useful in identifying an ovarian mass. By analogy, abdominal CT or MRI can additionally help locate a suspected adrenal mass. An associated biochemical test to rule out an adrenal tumor is the long-term (7-day) high-dose dexamethasone suppression test. If the DHEA-S suppresses on this regime, an adrenal tumor would be ruled out.

Laboratory features of PCOS are mild to moderate elevations of luteinizing hormone (the elevation is sustained and without the midcycle peak), testosterone, androstenedione, DHEA-S, prolactin, estradiol (elevation of the mean value with loss of cyclicity) and estrone. Follicle-stimulating hormone, however, is decreased.

3. The patient might have had exaggeration of her hirsutism only recently because she had been on the oral contraceptive pill. Use of the pill would have decreased ovarian androgen output (a particular feature of PCOS is the relative ability of the theca cells to produce androgens, the inability of granulosa cells to aromatize them to estrogens). Oral contraceptives also decrease dihydrotestosterone receptor binding and decrease adrenal

androgen production. Additionally, by increasing sex hormone binding globulin (SHBG), they decrease the level of 'free' testosterone, the 'active' testosterone component.

4. She was not virilized because virilization would require a higher circulating androgen level than is commonly associated with PCOS. Hirsutism and irregular menses are at one end of a spectrum of potential masculinizing features of the hyperandrogenic state. Virilization, on the other hand, might be an expected feature of a testosterone-producing ovarian tumor where both the concentration and potency of testosterone would produce overt masculinization.

5. Insulin resistance may play a role in the pathophysiology of PCOS. Theca cells may not be as resistant to insulin as other tissues and thus may be disproportionately stimulated. Likewise, acanthosis nigricans, frequently seen in this syndrome, may be another expression of heightened and focused insulin activity. The frequent association of obesity with PCOS may be related to the relative insulin resistance seen in the obese state. This patient is very likely to have a high insulin : glucose ratio.

# SELECTED BIBLIOGRAPHY

## ENDOCRINOLOGY OVERVIEW AND REFERENCE RESOURCES

American College of Physicians, *MKSAP Learning Program (Part C, Book 4 – Endocrinology and Metabolism)*, X edition, 1995.

Bardin, C.W. *Current Therapy in Endocrinology and Metabolism*, 5th edition. C.V. Mosby, 1994.

Becker, K.L. (ed.) *Principles and Practice of Endocrinology and Metabolism*, 2nd edition. Philadelphia: J.B. Lippincott, 1995.

DeGroot, L.J. (ed.) *Endocrinology*, 3rd edition. Philadelphia: W.B. Saunders, 1995.

Felig, P., Baxter, J.D., Frohman, L.A. (eds.) *Endocrinology and Metabolism*, 3rd edition. New York: McGraw Hill, 1995.

Greenspan, F.S., ed., *Basic and Clinical Endocrinology*, 3rd edition. Appleton and Lange, 1991.

Grinspoon, S.K., Bilezikian, J.P. HIV Disease and the Endocrine System. *N Engl J Med* 1992; 327: 1360.

Section on Endocrinology and Metabolism, *Harrison's Principles of Internal Medicine*, 12th edition. New York: McGraw Hill, 1991.

Section on Endocrinology and Metabolism, *Cecil: Textbook of Medicine*, 19th edition. Philadelphia: W.B. Saunders Company, 1992.

Wilson, J. D., Foster, D.W., eds., *Williams Textbook of Endocrinology*, 8th edition. Philadelphia: W. B. Saunders Company, 1992.

## 1. THE NATURE OF HORMONES

Gill, G.N. Principles of Endocrinology. In *Cecil: Textbook of Medicine*, 19th edition. Philadelphia: W.B. Saunders Company, 1992.

Reichlin, S. Neuroendocrine-Immune Interactions. *N Engl J Med* 1993; 329: 1246.

## 2. THE HYPOTHALAMUS AND ANTERIOR PITUITARY GLAND

Bateman, A., Singh, A., Kral, T. *et al.* The immune–hypothalamic–pituitary–adrenal axis. *Endocr Rev* 1989; 10: 92.

Daniels, G.H., Martin, J.B. Neuroendocrine regulation and diseases of the anterior pituitary and hypothalamus. In: *Harrison's Principles of Internal Medicine*, 12th edition. New York: McGraw Hill, 1991: Chapter 313, pp. 1655.

Martin, J.B., Reichlin, S. *Clinical Neuroendocrinology*, 2nd edition Davis, 1987.

Molitch, M.E., ed. Pituitary Tumors: Diagnosis and Management. *Endocrinol Metab Clin North Am* 1987; 16: 3

Streeten, D.H., Anderson, G.H. Jr, Dalakos, T.G. *et al.* Normal and abnormal function of the hypothalamic–pituitary–adrenal system in man. *Endocr Rev* 1984; 5: 371.

Wenzel, E., Comi, R.J. Use of octreotide in clinical endocrinology. *The Endocrinologist* 1991; 1: 256.

## 3. HYPOPITUITARISM

Abboud, C.F. Laboratory Diagnosis of Hypopituitarism. *Mayo Clin Proc* 1986; 61: 35.

Christensen, R.B., Matsumoto, A.M., Bremner, W. Idiopathic hypogonadotropic hypogonadism with anosmia (Kallman's syndrome). *The Endocrinologist* 1992; 2: 332.

Eddy, R.L., Gilliland, P.F., Ibarra, J.D., Jr., *et al.* Human growth hormone release: comparison of provocative test procedures. *Am J Med* 1974; 56: 179.

Edwards, O.M., Clark, J.D.A. Post-traumatic hypopituitarism. *Medicine* 1986; 65: 281.

Laws, E. R., Jr. Craniopharyngioma: Diagnosis and Treatment. *The Endocrinologist* 1992; 2: 184.

Loriaux, D.L., Nieman, L. Corticotropin-releasing hormone testing in pituitary disease. *Endocrinol Metab Clin North Am* 1991; 20: 363.

Oelkers, W. Hyponatremia and inappropriate secretion of vasopressin in patients with hypopituitarism. *N Engl J Med* 1989; 321: 492.

Vance, M. Hypopituitarism. *N Engl J Med* 1994; 330: 1651.

## 4. ACROMEGALY

Acromegaly Therapy Consensus Development Panel. Benefits versus risk of medical therapy for acromegaly. *Am J Med* 1994; 97: 468.

Barkan, A. Acromegaly: Diagnosis and Treatment. *Endocrinol Metab Clin N Am* 1989; 18: 277.

Barkan, A., Shenker, Y., Grekin, R. *et. al.* Acromegaly due to ectopic GHRH production: dynamic studies of GH and ectopic GHRH secretion. *J Clin Endocrinol Metab* 1986; 63: 1057.

Faglia, G., Arosio, M., Ambrosi, B. Recent advances in diagnosis and treatment of acromegaly. In: Imura, H. (ed.) *Pituitary Gland*. New York: Raven Press 1985: p. 363.

Lamberts, S.W. The role of somatostatin in the regulation of anterior pituitary hormone secretion and the use of its analogues in the treatment of human pituitary tumors. *Endocr Rev* 1989; 9: 417.

Melmed, S. Management choices in acromegaly. *The Endocrinologist* 1991; 1: 331.

Ross, D.A., Wilson, C.B. Results of transsphenoidal microsurgery for growth hormone-secreting pituitary adenoma in a series of 214 patients. *J Neurosurg* 1988; 68: 854.

## 5. PROLACTIN-PRODUCING ADENOMA

Klibanski, A., Greenspan, S.L. Increased bone mass in treated hyperprolactinemic amenorrheic women. *N Engl J Med* 1986; 315: 542.

Leong, D.A., Frawley, L.S., Neill, J.D. Neuroendocrine control of prolactin secretion. *Ann Rev Physiol* 1983; 109: 45.

Molitch, M. Hyperprolactinemia. *Med Grand Rounds* 1982; 1: 307.

Molitch, M. Pregnancy and the hyperprolactinemic woman. *N Engl J Med* 1985; 312: 1364.

Schlecte, J., Dolan, K., Sherman, B. *et al*. The natural history of untreated hyperprolactinemia: a prospective analysis. *J Clin Endocrinol Metab* 1989; 68: 412.

## 6. OTHER PRIMARY TUMORS OF THE ANTERIOR PITUITARY GLAND

Demura, R., Jibiki, K., Kubo, O. *et al.* The significance of alpha-subunit as a tumor marker for gonadotropin-producing adenomas. *J Clin Endocrinol Metab* 1986; 63: 564.

Katznelson, L., Alexander, J.M., Bikkal, H.A. *et al.* Imbalanced follicle stimulating hormone beta-subunit hormone biosynthesis in human pituitary adenomas. *J Clin Endocrinol Metab* 1992; 74: 1343.

Klibanski, A. Nonsecreting Pituitary tumors. *Endocrinol Metab Clin North Am* 1987; 16(3): 793.

Oppenheim, D.S., Klibanski, A. Medical therapy of glycoprotein hormone-secreting pituitary tumors. *Endocrinol Metab Clin North Am* 1989; 18(2): 339.

Ridgeway, E.C., Klibanski, A., Ladenson, P.W. *et al.* Pure alpha-secreting pituitary adenomas. *N Engl J Med* 1981; 304: 1254.

Smallridge, R.C. Thyrotropin-secreting pituitary tumors. *Endocrinol Metab Clin North Am* 1987; 16(3): 765.

## 7. THE POSTERIOR PITUITARY

Berl, T. Treating hyponatremia: damned if we do and damned if we don't. *Kidney Int* 1990; 37: 1006.

Holtzman, E.J., Ausiello, D.A. Nephrogenic diabetes insipidus: causes revealed. *Hosp Pract* 1994; 29: 89.

Kovács, L., Vokes, T., Robertson, G.L. Syndrome of inappropriate antidiuretic hormone secretion. In: *Medicine For the Practicing Physician*. J.W. Hurst ed. Boston: Butterworth-Heinemann, 1992; pp. 629.

Lohr, J.W. Osmotic demyelination syndrome following correction of hyponatremia: association with hypokalemia. *Am J Med* 1994; 96: 408.

Robertson, G.L. Posterior pituitary. In: *Endocrinology and Metabolism*, 3rd edition. P. Felig, J.D. Baxter and L. A. Frohman, eds. New York: McGraw-Hill, 1995; pp. 385.

Robertson, G.L., Harris, A. Clinical use of vasopressin analogs. *Hosp Pract* 1989; 15:114.

Vokes, T.J., Robertson, G.L. Disorders of antidiuretic hormone. *Endocrinol Metab Clin North Am* 1988; 17: 28.

Zerbe, R.L., Robertson, G.L. A comparison of plasma vasopressin measurements with a standard indirect test in the differential diagnosis of polyuria. *N Engl J Med* 1981; 305: 1539.

## 8. THE THYROID GLAND – INTRODUCTION AND CLINICAL PHYSIOLOGY

Greenspan, F.S., guest ed. 'Thyroid Diseases', *Med Clin North Am* 1991; 75: 1

Braverman, L.E, Utiger, R.D. *Werner and Ingbar's The Thyroid*, 6th edition. Philadelphia: J.B. Lippincott Company, 1991.

Brent, G.A. The molecular basis of thyroid hormone action. *N Engl J Med* 1994; 331: 847.

Burrow, G.N., Oppenheimer, J.H., Volpe, R. *Thyroid Function and Disease*. Philadelphia: W.B. Saunders, 1990.

Burrow, G.N., Fisher, D.A., Larsen, P.R. Maternal and fetal thyroid function. *N Engl J Med* 1994; 331: 1072.

Cavalieri, R.R. Thyroid radioiodine uptake: indications and interpretation. *The Endocrinologist* 1992; 2: 341.

Hay, I.D., Klee, G.G. Thyroid dysfunction in diagnostic evaluation of endocrine disorders. *Endocrinol Metab Clin North Am* 1988; 17: 473.

Kaplan, M.M. Clinical and laboratory assessment of thyroid abnormalities. *Med Clin North Am* 1985; 69: 863.

Martino, E., Bambini, C., Bartalena, L. *et al.* Human serum thyrotrophin measurement by ultrasensitive immunoradiometric assay as a first-line test in the evaluation of thyroid function. *Clin Endocrinol* 1986; 24: 141.

Polikar, R., Burger, A.G., Scherrer, U., Nicod, P. The thyroid and the heart. *Circulation* 1993; 87: 1435

Rosenbaum, D., Davies, T.F. The clinical use of thyroid autoantibodies. *The Endocrinologist* 1992; 2: 55.

Wilber, J. The current status of the TRH test. *The Endocrinologist* 1991; 1: 45.

## 9. HYPOTHYROIDISM

Bagchi, N., Brown, T.R., Parish, R.F. Thyroid dysfunction in adults over age 55 years. *Arch Int Med* 1990; 150: 785.

Bastenie, P.A., Bonnyns, M., Vanhaelst, L. Natural history of primary myxedema. *Am J Med* 1985; 79: 91.

Dussault, J.H., Rousseau, F. Immunologically mediated hypothyroidism. *Endocrinol Metab Clin North Am* 1987; 16: 417.

Ehrman, D.A., Sarne, D.H. Serum thyrotropin and the assessment of thyroid status. *Ann Int Med* 1989; 110: 179.

Hall, R., Scanlon, M.F. Hypothyroidism: clinical features and complications. *Clin Endocrinol Metab* 1979; 8: 29.

Helfand, M., Crapo, L.M. Monitoring therapy in patients taking levothyroxine. *Ann Int Med* 1990; 113: 450.

Refetoff, S. Clinical and genetic aspects of resistance to thyroid hormone. *The Endocrinologist* 1992; 2: 261.

Shapiro, L.E., Surks, M.I. Managing hypothyroidism. *The Endocrinologist* 1991; 1: 343.

Tachman, M.L., Guthrie, G.P. Hypothyroidism: diversity of presentation. *Endocr Rev* 1984; 5: 456.

Toft, A.D. Thyroxine therapy. *N Engl J Med* 1994; 331: 174.

## 10. THYROTOXICOSIS

Bahn, R.S., Heufelder, A.E. Pathogenesis of Graves' ophthalmopathy. *N Engl J Med* 1993; 329: 1468.

Cooper, D. S. Antithyroid drugs. *N Engl J Med* 1984; 311: 1353.

Emerson, C.H. Central hypothyroidism and hyperthyroidism. *Med Clin North Am* 1985; 69: 1019.

Farrar, J.J., Taft, A.D. Iodine-131 treatment of hyperthyroidism: current issues. *Clin Endocrinol* 1991; 35: 207.

Gossage, A.A.R., Munro, D.S. The pathogenesis of Graves' disease. *Clin Endocrinol Metab* 1985; 14: 299.

Klein, I., Becker, D.V., Levey, G.S. Treatment of hyperthyroid disease. *Ann Int Med* 1994; 121: 281.

Nikolai, T.F., Coombs, G.J., McKenzie, A.K. *et al.* Lymphocytic thyroiditis with spontaneously resolving hyperthyroidism and subacute thyroiditis. Long-term follow-up. *Arch Intern Med* 1981; 141: 1455.

Roti, E., Emerson, C.H. Postpartum thyroiditis. *J Clin Endocrinol Metab* 1992; 74: 3.

Seely, B.L., Burrow, G.N. Thyrotoxicosis in pregnancy. *The Endocrinologist* 1991; 1: 409.

Seth, J., Beckett, G. Diagnosis of hyperthyroidism: the newer biochemical tests. *Clin Endocrinol Metab* 1985; 14: 373.

Silva, J.E. Effects of iodine and iodine containing compounds on thyroid function. *Med Clin North Am* 1985; 69: 881.

Spaulding, S.W., Lippes, H. Hyperthyroidism: causes, clinical features and diagnosis. *Med Clin North Am* 1985; 69: 937.

Studer, H., Peter, H.J., Gerber, H. *et al.* Toxic nodular goiter. *Clin Endocrinol Metab* 1985; 14: 351.

Wartofsky, L. Bone disease in thyrotoxicosis. *Hosp Pract* 1994; 29:69.

## 11. NEOPLASTIC DISEASE OF THE THYROID

Cady, B., Rossi, R. An expanded view of risk group definition in differentiated thyroid carcinoma. *Surgery* 1988; 104: 947.

Caruso, D., Mazzaferri, E.L. Fine needle aspiration biopsy in the management of thyroid nodules. *The Endocrinologist* 1991; 1: 194.

Clark, O.H., Elmhed, J. Thyroid surgery – past, present and future. *Thyroid Today* 1995; 18(1): 1.

Ezzat, S., Sarti, D.A., Cain, D.R., Braunstein, G.D. Thyroid incidentalomas: prevalence by palpation and ultrasonography. *Arch Intern Med* 1994; 154: 1838.

Gharib, H., Goellner, J.R. Fine-needle aspiration biopsy of the thyroid: an appraisal. *Ann Intern Med* 1983; 118: 282.

Hay, I.D. Papillary thyroid carcinoma. *Endocrinol Metab Clin North Am* 1990; 19: 545.

Heufelder, A.E., Gorman, C.A. Radioiodine therapy in the treatment of differentiated thyroid cancer: guidelines and considerations. *The Endocrinologist* 1991; 1: 273.

Mazzaferri, E.L. Thyroid cancer in thyroid nodules: finding a needle in the haystack. *Am J Med* 1992; 93: 359.

Mazzaferri, E.L. Management of a solitary thyroid nodule. *N Engl J Med* 1993; 328: 553.

Rojeski, M.T., Gharib, H. Nodular thyroid disease: evaluation and management. *N Engl J Med* 1985; 313: 428.

Van Herle, A.J., moderator. The thyroid nodule. *Ann Intern Med* 1982; 96: 221.

## 12. THE ADRENAL CORTEX: OVERVIEW

Besser, G.M., Rees, L.H. The pituitary–adrenocortical axis. *Clin Endocrinol Metab* 1985; 14: 765.

Miller, W.L. Molecular biology of steroid hormone synthesis. *Endocr Rev* 1988; 9: 295.

Neville, A.M., O'Hare, M.J. Histopathology of the human adrenal cortex. *Clin Endocrinol Metab* 1985; 14: 791.

Streeten, D.H.P., Anderson, G.H. Jr, Dalakos, T.G. *et al.* Normal and abnormal function of the hypothalamic–pituitary–adrenocortical system in man. *Endocr Rev* 1984; 5: 371.

Taylor, A.L., Fishman, L.M. Corticotropin-releasing hormone. *N Engl J Med* 1988; 319: 213.

## 13. HYPERFUNCTION OF THE ADRENAL CORTEX

Aron, D.C., Findling, J.W., Fitzgerald, P.A. *et al.* Cushing's syndrome: problems in management. *Endocr Rev* 1982; 3: 229.

Aron, D.C., Finding, J.W., Tyrrell, J.B. Cushing's disease. *Endocrinol Metab Clin North Am* 1987; 16: 705.

Doppman, J.L. The search for occult ectopic ACTH-producing tumors. *The Endocrinologist* 1992; 2: 41.

Howlett, T.A., Rees, L.H., Besser, G.M. Cushing's Syndrome. *Clin Endocrinol Metab* 1985; 14: 911.

Jex, R.K., van Heerden, J.A., Carpenter, P.C., Grant, C.S. Ectopic ACTH syndrome: diagnostic and therapeutic aspects. *Am J Surg* 1985; 149: 276.

Magiakou, M.A., Mastorakos, G., Oldfield, E.H. *et al.* Cushing's syndrome in children and adolescents: presentation, diagnosis and therapy. *N Engl J Med* 1994; 331: 629.

Miller, J.W., Crapo, L. The medical treatment of Cushing's syndrome. *Endocr Rev* 1993; 14: 443.

Nadler, J.L., Radin, R. Evaluation and management of the incidentally discovered adrenal mass. *The Endocrinologist* 1991; 1: 5.

Oldfield, E.H., Doppman, J.L., Nieman, L.K. *et al.* Petrosal sinus sampling with and without corticotropin-releasing hormone for the differential diagnosis of Cushing's syndrome. *N Engl J Med* 1991; 325: 897.

Orth, D.N. Cushing's syndrome. *N Engl J Med* 1995; 332: 791.

Orth, D.N. The Cushing syndrome: quest for the holy grail (editorial). *Ann Int Med* 1994; 121: 377.

Schteingart, D.E. Treating adrenal cancer. *The Endocrinologist* 1992; 2: 149.

## 14. ADRENAL CORTICAL INSUFFICIENCY

Burke, C.W. Adrenocortical insufficiency. *Clin Endocrinol Metab* 1985; 14: 947.

Chrousos, G.P., Detera-Wadleigh, S.D., Karl, M. Syndromes of glucocorticoid resistance. *Ann Intern Med* 1993; 119: 1113.

Leshin, M. Polyglandular autoimmune syndromes. *Am J Med Sci* 1985; 290: 77.

Redman, B.G., Pazdur, R., Zingas, A.P., Loredo, R. Prospective evaluation of adrenal insufficiency in patients with adrenal metastasis. *Cancer* 1987; 60: 103.

Schulte, H.M., Chrousos, G.P., Booth, J.D. *et al.* The corticotropin-releasing hormone stimulation test: a possible aid in the evaluation of patients with adrenal insufficiency. *J Clin Endocrinol Metab* 1984; 58: 1064.

Siegel, R.D., Melby, J. Fatigue: the role of adrenal insufficiency. *Hosp Pract* 1994; 29: 59.

Vita, J.A., Silverberg, S.J., Goland, R.S. *et al.* Clinical clues to the cause of Addison's disease. *Am J Med* 1985; 78: 461.

## 15. CONGENITAL ADRENAL HYPERPLASIA

Birnbaum, M.D., Rose, L.I. Late onset adrenocortical hydroxylase deficiencies associated with menstrual dysfunction. *Obstet Gynecol* 1985; 63: 445.

Horrocks, P.M., London, D.R. Effects of long term dexamethasone treatment in adult patients with congenital adrenal hyperplasia. *Clin Endocr* 1987; 27: 635.

Laue, L., Cutler, G.B. Jr. 21-Hydroxylase deficiency: overview of treatment. *The Endocrinologist* 1992; 2: 291.

New, M.I., ed. Congenital adrenal hyperplasia. *Ann NY Acad Sci* 1985; 458: 1.

White, P.C., New, M.I., Dupont, B. Congenital adrenal hyperplasia. Part 1. *N Engl J Med* 1987; 316: 1519.

White, P.C., New, M.I., Dupont, B. Congenital adrenal hyperplasia. Part 2. *N Engl J Med* 1987; 316: 1580.

## 16. PRIMARY HYPERALDOSTERONISM

Blumenfeld, J.D., Sealey, J.E., Schlussel, Y. *et al.* Diagnosis and treatment of primary hyperaldosteronism. *Ann Int Med* 1994; 121: 877.

Bravo, E.L., Tarazi, R.C., Dustan, H.P. *et al.* The changing clinical spectrum of primary aldosteronism. *Am J Med* 1983; 74: 641.

Gill, J.R., Jr. Primary hyperaldosteronism: strategies for diagnosis and treatment. *The Endocrinologist* 1991; 1: 365.

Melby, J.C. Primary aldosteronism. *Kidney Int* 1984; 26: 769.

Warnock, D.G., Bubien, J.K. Liddle Syndrome: Clinical and Cellular Abnormalities. *Hosp Pract* 1994; 29: 95.

White, P.C. Disorders of Aldosterone Biosynthesis and Action. *N Engl J Med* 1994; 331: 250.

Young, W.F., Klee, G.G. Primary aldosteronism: diagnostic evaluation. *Endocrinol Metab Clin North Am* 1988; 17: 367.

## 17. PHEOCHROMOCYTOMA

Bravo, E., Gifford, R.W., Jr. Pheochromocytoma: diagnosis, localization and management. *N Engl J Med* 1984; 311: 1298.

Cryer, P.E. Physiology and pathophysiology of the human sympathoadrenal neuroendocrine system. *N Engl J Med* 1980; 303: 436.

Golub, M.S., Tuck, M.L. Diagnostic and therapeutic strategies in pheochromocytoma. *The Endocrinologist* 1992; 2: 101.

Manger, W. M. Pheochromocytoma. *West J Med* 1986; 145: 382.

Ponder, B.A., Jackson, C.E., eds. The second international workshop on multiple endocrine neoplasia type 2 syndromes. *Henry Ford Hosp Med J* 1987; 35: 1.

## 18. GLUCOSE METABOLISM: NORMAL PHYSIOLOGY AND OVERVIEW

Hellerstrom, C. The life story of the pancreatic B cell. *Diabetologia* 1984; 26: 393.

Howell, S.L. The mechanism of insulin secretion. *Diabetologia* 1984; 26: 319.

Pandit, M., Burke, J., Gustafson, A. *et al*. Drug-induced disorders of glucose metabolism. *Ann Intern Med* 1993; 118: 529.

Pipeleers, G. The biosociology of pancreatic B cells. *Diabetologia* 1987; 30: 277.

Unger, R.H., Orci, L. Glucagon and the A cell. Physiology and pathophysiology. *N Engl J Med* 1981; 304: 1518.

## 19. HYPOGLYCEMIA

Cryer, P.E., Gerich, J.E. Glucose counterregulation, hypoglycemia, and intensive therapy in diabetes mellitus. *N Engl J Med* 1985; 313: 232.

Field, J.B. ed. Hypoglycemia. *Endocrinol Metab Clin North Am* 1989; (entire issue) 18.

Madison, L.L. Ethanol-induced hypoglycemia. *Adv Metabol Dis* 1968; 3: 85.

Norton, J.A., Whitman, E.D. Insulinoma. *The Endocrinologist* 1993; 3: 258.

Ron, D., Powers, A.C., Pandian, M.R. *et al.* Increased insulin-like growth factor II production and consequent suppression of growth hormone secretion: a dual mechanism for tumor-induced hypoglycemia. *J Clin Endocrinol Metab* 1989; 68: 701.

Service, F.J. Factitial hypoglycemia. *The Endocrinologist* 1992; 2: 173.

Service, F.J. Hypoglycemic disorders. *N Engl J Med* 1995; 332: 1144

## 20.  DIABETES MELLITUS

AACE Guidelines for the Management of Diabetes Mellitus. American Association of Clinical Endocrinologists. Jacksonville: American College of Endocrinology 1994.

Atkinson, M.A., MacLaren, N.K. The pathogenesis of insulin-dependent diabetes mellitus. *N Engl J Med* 1995; 331: 1428.

Bailey, C.J. Biguanides and NIDDM. *Diabetes Care* 1992; 15: 755.

Bennett, P.H. The diagnosis of diabetes: new international classification and diagnostic criteria. *Annu Rev Med* 1983; 34: 295.

Carroll, P.B., Eastman, R.C. Insulin resistance: diagnosis and treatment. *The Endocrinologist* 1991; 1:89.

Clark, C.M., Lee, D.A. Prevention and treatment of the complications of diabetes mellitus. *N Engl J Med* 1995; 332: 1210.

Cogan, D.G., Kinashita, J.H., Kador, P.F. *et al.* Aldose reductase and complications of diabetes. *Ann Intern Med* 1984; 101: 82.

Coustan, D.R., guest ed. Diabetes in pregnancy and the newborn. *Seminars in Perinatology,* Volume 18, Number 5. W.B. Saunders Company 1994; pp. 399.

Cranston, I., Lomas, J., Maran, A. *et al.* Restoration of hypoglycemia awareness in patients with long-duration insulin-dependent diabetes. *Lancet* 1994; 344: 283.

De Fronzo, R.A., Goodman, A.M. and the Multicenter Metformin

Study Group. Efficacy of metformin in patients with non-insulin-dependent diabetes mellitus. *N Engl J Med* 1995; 333: 541.

The Diabetes Control and Complications Trial Research Group. The effect of intensive diabetes therapy on the development and progression of neuropathy. *Ann Intern Med* 1995; 122: 561.

The Diabetes Control and Complications Trial Research Group. The effect of intensive treatment of diabetes on the development and progression of long-term complications in insulin-dependent diabetes mellitus. *N Engl J Med* 1995; 329: 977.

Dunn, F.L. Hyperlipidemia and diabetes. *Med Clin North Am* 1982; 66: 1347.

Feingold, K.R., Siperstein, M.D. Diabetic vascular disease. *Adv Intern Med* 1986; 31: 309.

Froguel, P., Zouali, H., Vionnet, N. *et al.* Familial hyperglycemia due to mutations in glucokinase. *N Engl J Med* 1993; 328: 697.

Fulop, M. The treatment of severely uncontrolled diabetes mellitus. *Adv Intern Med* 1984; 29: 327.

Groop, L.C., Kankuri, M., Schalin-Jäntti, C. *et al.* Association between polymorphism of the glycogen synthase gene and non-insulin-dependent diabetes mellitus. *N Engl J Med* 1993; 328: 10.

Jovanovic-Peterson, L., Peterson, C.M. Managing the pregnant diabetic woman. *The Endocrinologist* 1991; 1:301.

Ketchum, R.J., Moore, W.V. Islet transplantation for the treatment of diabetes mellitus. *The Endocrinologist* 1992; 2: 301.

Kolaczynski, J.W., Caro, J.F. Insulin-like growth factor-I therapy in diabetes: physiologic basis, clinical benefits, and risks. *Ann Intern Med* 1994; 120:47.

Kreisberg, R.A. Pathogenesis and management of lactic acidosis. *Annu Rev Med* 1984; 35: 181.

Little, R.R., England, J.D., Wiedmeyer, H.M. *et al.* Relationship of glycosylated hemoglobin to oral glucose tolerance: implications for diabetes screening. *Diabetes* 1988; 37: 60.

Mecklenburg, R.S. The acute complications associated with the use of insulin infusion pumps. *The Endocrinologist* 1991; 1: 19.

Melander, A. Clinical pharmacology of sulfonylureas. *Metabolism* 1987; 36 (2 Suppl. 1): 12.

Mogensen, C.E. Management of diabetic renal involvement and disease. *Lancet* 1988; 1:867.

Nathan, D.M. Long-term complications of diabetes mellitus. *N Engl J Med* 1993; 328: 1676.

Nathan, D.M., Roussell, A., Godine, J.E. Glyburide or insulin for metabolic control in non-insulin-dependent diabetes mellitus: a randomized, double-blind study. *Ann Intern Med* 1988; 108: 334.

Nuttal, F.Q. The high-carbohydrate diet in diabetes management. *Adv Intern Med* 1988; 33: 165.

Proietto, J. Treatment options in Type II diabetes. *The Endocrinologist* 1992; 2: 107.

Reichard, P., Nilsson, B., Rosenqvist, U. The effect of long-term intensified insulin treatment on the development of microvascular complications of diabetes mellitus. *N Engl J Med* 1993; 329: 304.

Remuzzi, G., Ruggenenti, P., Mauer, S.M. Pancreas and kidney/pancreas transplants: experimental medicine or real improvement? *Lancet* 1994; 343: 27.

Rotter, J.I., Anderson, C.E., Rimoin, D.L. Genetics of diabetes mellitus. In Ellenberg, M., Rifkin, H., eds. *Diabetes Mellitus. Theory and Practice,* 3rd edition. New Hyde Park, NY: Medical Examination Publishing Company 1983; 481.

Schade, D.W., Eaton, R.P. Diabetic ketoacidosis: pathogenesis, prevention, and therapy. *Clin Endocrinol Metab* 1983; 13: 332.

Schade, D.S., Drumm, D.A., Duckworth, W.C., Eaton, R.P. The etiology of incapacitating, brittle diabetes. *Diabetes Care* 1985; 8: 12.

Soon-Shiong, P., Heintz, R.E. Merideth, N. *et al.* Insulin independence in a type I diabetic patient after encapsulated islet transplantation. *Lancet* 1994; 343: 950.

Vora, J.P., Anderson, S. Diabetic renal disease: an overview with therapeutic implications. *The Endocrinologist* 1992; 2: 223.

Wachtel, T.J., Silliman, R.A., Lamberton, P. Predisposing factors for the diabetic hyperosmolar state. *Arch Intern Med* 1988; 148: 747.

Ward, J.D. The diabetic leg. *Diabetologia* 1982; 22: 141.

Williams, G. Management of non-insulin-dependent diabetes mellitus. *Lancet* 1994; 343: 95.

Yki-Jarvinen, H. Pathogenesis of non-insulin-dependent diabetes mellitus. *Lancet* 1994; 343: 91.

Yki-Jarvinen, H., Kauppila, M., Kujansuu, E. *et al.* Comparison of insulin regimens in patients with non-insulin-dependent diabetes mellitus. *N Engl J Med* 1992; 327: 1426.

Young, C.W. Rationale for glycemic control. *Am J Med* 1985; 79 (Suppl. 3B): 8.

Zata, R., Brenner, B.M. Pathogenesis of diabetic microangiopathy. *Am J Med* 1986; 80: 443.

## 21. MINERAL METABOLISM: NORMAL PHYSIOLOGY AND PATHOPHYSIOLOGY

Audran, M., Kumar, R. The physiology and pathophysiology of vitamin D. *Mayo Clin Proc* 1985; 60: 851.

Austin, L.A., Heath, H.H., III. Calcitonin: physiology and pathophysiology. *N Engl J Med* 1981; 304: 269.

Habener, J.F., Rosenblatt, M., Potts, J.T. Jr. Parathyroid hormone: biochemical aspects of biosynthesis, secretion, action, and metabolism. *Physiol Rev* 1984; 64: 985.

Holick, M.F., Vitamin D: photobiology, metabolism and clinical applications. In: DeGroot, L.J. ed. *Endocrinology*, 3rd edition. W.B. Saunders 1995; 2: 90

McLean, R.M. Magnesium and its therapeutic uses: a review. *Am J Med* 1994; 96: 63.

Matz, R. Magnesium: deficiencies and therapeutic uses. *Hosp Pract* 1993; 28: 79.

Norman, A.W. The vitamin D endocrine system. *Physiologist* 1985; 28: 219.

Potts, J.T. Jr, Bringhurst, F.R., Gardella, T. *et al.* Parathyroid hormone: physiology, chemistry, biosynthesis, secretion, metabolism, and mode of action. In: DeGroot, L.J. *et al.* eds. *Endocrinology*, 3rd edition. W.B. Saunders 1995; 2: 920.

Strewler, G.J., Rosenblatt, M. Mineral metabolism. In: Felig, P., Baxter, J.D., Frohman, L.A. eds. *Endocrinology and Metabolism*, 3rd edition. New York: McGraw-Hill 1995; pp. 1407.

## 22. HYPERCALCEMIA

Attie, M.F. Treatment of hypercalcemia. *Endocrinol Metab Clin North Am* 1989; 18: 807.

Attie, M.F., Gill, J.R., Jr., Stock, J.L. *et al.* Urinary calcium excretion in familial hypocalciuric hypercalcemia: persistence of relative hypocalciuria after induction of hypoparathyroidism. *J Clin Invest* 1983; 72: 667.

Bilezikian, J.P. Etiologies and therapy of hypercalcemia. Endocrinol *Metab Clin North Am* 1989; 18: 389.

Broadus, A.E., Mangin, M., Ikeda, K. *et al.* Humoral hypercalcemia of cancer. *N Engl J Med* 1988; 319: 556.

Gaich, G., Burtis, W.J. The diagnosis and treatment of malignancy-associated hypercalcemia. *The Endocrinologist* 1991; 1: 371.

Mundy, G.R. Hypercalcemic factors other than parathyroid hormone-related protein. *Endocrinol Metab Clin North Am* 1989; 18: 741.

Mundy, G.R., Mazzaferri, E.L. Evaluation and treatment of hypercalcemia. *Hosp Pract* 1994; 29: 79.

Nussbaum, S.R., Zahradnik, R.J., Lavigne, J.R. *et al.* Highly sensitive two-site immunoradiometric assay of parathyrin and its clinical utility in evaluating patients with hypercalcemia. *Clin Chem* 1987; 8: 1364.

Singer, F.R., Adams, J.S. Abnormal calcium homeostasis in sarcoidosis. *N Engl J Med* 1986; 315: 755.

## 23. PRIMARY HYPERPARATHYROIDISM

Fitzpatrick, L.A., Bilezikian, J.P. Acute primary hyperparathyroidism. *Am J Med* 1987; 82: 275.

Kleerekoper, M., Bilezekian, J.P. A cure in search of a disease: parathyroidectomy for non-traditional features of primary hyperparathyroidism. *Am J Med* 1994; 96: 99.

NIH Consensus Development Conference Panel. Diagnosis and

management of asymptomatic primary hyperparathyroidism. *Ann Intern Med* 1991; 114 (7): 593.

Palmer, M., Adami, H.O., Berstrom, R. *et al.* Mortality after surgery for primary hyperparathyroidism: a follow-up of 441 patients operated on from 1956 to 1979. *Surgery* 1987; 102(1): 1.

Potts, J.T. Jr. Clinical review 9: management of asymptomatic hyperparathyroidism. *J Clin Endocrinol Metab* 1990; 70(6): 1489.

Solomon, B.L., Schaaf, M., Smallridge, R.C. Psychologic symptoms before and after parathyroid surgery. *Am J Med* 1994; 96: 101.

Wilson, R.J., Sudhaker, D., Ellis, B. *et al.* Mild asymptomatic primary hyperparathyroidism is not a risk factor for vertebral fractures. *Ann Intern Med* 1988; 109: 959.

Winzelberg, G.G. Parathyroid imaging. *Ann Intern Med* 1987; 107: 64.

## 24. HYPOCALCEMIA

Breslau, N. A., Pak, C.Y.C. Hypoparathyroidism. *Metabolism* 1979; 28: 1261.

Connor, T.B., Rosen, B.L., Blaustein, M.B. *et al.* Hypocalcemia precipitating congestive heart failure. *N Engl J Med* 1982; 307: 869.

Heubi, J. E., Partin, J.C., Schubert, W.K. *et al.* Hypocalcemia and steatorrhea: clues to etiology. *Dig Dis Sci* 1983; 28: 124.

Rude, R.K., Oldham, S.B., Sharp, C.F., Jr., *et al.* Parathyroid hormone secretion in magnesium deficiency. *J Clin Endocrinol Metab* 1978; 47: 800.

Van Dop, C., Bourne, H.R. Pseudohypoparathyroidism. *Annu Rev Med* 1983; 34: 259.

## 25. METABOLIC BONE DISEASE

### Paget's Disease

Avioli, L.V. Paget's disease: state of the art. *Clin Ther* 1987; 9: 567.

Freeman, D.A. Paget's disease of bone. *Am J Med Sci* 1988; 295: 144.

Krane, S.M.: Paget's disease of bone. *Calcif Tissue Res* 1986; 38: 309.

McClung, M. Treating Paget's disease of bone. *The Endocrinologist* 1992; 2: 22.

Rebel, A. ed. Symposium: Paget's disease. *Clin Orthoped* 1987; 217: 2.

**Rickets and Osteomalacia**
Christensen, C.K., Lund, B., Lund, B. J. *et al*. Reduced 1, 25-dihydroxyvitamin D and 24, 25-dihydroxyvitamin D in epileptic patients receiving chronic combined anticonvulsant therapy. *Metab Bone Dis Rel Res* 1981; 3: 17.

Econs, M.J., Drezner, M.D. Tumor-induced osteomalacia – unveiling a new hormone. *N Engl J Med* 1994; 330: 1679.

Glorieux, F.H., ed. *Rickets*. New York: Raven Press, 1991.

Marel, G.M., McKenna, M.J., Frame, B. Osteomalacia. *Bone Mineral Res* 1986; 4: 335.

Parfitt, A.M., Gallagher, J.C., Heaney, R.P. *et al*. Vitamin D and bone health in the elderly. *Am J Clin Nutr* 1982; 36: 1014.

Ryan, E.Q., Reiss, E. Oncogenous osteomalacia: a review of the world literature of 42 cases and report of two new cases. *Am J Med* 1984; 77: 501.

**Osteoporosis**
Aloia, J.F., Vaswani, A., Yeh, J.K. *et al*. Calcium supplementation with and without hormone replacement therapy to prevent postmenopausal bone loss. *Ann Intern Med* 1994; 120: 97.

Chapuy, M., Arlot, M.E., Duboeuf, F. *et al*. Vitamin $D_3$ and calcium to prevent hip fractures in elderly women. *N Engl J Med* 1992; 327: 1637.

Ettinger, B., Genant, H.K., Cann, C.E. Long-term estrogen replacement therapy prevents bone loss and fractures. *Ann Intern Med* 1985; 102: 319.

Jackson, J.A., Kleerekoper, M. Osteoporosis in men: diagnosis, pathophysiology, and prevention. *Medicine* 1990; 69: 137.

Johnston, C.C., Jr., Slemenda, C.W. Measuring bone density and what it means. *The Endocrinologist* 1991; 1: 83.

Kraut, J.A., Coburn, J.W. Bone, acid,and osteoporosis (editorial). *N Engl J Med* 1994; 330: 1821.

Marcus, R. Cyclic etidronate: has the rose lost its bloom? *Am J Med* 1993; 95: 555.

Raisz, L.G. Therapeutic options for the patient with osteoporosis. *The Endocrinologist* 1991; 1: 11.

Reid, I.R., Ames, R., Evans, M.C. *et al.* Effect of calcium supplementation on bone loss in postmenopausal women. *N Engl J Med* 1993; 328: 460.

Richelson, L.S., Wahner, H.W., Melton, L.J., III, Riggs, B.L. Relative contributions of aging and estrogen deficiency to postmenopausal bone loss. *N Engl J Med* 1984; 311: 1273.

Riggs, B.L., Melton, L.J., III. Involutional osteoporosis. *N Engl J Med* 1986; 314: 1676.

Rigotti, N.A., Nussbaum, S.R., Herzog, D.B., Neer, R.M. Osteoporosis in women with anorexia nervosa. *N Engl J Med* 1984; 311: 1601.

Riis, B., Thomsen, K., Christiansen, C. Does calcium supplementation prevent postmenopausal bone loss? *N Engl J Med* 1987; 316: 173.

Sambook, P., Birmingham, J., Kelly, P. *et al.* Prevention of corticosteroid osteoporosis. *N Engl J Med* 1993; 238: 1747.

## 26. RENAL STONE DISEASE

Coe, F.L., Parks, J.H., Asplin, J.R. The pathogenesis and treatment of kidney stones. *N Engl J Med* 1992; 327: 1141.

Curhan, G., Willett, W., Rimm, E., Stampfer, M. A prospective study of dietary calcium and other nutrients and the risk of symptomatic kidney stones. *N Engl J Med* 1993; 328: 833.

NIH Consensus Conference: Prevention and treatment of kidney stones. *J Urol* 1989; 141: 804.

Pak, C.Y.C., Sakhaee, K., Crowther, C., Brinkley, L. Evidence justifying a high fluid intake in treatment of nephrolithiasis. *Ann Intern Med* 1980; 93: 36.

Pak, C.Y.C. The management of recurrent idiopathic urolithiasis. *The Endocrinologist* 1991; 1: 233.

Silverberg, S.J., Shane, E., Jacobs, T.P. *et al.* Nephrolithiasis and bone involvement in primary hyperparathyroidism. *Am J Med* 1990; 89: 327.

Smith, L.H. The pathophysiology and medical treatment of urolithiasis. *Seminars in Nephrology* 1990; 10: 31.

Trinchieri, A., Mandressi, A., Luongo, P. et al. Familial aggregation of renal calcium stone disease. J Urol 1988; 139: 478.

Uribarri, J., Oh, M.S., Carroll, H.J. The first kidney stone. Ann Intern Med 1989; 111: 1006.

Wilson, D.M. Clinical and laboratory approaches for evaluation of nephrolithiasis. J Urol 1989; 141: 770.

## 27. THE RELATIONSHIP BETWEEN ENDOCRINOLOGY AND NEOPLASTIC DISEASE

Bates, S.E., Longo, D.L. Use of serum tumor markers in cancer diagnosis and management. Semin Oncol 1987; 14: 102.

Baylin, S.B., Mendelsohn, G. Ectopic (inappropriate) hormone production by tumors: mechanisms involved and the biological and clinical implications. Endocr Rev 1980; 1: 45.

Deftos, L.J., Catherwood, B.D., Bone, H.G., III. Multliglandular endocrine disorders. In Felig, P., Baxter, J.D., Broadus, A.E., Frohman, L.A. eds. Endocrinology and Metabolism, 3rd edition New York: McGraw-Hill 1995; pp. 1703.

Genetic markers in multiple endocrine neoplasia type 2 (editorial). Lancet 1988; 1: 396.

Kloos, R.T., Gross, M.D., Francis, I.R. et al. Incidentally discovered adrenal masses. Endocr Rev 1995; 16: 460.

Lippman, M.E., Swain, S. Endocrine responsive cancers of humans. In: Williams Textbook of Endocrinology, 8th edition. Philadelphia: W.B. Saunders, 1992.

Melmed, S., Rushakoff, R.J. Ectopic pituitary and hypothalamic hormone syndromes. Endocrinol Metab Clin North Am 1987; 16: 805.

Samaan, N.A., Castillo, S., Schultz, P.N. et al. Serum calcitonin after pentagastrin stimulation in patients with bronchogenic and breast cancer compared to that in patients with medullary thyroid carcinoma. J Clin Endocrinol Metab 1980; 51: 237.

Sizemore, G.W., Heath, H. III, Carney, J.A. Multiple endocrine neoplasia type 2. Clin Endocrinol Metab 1980; 9: 299.

## 28. NORMAL LIPID METABOLISM AND RELATED DISEASE STATES

Albers, J.J., Tollefson, J.H., Raust, R.A., Nishide, T. Plasma cholesterol (ester) and phospholipid (transfer proteins) and their regulation. *Adv Exp Med Biol* 1988; 243: 213.

Brown, G., Albers, J., Fisher, L. *et al.* Regression of coronary artery disease as a result of intensive lipid lowering therapy in men with high levels of apolipoprotein B. *N Engl J Med* 1990; 323: 1289.

Castelli, W.P. The triglyceride issue: a view from Framingham. *Am Heart J* 1986; 112: 432.

Castelli, W.P. Cardiovascular disease in women. *Am J Obstet Gynecol* 1988; 158: 1553.

Castelli, W.P. Cholesterol and lipids in the risk of coronary artery disease – The Framingham Heart Study. *Can J Cardiol* Suppl A 1988; 4.

Connor, W.E., Connor, S.L. Dietary treatment of hyperlipidemia: rationale and benefit. *The Endocrinologist* 1991; 1: 33.

Consensus conference. Lowering blood cholesterol to prevent heart disease. *J Am Med Assoc* 1985; 253: 2080.

Duell, P.B. Hypertriglyceridemia: pathophysiology, diagnosis, and treatment. *The Endocrinologist* 1992; 2: 321.

Henkin, Y., Kreisberg, R.A. HDL: the underdog in the battle against atherosclerosis. *The Endocrinologist* 1992; 2: 122.

Havel, R.J., Rapaport, E. Management of primary hyperlipidemia. *N Engl J Med* 1995; 332: 1491.

Hunninghake, D.B., guest ed. 'Lipid Disorders' *Med Clin North Am* 1994; 78: 1.

Illingworth, D.R. Use and abuse of lovastatin. *The Endocrinologist* 1991; 1: 323.

Jones, P.H. A clinical overview of dyslipidemias: treatment strategies. *Am J Med* 1992; 93: 187.

Kato, H., Tillotson, J., Nichaman, N.J. *et al.* Epidemiologic studies of coronary heart disease and stroke in Japanese men living in Japan, Hawaii and California. *Am J Epidemiol* 1973; 97: 372.

Keys, A. Coronary heart disease in seven countries. Circulation (Suppl 1) 1970; 41: I-1–I-8.

LaRosa, J.C. Combinations of drugs in lipid-lowering therapy. *Am J Med* 1994; 96: 399.

Levine, G.N., Keaney, J.F., Vita, J.A. Cholesterol reduction in cardiovascular disease: clinical benefits and possible mechanisms. *N Engl J Med* 1995; 332: 512.

*National Cholesterol Education Program: Highlights of the Report of the Expert Panel on Blood Cholesterol Levels in Children and Adolescents.* Bethesda: U.S. Department of Health and Human Services, Public Health Service, National Institutes of Health 1992.

Pearson, T.A., Patel, R.V. The quest for a cholesterol-decreasing diet: should we subtract, substitute or supplement? *Ann Intern Med* 1993; 119: 627.

Scandinavian Simvastatin Survival Study Group. Randomised trial of cholesterol lowering in 4444 patients with coronary heart disease: the Scandinavian Simvastatin Survival Study (4S). *Lancet* 1994; 344: 1383.

Schaefer, E.J., Levy, R.I. Pathogenesis and management of lipoprotein disorders. *N Engl J Med* 1985; 312: 1300.

Utermann, G. The mysteries of lipoprotein (a). *Science* 1989; 246: 904.

## 29.   OBESITY

Amatruda, J.M. Very low energy diets for the treatment of simple and complicated obesity. *The Endocrinologist* 1991; 1: 171.

Bjorntorp, P. Metabolic implications of body fat distribution. *Diabetes Care* 1991; 14: 1132.

Bray, G.A. ed. Obesity. *Med Clin North Am* (entire issue) 1989; 73: 1.

Bray, G.A., Bray, D.S. Obesity. *Western J Med* 1988; 149: 429–41 (Part I), 555–71 (Part II).

Kaplan, N.M. The deadly quartet: upper body obesity, glucose intolerance, hypertriglyceridemia and hypertension. *Arch Intern Med* 1989; 149: 1514.

Kuller, L., Wing, R. Weight loss and mortality (editorial). *Ann Intern Med* 1993; 119: 630.

Pi-Sunyer, F.X. Medical hazards of obesity. *Ann Intern Med* 1993; 119: 655.

Weigle, D.S. The pathophysiology of obesity: implications for treatment. *The Endocrinologist* 1991; 1: 385.

Weintraub, M., Sundaresan, P.R., Madan, M. *et al.* Long-term weight control study I (weeks 0 to 34). The enhancement of behavior modification, caloric restriction, and exercise by fenfluramine plus phentermine versus placebo. *Clin Pharmacol Ther* 1992; 51: 586.

## 30. ANOREXIA NERVOSA AND BULIMIA NERVOSA

Ben-Tovim, D.I., Subbiah, N., Scheutz, B. *et al.* Bulimia: symptoms and syndromes in an urban population. *Aust NZ J Psychiatr* 1989; 23: 73.

Devlin, M.J., Walsh, B.T., Katz, J.L., *et al.* Hypothalamic–pituitary–gonadal function in anorexia nervosa and bulimia. *Psychiatr Res* 1989; 28: 11.

Herzog, D. B. Bulimia: the secretive syndrome. *Psychosomatics* 1982; 23: 481.

Herzog, D.B., Copeland, P.M. Bulimia nervosa – psyche and satiety. *N Engl J Med* 1988; 319: 716.

Issacs, A.J., Leslie, R.D.G., Gomez, J. *et al.* The effect of weight gain on gonadotrophins and prolactin in anorexia nervosa. *Acta Endocrinol* 1980; 94: 145.

Lucas, A.R., Beard, C.M., O'Fallon, W.M. *et al.* Anorexia nervosa in Rochester, Minnesota: a 45 year study. *Mayo Clin Proc* 1988; 63: 433.

Mitchell, J.E., Seim, H.C., Colon, E. *et al.* Medical complications and medical management of bulimia. *Ann Intern Med* 1987; 107: 71.

Newman, M.M., Halmi, K.A. The endocrinology of anorexia nervosa and bulimia nervosa. *Endocrinol Metab Clin North Am* 1988; 17: 195.

Schwabe, A.D., Lippe, B.M., Chang, R.J. *et al.* Anorexia nervosa. *Ann Intern Med* 1981; 94: 371.

## 31. NORMAL MALE REPRODUCTIVE ENDOCRINOLOGY AND RELATED DISEASE STATES

Braunstein, G.D. Gynecomastia. *N Engl J Med* 1993; 328:490.

Federman, D.D. Life without estrogen (editorial). *N Engl J Med* 1994; 331: 1088.

Ghusn, H.F., Cunningham, G.R. Evaluation and treatment of androgen deficiency in males. *The Endocrinologist* 1991; 1: 399.

Klinefelter, H.F. Klinefelter's syndrome: historical background and development. *South Med J* 1986; 79: 1089.

Morley, J.E. Impotence. *Am J Med* 1986; 80: 897.

Nelson, R.P. Male sexual dysfunction: evaluation and treatment. *South Med J* 1987; 80: 69.

Niewoehner, C.B., Nuttall, F.Q. Gynecomastia in a hospitalized male population. *Am J Med* 1984; 77: 633.

NIH Consensus Statement on Impotence. Volume 10, Number 4. Bethesda, MD: National Institutes of Health. December 7–9, 1992.

Padma-Nathan, H., Goldstein, I., Krane, R.J. Evaluation of the impotent patient. *Semin Urol* 1986; 4: 225.

Rittmaster, R.S. Finasteride. *N Engl J Med* 1994; 330: 120.

Skakkebaek, N.E. Pathogenesis and management of male infertility. *Lancet* 1994; 343: 1473.

Snyder, P.J. Clinical use of androgens. *Annu Rev Med* 1984; 35: 207.

Tsitouras, P.D. Effects of age on testicular function. *Endocrinol Metab Clin North Am* 1987; 16: 1045.

Whitcomb, R.W. The approach to the oligo/azoospermic male. *The Endocrinologist* 1991; 1: 125.

Wilson, J.D., Aiman, J., McDonald, P.C. The pathogenesis of gynecomastia. *Adv Intern Med* 1980; 25: 1.

Winter, J.S.D. Ambiguous genitalia: a clinician's approach. *The Endocrinologist* 1992; 2: 312.

Wu, F.C. Male hypogonadism: current concepts and trends. *Clin Obstet Gynaecol* 1985; 12: 531.

## 32. NORMAL FEMALE REPRODUCTIVE ENDOCRINOLOGY AND RELATED DISEASE STATES

Alper, M.M., Garner, P., Chir, B., Seibel, M.M. Premature ovarian failure – current concepts. *J Reprod Med* 1986; 31: 699.

Baird, D.T., Glasier, A.F. Hormonal contraception. *N Engl J Med* 1993; 328: 1543.

Barth, J.H. Alopecia and hirsuties: current concepts in pathogenesis and management. *Practical Therapeutics* 1988; 35: 83.

Belchetz, P.E. Hormonal treatment of postmenopausal women. *N Engl J Med* 1994; 330: 1062.

Biller, B.M.K., Klibanski, A. Amenorrhea and osteoporosis. *The Endocrinologist* 1991; 1: 294.

Burger, H.G. Inhibin and its implications for clinical practice. *The Endocrinologist* 1992; 2: 249.

Cobleigh, M.A., Berris, R.F., Bush, T. *et al.* Estrogen replacement therapy in breast cancer survivors: a time for change. *J Am Med Assoc* 1994; 272: 540.

Dunaif, A. Insulin resistance and ovarian hyperandrogenism. *The Endocrinologist* 1992; 2: 248.

Dunaif, A., Givens, J.R., Haseltine, F.P., Merrian, G.R. *Current Issues in Endocrinology and Metabolism – Polycystic Ovary Syndrome*. Boston: Blackwell Scientific Publications 1992.

Jaffe, R. The menopause and perimenopausal period. In: Yen, S.S.C., Jaffe, R. eds. *Reproductive Endocrinology*. Philadelphia: W.B. Saunders, 1986; 406.

Loprinzi, C.L., Michalak, J.C., Quella, S.K. *et al.* Megestrol acetate for the prevention of hot flashes. *N Engl J Med* 1994; 331: 347.

Lufkin, E.G., Carpenter, P.C., Ory, S.J. *et al.* Estrogen replacement therapy: current recommendations. *Mayo Clin Proc* 1988; 63: 453.

Martin, K.A., Freeman, M.W. Postmenopausal hormone-replacement therapy (editorial). *N Engl J Med* 1993; 328: 1115.

Moorman, P.G., Hulka, B.S. Menopausal hormones and the risk of breast cancer. *The Endocrinologist* 1992; 2: 189.

Rittmaster, R.S., Loriaux, D.L. Hirsutism. *Ann Intern Med* 1987; 106: 95.

Ross, J.L., Cutler, G.B. The optimal use of estrogen in the treatment of Turner's syndrome. *The Endocrinologist* 1992; 2: 119.

Soules, M.R. Adolescent amenorrhea. *Ped Clin North Am* 1987; 334: 1083.

Speroff, L. Cardiovascular disease and postmenopausal hormone replacement therapy. *The Endocrinologist* 1991; 1: 49.

Speroff, L., Glass, R.H., Kase, N.G. *Clinical Gynecologic Endocrinology and Infertility*, 5th edition. Baltimore: Williams and Wilkins, 1995.

teVelde, E.R. Hormonal treatment for the climacteric: alleviation of symptoms and prevention of postmenopausal disease. *Lancet* 1994; 343: 654.

van der Spuy, Z.M. Nutrition and reproduction. *Clin Obstet Gynecol* 1985; 12: 579.

# INDEX